Providing HIV Care: Lessons from the Field for Nurses and Healthcare Practitioners

Michelle Croston • Ian Hodgson
Editors

Providing HIV Care: Lessons from the Field for Nurses and Healthcare Practitioners

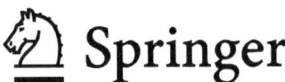 Springer

Editors
Michelle Croston (iD)
Department of Nursing
Manchester Metropolitan University
Manchester
UK

Ian Hodgson
Independent Consultant in Global Health
Sheffield
UK

ISBN 978-3-030-71294-5   ISBN 978-3-030-71295-2   (eBook)
https://doi.org/10.1007/978-3-030-71295-2

This Springer imprint is published by the registered company Springer Nature Switzerland AG
The registered company address is: Gewerbestrasse 11, 6330 Cham, Switzerland

Acknowledgements

We would like to thank all the authors who devoted hours of their precious time to contribute to this book, during a year that was especially clinically and personally demanding due to the COVID-19 pandemic. The world is a better place, and patient care a higher quality, because of your dedication and tireless work to improve outcomes for people living with HIV. We are grateful to Springer for support, patience, words of encouragement, and assistance in publishing our work.

Ian would like to thank his daughter Carrie for endless patience and support, and for always taking an active interest in his work. He would also like to thank the many people he has met over the years, on many continents, for their inspiration and wisdom.

Michelle would like to thank her daughter Harriet, son Louis, mum Pauline, and dad Mike, for their endless support, cups of tea, and gentle words of encouragement.

Ian and Michelle would also like to acknowledge each other in terms of their mutual support, professional respect, sense of humour, and determination that has spanned over 20 years to make this a resilient friendship.

Finally, we would both like to thank all the people living with HIV for sharing your stories, experiences, and journey with us. You continue to inspire us to provide the best care possible.

Contents

About the Authors

Christina Antoniadi was born and raised in Greece where she gained bachelor's degrees in nursing and communications. She has been working in HIV care since 2013. Her current role is Junior Sister/Charge Nurse at the inpatient HIV ward Ron Johnson of Chelsea and Westminster Hospital. She has worked in a variety of settings, but particularly enjoyed working in the Drug Consumption Room, "Ulysses" (2013–2015), and coordinating the women's group "EATG4Women" (2017–2018) at the European AIDS Treatment Group (EATG). She is currently a member of the executive committee of NHIVNA, and inspired the "AskTheHIVNurse/Talk2TheHIVNurse" campaign that ran in 2020, the Year of the Nurse.

Jane Bruton has worked in HIV and sexual health for 28 years. She started in HIV in 1987 as the Sister of an Infectious Disease Unit in Leicester, the admitting ward for HIV. In 1989, she was briefly a Health Advisor in London before becoming Sister on Broderip Ward, Middlesex Hospital, the first purpose-built HIV ward. In 1996, she took a sabbatical to work in HIV in Uganda and completed a master's degree in medical anthropology. In 1999, Jane returned to London to work at the Chelsea and Westminster hospital, first as a Practice Development Advisor for HIV and Sexual Health, covering inpatients, outpatients, and day care, and finally as Nurse Consultant. Her primary focus was developing the nurses' role, competency frameworks, and patient involvement in their care and service development. She was an Executive committee member of NHIVNA for several years. Having retired in 2013, she works part-time in the Patient Experience Research Centre at Imperial College London, undertaking qualitative research in HIV, Hepatitis C, COVID-19, Patient and Public Involvement and Engagement. She teaches on Civil Society and HIV and qualitative research. Jane was a project team member and interviewer in the "AIDS Era: an oral history of UK healthcare workers" project, 2016–2019. She runs NURSETRI workshops for HIV nurses in South-East Europe and is acting Chair of the Trustees Board, Positively UK.

Tomás Campbell is a chartered clinical psychologist, an Associate Fellow of the British Psychological Society (BPS), a chartered scientist, and a Fellow of the Royal

Society of Medicine. He is a member of the BPS Division of Clinical Psychology (DCP) and of Neuropsychology as well as being an active committee member of the Faculty for HIV and Sexual Health. He is an independent consultant for UNICEF and a guest lecturer on the University of Glasgow clinical neuropsychology course. Tomás spent 2 years working in a HIV programme in Zambia and is now chair of the UK board of trustees of a charity that supports HIV and reproductive health services for young people with HIV in South Africa and Ghana. His research interests have focused on African people with HIV in London and particularly on how families have developed HIV-coping mechanisms. He is especially interested in the neuropsychological aspects of HIV disease and in efforts to address the effects of HIV stigma. At the moment, he works currently as an independent clinical neuropsychologist with young people, adults, and their families who have an acquired brain injury.

Michelle Croston is a senior lecturer at the Faculty of Health, Psychology, and Social Care, Manchester Metropolitan University. She has a clinical background in HIV care working at national and international level to improve outcomes for people living with HIV. She holds a fellowship with European Society for Person Centered Healthcare (ESPCH). Michelle has extensive postgraduate qualifications in mental health and psychological trauma, alongside her role as a senior lecturer she is a qualified Mental Health First Aid Instructor and Crisis Counsellor for a Mental Health charity that specialises in working with healthcare workers. Michelle is passionate about develop teaching and learning strategies to prevent compassion fatigue and secondary trauma.

Catarina Esteves Santos has been working since 2005 with people living with HIV in the ambulatory clinic of Cascais Hospital, Portugal. She has authored several scientific publications and is a trainer and lecturer for various courses and events in around nursing adults living with HIV, ageing with HIV, and paediatrics, including for the Portuguese Council of Nurses. She has been a coordinator for the European HIV Nursing Networking (EHNN) since 2007, proud to have taken a role in bringing together a group of expert HIV nurses to standardise and value the nursing role. Since 2018, she has been on the executive board of the Portuguese association for the study of AIDS. Catarina is also one of the coordinators of the European HIV Nursing Network.

Stuart Gibson is a clinical psychologist from Canada who has been teaching, conducting research and providing clinical services in HIV and sexual health for nearly 25 years. Stuart served as the Chair of the Faculty for HIV & Sexual Health with the British Psychological Society for many years. His current NHS appointment is at Barts Health in East London, where he works as a Consultant Clinical Psychologist and serves as the Head of Psychology in Infection & Immunity - one of the country's largest psychology services for HIV and sexual health.

Matthew Grundy-Bowers has been the consultant nurse (HIV/Sexual Health) at Imperial College Healthcare NHS Trust since 2005, Trust Lead for Advancing Practice since 2018, and is a senior lecturer in Advanced Clinical Practice at City, University of London. In 2020 he was awarded the prestigious Fellowship of the RCN for his contribution to HIV/Sexual Health, advanced clinical practice, and interdisciplinary education. Matthew has a national leadership profile in HIV/Sexual Health, he is the current chair of the BASHH/STIF Competencies Committee and was a member of the NHIVNA executive. He is actively involved with various Advanced Practice projects with Health Education England and is currently leading the joint project between BASHH, FSRH and NHIVNA to develop a curriculum (which was launched in 2019) and credentialing for ACPs in Integrated Sexual Health and HIV.

Ian Hodgson has been involved in the international health sector for over 20 years. Areas of interest include HIV and TB stigma, sexual and reproductive health and rights, cultural determinants of HIV prevention, advocacy for HIV treatment access, and adolescents living with HIV. He has worked on a range of projects in Asia, Africa, and Europe, and much of his work involves the monitoring and evaluation of HIV community projects using a systematic qualitative approach.

Ian is a member of the European AIDS Treatment Group (EATG), and currently on the board of directors. He is also a coordinator of the European HIV Nursing Network. He is an Associate Editor of the journal Ethnicity and Health, supervisor for international health-based research studies, and visiting lecturer at universities in Belgium, Ireland, the UK, and the US.

Chris Irons is a clinical psychologist, researcher, writer and trainer specialising in Compassion Focused Therapy. He is co-director of Balanced Minds (www.balancedminds.com), a London based organisation providing compassion-focused psychological interventions for individuals and organisations. He also works for the Compassionate Mind Foundation, and as a Visiting Lecturer at the University of Derby.

For almost two decades, Chris has worked with Professor Paul Gilbert and other colleagues on research and clinical developments linked to CFT. He was involved in some of the initial research papers and book chapters on CFT (Gilbert & Irons, 2004, 2005), and has published many articles and book chapters on compassion, attachment, shame and self-criticism. He has authored five books, including "The Compassionate Mind Workbook" (with Dr Elaine Beaumont) and "CFT from the Inside Out" (with Russell Kolts, James Bennett-Levy, and Tobyn Bell), and "The Compassionate Mind Approach for Difficult Emotions".

Jeffrey Kwong is a professor in the Division of Advanced Nursing Practice at Rutgers University School of Nursing. He is a certified Adult-Gerontology Primary Care Nurse Practitioner and maintains a clinical practice in New York City where he provides care to adults living with HIV across the age continuum. He is the Co-Medical Director of the HIV & Ageing Initiative sponsored by the American

Academy of HIV Medicine and the American Geriatrics Society. He has served as the previous president for the National Association of Nurses in AIDS Care and an educational consultant for the New York State AIDS Institute's HIV Clinical Education Initiative. Dr. Kwong is a fellow of the American Academy of Nurse Practitioners and the American Academy of Nursing.

Alexander Margetts is a Clinical Psychologist and BABCP accredited CBT therapist with experience in working with individuals presenting with common mental health difficulties, especially in the context of physical health and neurocognitive issues. He has worked in HIV and Sexual Health at Chelsea and Westminster Hospital for the past decade and has a special interest in the training and supervision of psychologists and other mental health professionals and their continuing professional development. He completed his Doctorate in Clinical Psychology at Oxford University (2008), and Postgraduate Diplomas in CBT at Royal Holloway University (2011), and Neuropsychology at Glasgow University (2015). Alex currently works as a Clinical Tutor for the University of Leicester Doctorate in Clinical Psychology and the CNWL/RHUL CBT Postgraduate Diploma (IAPT High Intensity Training), as well as being an active committee member of the British Psychological Society Division of Clinical Psychology Faculty for HIV and Sexual Health.

Jackie Morton qualified as a Registered Nurse, District Nurse with a master's degree in Business Administration. She retired from the NHS in 2011, following a 40-year career in several senior management positions and high-level nursing roles in England and Scotland. From 2010, following a diagnosis of HIV, she has used her knowledge of the NHS to strive for the rights of PLHIV, influencing those in power at a national and government level. She has been the chair of national and international charities, HIV Scotland, and European Aids Treatment Group (EATG), and interim Chief Executive of Terrence Higgins Trust, London during 2015–16. She has been actively engaged in leading patient advocacy roles; on the British HIV Association's primary care project; the advisory group of the 2015 UK Stigma Index and a Patient Public Voice for three years on the HIV Clinical Reference Group until 2019. She has presented at national and international HIV forums in Europe and the UK and has been involved in the writing of articles on HIV over the past ten years. From 2018 to 2020 she has been the director of her own company, health podcasts.

Hilary Piercy is an associate professor and works at Sheffield Hallam University, England. Hilary has a clinical background in nursing and midwifery and a long academic career that has combined teaching, research and clinical practice around her specialist area of sexual and reproductive health. A substantial proportion of Hilary's current research portfolio is concerned with aspects of healthcare service delivery and workforce development in response to changing expectations around the way that services are organised and delivered and has a specific focus on sexual health and HIV services.

Sarah Rutter is a Clinical Psychologist with a particular interest in complex psychological issues within HIV. As well as her present role as psychology lead in the HIV service at North Manchester General Hospital, Sarah is also the current chair of the British Psychological Society's Faculty for HIV and Sexual Health. Sarah is also an honorary lecturer at the University of Liverpool.

Fiona Wallis has worked in HIV care since 1988, as the Senior Sister on the Inpatient Unit at St. Mary's Hospital in London before relocating to York in 1992, where she was the Lead Nurse for HIV in York and Scarborough until she retired in 2018.

Fiona has been central to leading the development of HIV services across York and North Yorkshire which provides HIV care within the Acute Hospital setting, Outpatient Clinics, and in the Community. The nursing and medical teams are integrated and use a case management model of care. Fiona's areas of interest are HIV Late Presenters, HIV Testing in Primary Care, and Rural Healthcare Issues.

Jane Vosper is a Clinical Psychologist who has been working clinically in the field of Sexual Health and HIV for 9 years. She also works as a Lecturer in Clinical Psychology at Royal Holloway University of London on the Doctorate in Clinical Psychology Programme. Her clinical and research work have focused on psychosexual problems, HIV, sexual assault, health services research, with recent projects linked to Compassion-Focused Therapy.

Anna Maria Żakowicz is Deputy Bureau Chief and Director of Programs at AHF (AIDS Healthcare Foundation) Europe in Amsterdam, the Netherlands. In her work, she focuses on implementation of people-centred care approaches in HIV testing, treatment and care, and prevention. She is committed to putting into practice concepts of integration, taskshifting, user-driven care, and patients' involvement in co-production of care. She believes that every person should receive loving and caring health services. She works across Europe; Eastern Europe has a special place in her heart. She serves on the Board of Trustees of AIDSFonds. Equity and access to quality HIV treatment and care were the issues she was addressing while serving as a co-chair of Global Network of People Who Live with HIV (GNP+), Civil Society Forum on HIV (CSF), a chair of European AIDS Treatment Group (EATG), and a board member of Medicines Patent Pool (MPP). Żakowicz has a background in humanities and public health. She received her MA from Silesian University and MIH from the University of Copenhagen.

Introduction

At the time of writing this book, based on data from 2019, 38 million people globally live with HIV [1]. The burden of the epidemic varies considerably between countries and regions, yet healthcare professionals continue to rise to the challenge by adapting new ways of working. Pioneering nurses and healthcare professionals continually champion creative solutions to deliver exemplary models of care in HIV services in response to the ever-evolving needs of people living with HIV.

Advances in HIV treatment mean people diagnosed with HIV now live much longer, healthier lives. In many countries, there has been rapid progress in timely HIV diagnosis, access to treatment, and viral suppression, as advocated by the UNAIDS worldwide targets of 90-90-90 (90% of people living with HIV to be diagnosed, 90% of those diagnosed to be on treatment, and 90% of those treated to have an undetectable viral load) [2]. This has also resulted in a significant proportion of people living with HIV now being unable to transmit the virus to others. This is based on evidence that an undetectable viral load means the virus is untransmittable, reflected in the U=U campaign [3]. Whereas these scientific advances are hugely welcome, new challenges have emerged in HIV care. Many of these are psychosocial in nature and include factors that impact on a person's quality of life such as lifelong adherence to treatment, ageing, stigma, and disclosure. The landscape of HIV care is therefore in a constant state of flux, never more evident than during the recent COVID-19 pandemic. There has been immense stress on the capacity for HIV care to maintain services. Healthcare professionals working in HIV care are striving to deliver high standard, person-centred care whilst facing the uncertainty of what this might mean in light of global health challenges. That said, services are now beginning to respond, giving rise to innovative thinking and opportunities to reflect on how services can be delivered in different ways. Ongoing reflection is crucial in all areas of nursing care, and the chapters in this book are designed to help people consider their own practice. It offers an opportunity to explore alternative ways to deliver high-quality care to meet the ever-changing needs of people living with HIV and the evolving capacity of health systems in which they work.

Features of the Book

Within this book, each of the chapters is structured so as to enable the reader to consider their own clinical practice by reflecting on the theories and concepts discussed by the authors. Within the main body of the chapter, the authors include a mixture of reflection points, activities boxes, cases studies, and resources boxes designed to support your learning. The book has not been designed to be used as a workbook, so we recommend you to use a separate notebook for any written reflections or activities, so you can refer to them at a later date.

The book can be used in a variety of different ways. You may choose to focus on the chapters relevant to your particular area of practice or development need or you may choose to read the book in its entirety. Where possible, we have grouped chapters by broad topic to facilitate your learning. Whatever approach you take, we do hope you enjoy the chapters, and that the material adds value to your clinical practice.

Chapter Overviews

Chapter 1: We Broke the Rules: Building the Foundation of HIV Nursing

HIV nursing has had, and will continue to have, a critical role in the treatment and care of people living with HIV (PLHIV). In the 1980s and 1990s, HIV was a devastating, stigmatised disease with no cure. In response to this crisis, HIV nurses transformed the fundamentals of care. Within this chapter, Jane examines how and why these changes occurred and tells the stories of the nurses' experiences on the front line. Jane starts the historical journey in the 1960s with the radicalising social, cultural, and economic landscape which stimulated nurse academics to challenge the biomedical model and develop new nursing theories and innovative practices based on holism. These theories inspired the new HIV nurses to develop nurse–patient partnerships based in person-centred models which became the central element of the HIV nursing legacy. As HIV transformed into a chronic condition with new treatments, nurses transformed their role to meet the changing needs of people living with HIV, never losing sight of the person-centred approach. This history has implications for today's HIV nurses. It is a history we share with those diagnosed before treatment was available, some of whom are still alive today. We witnessed their pain and loss, their anger and determination, their humour; all of which has shaped their journey and ours.

Keywords

HIV nursing; HIV 1980s; Person-centred care; Nurse–patient partnerships; Nursing models; Holism; Biomedical model

Chapter 2: Understanding and Expanding HIV Nursing Roles

Following on from the historical background of HIV nursing, in this chapter Hilary Piercy encourages the reader to explore the clinical component of the HIV nursing role. Hilary shares with the reader her research experiences as she examines what we know about the nursing role and how it operates in different services across England. The reflection points and case studies encourage the reader to consider their current role and how this might meet the current needs of people living with HIV.

Keywords

HIV; Nursing workforce; Nurse led; Advance practice; Person-centred care

Chapter 3: Nurse Leadership in HIV Care

Within this chapter, Jackie explores the history of nurse leadership in the care of people living with HIV and AIDS and explains how nurses have led and driven health and care provision. Jackie also considers the leadership qualities required to adapt nursing practice to meet the changing needs of people living with HIV and makes recommendations for nursing practice and nurse educators. It concludes with a proposed model of nurse leadership within the modern and dynamic environment of HIV services, expanded for clarity by examples where necessary.

Keywords

Nursing history; Leadership and governance; Care models and nurse leadership; Adaption and learning in leadership; Personal reflection

Chapter 4: HIV Is a Small Word with a Big Impact: Psychosocial Interventions to Support Children, Young People, and Families with HIV

The focus of this chapter explores the advances in HIV treatment and the significant impact that this has had on families living with HIV. Tomás outlines a comprehensive psychosocial support strategy for children, young people, and families living with HIV. Within the chapter, the concept of stigma is explored, and the reader is introduced to the concept of family-centered care.

Keywords

HIV; Stigma; Young people; Children; Families with HIV

Chapter 5: Advancing the Role of the Nurse: Sexual Health for People Living with HIV

Within this chapter, Matthew provides a comprehensive overview of HIV-advanced clinical practitioners (ACP) with regard to providing person-centred care to improve and maintain their sexual health (SH) for people living with HIV. The chapter draws on the knowledge, skills, and behaviours that advanced clinical practitioner should have in relation to sexual health, considering not just Sexually Transmitted Infections (STIs) and contraception, but other aspects of sexual health, including sexual dysfunction (SD) and sexualised drug use (SDU).

Keywords

HIV; Sexual health; MSM; Advanced clinical practice; Nurse

Chapter 6: Nurses in HIV Care in Eastern Europe, Past, Present, and Future

The chapter focuses on the role of nurses in Eastern European healthcare system with specific focus on HIV care. It refers to the beginnings of Soviet healthcare, describes the system and formation of cadres of nurses, addresses changes that happened in mid 1990s in the region and the need to strengthen the role of nurses in medical community related to ageing population, increase of chronic diseases, and appearance of new diseases like HIV. The chapter describes the functions of nurses in the healthcare system, discusses the need to increase the role of the nurses, boosts the prestige of the profession, and points to the areas of education and training that would be needed for the future. The chapter refers to the ongoing work of the World Health Organization (WHO) to strengthen the role of nurses through task-shifting and task sharing to implement people-centred care for people who live with HIV.

Keywords

HIV; Eastern Europe; Nurses; Healthcare; HIV care; People-centred care

Chapter 7: Access to HIV Services for Key Populations: Leaving No One Behind

As a virus, HIV can potentially pose a threat to any person. However, since the beginning of the epidemic in the early 1980s, certain groups have been at higher risk of infection due to biological, personal or interpersonal, or sociocultural and structural factors. These key-affected and vulnerable populations also face significant barriers in gaining access to important health and support services because of factors such as stigma and discrimination, the political and legal contexts, and because healthcare workers do not always possess the necessary skills to provide the necessary support. Healthcare is not always a "safe haven". In order to improve access, it is necessary to ensure that healthcare services are underpinned by a robust rights-based approach, engage with affected communities, and prepare healthcare workers with the sufficient aptitude, attitude, and skillset. This will ensure that all people affected by HIV, and especially key and vulnerable populations, are able to keep themselves and others safe, and protect their quality of life.

Keywords

HIV; AIDS; Key-affected populations; Healthcare; Equality; Equity; Human rights; Stigma

Chapter 8: HIV Care in Rural Areas

Based on long career as a HIV nurse, within this chapter Fiona explores the challenges of providing care in a rural setting. Within this chapter, Fiona skilfully discusses the challenges that providing care in a rural setting can provide for nurses exploring issues such as confidentiality and stigma. Throughout the chapter Fiona reflects on the challenges she faced as a nurse providing care and offers some practical solutions for the reader to consider when thinking about their own clinical practices

Keywords

Rural; HIV; Nursing care; Stigma; Long-term condition

Chapter 9: Care Considerations for Ageing with HIV

This chapter provides an overview of care considerations for older adults living with HIV. With the success of effective HIV antiretroviral therapy, persons living with HIV are now ageing into older adulthood. In the UK, approximately one-third of all persons living with HIV are aged 50 or older. Similar trends are seen in other countries, including the United States, where it has been estimated that more than half of all persons living with HIV are 50 years or older. As this population continues to grow, chronic conditions, such as cardiovascular disease, metabolic complications, and malignancy will become priorities. Nurses caring for this population should be familiar with how these other conditions manifest in the context of HIV.

Keywords

HIV; Ageing with HIV; Ageing; Chronic conditions; Non-communicable disease; Polypharmacy

Chapter 10: Women Living with or Affected by HIV: Frugality and the Politics of Deprivation

Women have always been present in the HIV epidemic either as healthcare workers, support networks (mothers, carers, partners, friends) for the people living with HIV or living with HIV themselves. As HIV was originally considered to affect mostly Men who are having Sex with Men (MSM), women were overlooked; however, today they represent 51% of the people living with HIV globally. In recent years, Eastern Europe and Central Asia are one of the two regions that the overall prevalence of HIV has not declined with adolescent girls and young women facing double the risk of HIV acquisition compared to their male counterparts. The chapter presents literature highlighting the areas where the HIV response has left women behind or is inadequate to address their needs. Areas of interest include: the biological differences, the identified need for better inclusion in research, the socio-economic factors leading to health disparities and the pleasure deficit that has guided the HIV response, leading to poor health outcomes and questionable well-being for the women living with HIV (WLHIV).

Keywords

HIV; Women living with HIV; Inequality; Clinical research; Politics

Chapter 11: Ageing with HIV: Lifestyle Interventions Towards Health

The care paradigm has changed in HIV infection as it has become a chronic condition. Comorbidities have increased and are happening at earlier ages. For the first time in the history of the disease, there is a first generation of people who are ageing with HIV.

Health is a fundamental factor for human development, training, and adaptability to change. Its promotion takes on a variety of outlines, dimensions, and responsibilities, including surveillance and individual investment, through the positive valuation of the factors that determine it—health promotion and health education both fall within the responsibility of nursing.

The quality of care provided to people with HIV is directly related and depends on the appropriate preparation of health professionals. Adequate skills support the capacity of nursing to provide holistic care to individuals, families, and communities, as well as a basis for supporting practice development and resources for strengthening nursing capacity in the context of HIV.

Nurses should have the knowledge, skills, and understanding that will allow them to help the person in their unique situation, as well as accompanying them in their life path.

Keywords

HIV; Nursing; Health promotion; Health protective factors; Ageing

Chapter 12: Bringing Compassion into HIV Care: Applying the Compassion-Focused Therapy Model to Healthcare Delivery

This chapter introduced compassion-focused therapy (CFT) with the goal of improving our understanding and compassion for the psychological difficulties that humans can face. Since this approach aims to normalise and de-shame psychological suffering, CFT appears useful for people living with HIV where stigma and discrimination leading to psychological distress and shame prevail. On understanding the role of individual histories, it is clear that difficult early lives characterised by a lack of love and support can place people at higher risk of falling into detrimental patterns of coping. As negative views of the self can be central to these patterns, we considered how compassionate approaches to supporting people living with HIV might begin to increase self-worth, relieve distress and improve coping. Within this chapter, Jane, Sarah, Stuart, and Chris look at different "flows of compassion": providing compassion to others, receiving it from others, and directing compassion towards oneself (self-compassion). Additionally, Jane, Sarah, Stuart, and Chris discussed the role of compassion for health professionals, as working in the complex area of HIV can be as challenging as it is rewarding. We discussed the concept of compassion fatigue with its negative impact on health professionals and highlighted the importance of self-care.

Keywords

HIV; Compassion; Psychological distress; Health outcomes; Staff self-care; Compassion fatigue; Shame

Chapter 13: Wounded Healers in a Shared Traumatic Reality: Why and How We Should Engage in Stepped-Care, Self-Care for Ourselves

Following on from Jane, Sarah, Stuart, and Chris chapter exploring Compassion-Focused Therapy, Alex and Michelle within this chapter explore practical solution to developing different flows of compassion. Throughout the chapter the readers are encouraged to find ways to support their own well-being in order to prevent compassion fatigue. Working through the chapter, the readers are invited to consider their own well-being and devise ways to promote a step-care approach to obtain support for life's challenges.

Keywords

Self-care; Nurses; Compassion fatigue; Well-being; Burnout

Overall Aim of the Book

The overall aim of the book is to explore a wide range of issues relevant to HIV care. It has been designed to be accessible to as many healthcare professionals as possible. The book does not claim to be exhaustive and readers may wish to deepen their knowledge by following up on relevant references, exploring the theories mentioned in more depth, and accessing the relevant resources mentioned. The chapters have been written by leading experts within the global field of HIV care and are, in some cases, co-written to enable different perspectives to be shared. The book has been designed to encourage the reader to think about HIV care and offer some practical ideas about how to continue to be innovative. Whether the reader works within a HIV care setting or would just like to learn more about HIV-related issues, the book provides a helpful framework for consider person-centred care for people living with HIV.

References

1. UNAIDS. Global HIV & AIDS statistics — 2020 fact sheet. 2020. https://www.unaids.org/en/resources/fact-sheet. Accessed January 2021.
2. UNAIDS. 90-90-90: An ambitious treatment target to help end the AIDS epidemic. Geneva: UNAIDS; 2014.
3. The Lancet H. U=U taking off in 2017. Lancet HIV. 2017;4(11):e475.

Chapter 1
We Broke the Rules: Building the Foundations of HIV Nursing

Jane Bruton

> *The movement to confront the HIV epidemic … has radically changed the world's understanding and response to health challenges and has been said to have created the concept of global health.* [1]

1.1 Chapter Overview

At time of writing, the world is six months into the COVID-19 pandemic. Globally, we are experiencing the uncertainty and fear of a new viral infection. Stories of courage and compassion in hospitals, care homes, and the community abound. Nurses hold the hands of dying patients in the absence of their loved ones, clinical staff look after dying colleagues, and clinical teams form new bonds in the face of this crisis. And misinformation is prevalent. All of this is very reminiscent of the early days of HIV care in the 1980s and 1990s.

Nursing has had, and will continue to have, a critical role in both pandemics. This chapter will examine how the advent of HIV changed nursing, why nursing became so central in HIV care and how the nurse role has changed as HIV was transformed from an acute, life-threatening disease into a chronic, manageable condition.

There are obvious reasons to re-explore this history: to educate future nurses and doctors about the values that underpinned our response to HIV; and to better prepare nurses facing new epidemics such as COVID-19. But another reason, less obvious, is that we share that history with those diagnosed before effective treatment was available some of whom are still alive today. We witnessed their pain and loss, their anger and determination, their humour; all of which has shaped their journey and ours.

J. Bruton (✉)
Imperial College London, London, UK

© The Author(s), under exclusive license to Springer Nature
Switzerland AG 2021
M. Croston, I. Hodgson (eds.), *Providing HIV Care: Lessons from the Field for Nurses and Healthcare Practitioners*,
https://doi.org/10.1007/978-3-030-71295-2_1

The chapter will outline the social, cultural, and economic context which, from the late 1960s, gave rise to communities of gay, women and black activists, and stimulated nurses to challenge the biomedical model, resulting in the development of new nursing theories and practices based on holism. It will examine the problems with the biomedical model, the nurse theorists' critique of it and how the nurse–patient partnership in a person-centred approach to care became one of the central elements of the HIV nursing legacy.

It will explore how HIV nursing carved a unique pathway in the context of a devastating, stigmatised disease for which there was no cure. It consisted of a commitment to person-centred care; a non-judgemental approach; nurse–patient partnerships both in care and activism; multidisciplinary working and support; innovative models of care; and the transformation of the clinical environment.

Using oral histories, written accounts, and interviews, it will illustrate how nurses implemented these new tenets of nursing care practically, in the pioneering HIV facilities in the UK and the USA.

It will describe the impact, from 1996, of effective antiretroviral therapy (ART), and from 2018 effective prevention, which offered new biomedical solutions. The consequent transformation of care drove nurses working in HIV to re-evaluate their role in order to meet the changing needs of people living with HIV, while maintaining a commitment to a person-centred approach. Finally, it will explore the implications of this history for today's nurses working with people living with HIV.

1.1.1 Social Turmoil

From the mid-1960s onwards, almost every aspect of life—from legal and political rights through to sexuality and the family—were called into question by social movements emerging from diverse communities: student and youth protests, the US Civil Rights movement, anti-colonial struggles, feminism, movements for gay liberation, and struggles for democracy in Eastern Europe. A generation emerged wanting to live in a better world, with an end to discrimination and inequality, and with universal human rights, dramatically changing the political culture [2, 3]. Those social movements, and the wider cultural change they stimulated, would influence the direction of HIV nursing in three ways.

First, the fight for gay rights and liberation in the UK, the USA, and other parts of the Global North established a defined, more visible, and organised community of activists. When the AIDS crisis broke in the 1980s, there was an already established community with experience of activism and self-help so critical to the response [4].

Second, women were challenging years of oppression and inequality within society. As a predominantly female profession, this had a deep resonance with nurses and nurse theorists, particularly in the USA, who were beginning to question the biomedical model and the highly gendered division of labour within healthcare [5].

Third, US nurse theorists' criticism of the biomedical model during the 1960s was gaining prominence. The biomedical model was seen as disease-focused, not patient- or person-focused [6, 7], and with cure more highly valued than care [8]. In turn, the hierarchy of cure over care reflected the prevailing gender stereotypes within the hospital as an institution: a male doctor as decision-maker, a female nurse as "handmaiden" receiving instructions, and a passive patient. This was rather like the prevailing family structure: mother, father, and the patient as child [5, 9, 10]. Stein [11], in his seminal work "The Doctor Nurse Game," described the inequality of professional power in healthcare in which nurses were "subordinate" to doctors.

Nurse theorists recognised that nursing needed to develop a body of knowledge as a foundation for its unique contribution within healthcare and to establish nursing as a recognised and valued profession [12, 13].

Despite changes to the doctor–nurse relationship, this critique of the power dynamic remains relevant today, particularly in the area of diagnosis and decision-making, where medical work continues to be deemed as having greater value [14, 15]. Studies have shown that the clinical environment is often determined by the professionals' relationships and if hierarchical can impact negatively on the quality of care and outcomes for patients. It also affects nurses, contributing to the level of their job satisfaction [16, 17].

1.1.2 Why Does Biomedicine Foster Inequalities?

It is useful to critique the traditional structure of healthcare using medical anthropology. This is the study of how people in different cultures and social groups experience and make sense of health and ill health. It explores how meaning is attributed to symptoms, the types of treatments people believe in, and who they consult when ill [18, 19]. Emerging formally in the 1960s, medical anthropology critically analysed the assumptions underpinning the biomedical model and the healthcare inequalities it creates.

Cassell [20] explained that while "illness" is what a patient feels when they go to the doctor, "disease" is what they have when they leave the surgery. He concludes that disease is something an organ has, while illness is something a human being has. Biomedicine had largely ignored the subjective experience of illness, whereas disease is something "real" and the biomedical search for its causes is based on a scientific, rational, and objective approach. Clinical research objectively and empirically tests hypotheses. The phenomenon or symptoms of disease are measured, quantified, and become facts and the accepted truth.

Unlike pre-industrial and folk medical systems, biomedicine separates mind and body. In doing so, the body is framed as a machine to be repaired. Modern technology increasingly divides the body into ever smaller parts moving the clinician even further away from the whole patient. Finally, biomedicine focuses on the individual patient rather than viewing them within their family and community [19].

Biomedicine confidently assumes that it can and will solve the problems of ill health [21].

While the biomedical model was being challenged theoretically from the 1960s onwards, the HIV epidemic led to it becoming further challenged in practice. Biomedicine's assumption that with the end of smallpox, it could finally conquer infectious diseases, was now called into question [22].

We should, of course, value the incredible achievements of biomedicine. It led to the development of antiretroviral therapy (ART), which can not only maintain an undetectable viral load but prevent onwards transmission at the same time. However, the quest for the "magic bullet"—a pill, a vaccine or a transplant—is not the complete answer. Why might this be?

First because, as we are experiencing today with COVID-19, biomedicine can rarely account for the differential impact of communicable diseases on different social groups. A purely biomedical response fails to acknowledge the social, cultural, economic, and political status of affected groups. As with HIV, biomedicine is a blunt instrument with little chance of eradicating the infections [23].

Second, because biomedicine has a blind spot regarding the validity and relevance of the subjective lived experience of patients and their significant others. It was this problem that inspired nurse theorists into action.

Helman [24], a doctor and anthropologist, laments that, "despite all these achievements [of biomedicine], I still feel that something is being lost from medicine today or is in danger of being lost, some precious, elusive quality of human interaction, something invisible and yet at the same time very real."

1.1.3   Nurses' Responses: Theory, Models, and Conceptual Frameworks for a New Nursing Care

Early nurse theorists in the USA wanted nurses to complement the medical model with a more holistic approach. Traditionally, nursing care delivery was known as 'functional" or task nursing, usually directed by a ward sister and based on the biomedical model. Each nurse would be allocated a task, rather than a group of patients, such as a bowel nurse or bed bath nurse. Team nursing was introduced in the mid-twentieth century, yet despite the growing popularity of new nursing concepts, task allocation prevailed for decades in many areas [25, 26].

Nurse theorists posed a fundamental question—'What is nursing?" [27, 28]. For an answer, they explored contemporary social scientific theories and frameworks around patient-hood, holism, and the lived experience of health and illness [6]. Two important writers emerged: Virginia Henderson, who created the Activities of Living model (see Box 1.1) and Ida Orlando's concept of the Nursing Process [25]. These theories are now familiar to most nurses, and together they provided a new framework for care and the role of the nurse. Both are based on a set of assumptions about care:

- the patient is the centre of care,
- the patient's needs must be assessed and understood,
- appropriate care for each patient must be planned and individualised,
- a 'whole patient' includes their family, friends, and community,
- nurse self-awareness is essential to empathise and understand other diverse human beings.

They recognised the therapeutic nature of the nurse/patient relationship and rejected the mind–body split. They also acknowledge the complexity and creativity of nursing, calling for the development of critical thinking skills based on the independence of the nurse [29–31].

These innovations, rooted in a holistic approach to care, paved the way for other theorists in the USA and Europe. Together, they created a body of knowledge that began to define the uniqueness of nursing (Box 1.1).

Box 1.1:
The unique function of the nurse is to assist the individual, sick or well, in the performance of those activities contributing to health or its recovery (or to a peaceful death) that he would perform unaided if he had the necessary strength, will or knowledge. And to do this in such a way as to help him gain independence as rapidly as possible. Virginia Henderson [32]

These developments soon reached the UK's shores. There was a mixed reception but, with some adaptations to the UK situation, the Nursing Process was embedded within the nurse curriculum by 1977 and rolled out to the wards. The challenge was to overcome the gap between the theories and the practical application [13, 28].

As a student nurse between 1978 and 1981, I was inspired by the Nursing Process and individualised nursing care. But any hopes of implementing it were quickly squashed by the reality of task allocation, which continued on the wards. However, by the early 1980s there were some champions of this approach among individual ward sisters, academics, and projects like the Oxford Burford Model [33, 34]. Then, in 1982, AIDS hit the headlines.

1.2   HIV/AIDS: The Chance to Turn Theory into Practice

In mid-1981 reports of a cluster of young men who have sex with men (MSM) were presenting with fatal pneumocystis carinii pneumonia (PCP) and Kaposi's sarcoma in both California and New York. By mid 1982 the disease was officially named as acquired immune deficiency syndrome (AIDS). The causative virus was found and eventually named HIV-1 in 1986 [35].

There was no cure. Care and treatment for opportunistic infections were the only clinical management options. Moral panic and hysteria were widespread in the face of this new disease, linked as it was to taboo subjects such as sex, sexuality, and death. It affected primarily MSM whose behaviour was already stigmatised as deviant, 'other,' and unacceptable. The media and wider society stigmatised and discriminated against people living with HIV (PLHIV) despite the fact that they were dying. There were reports of clinical staff refusing to care for 'these patients' [36].

This toxic mix mobilised clinicians, nurses, the "expert patient" and activists, who were outraged at this tirade of hate and united both in activism and as partners in care [37–39]. There was now no excuse for avoiding the "social" and "cultural" context of the disease. Science itself was subjected to cultural analysis, mainly because of the crisis of the biomedical and scientific response to HIV [37, 40].

In the UK, the epidemic coincided with growing aspirations in nursing to turn theory of individualised patient care into practice. HIV/AIDS became a vehicle for changing nursing practice. Richard Wells, a UK nurse, summed up the sentiments of those wanting change:

> If we get it right for AIDS we'll get it right for the whole of nursing. [38, 41]

Despite the commitment to show that HIV nurses could put nursing theory into practice, relatively little was written about the experience at the time. Jacqui Elliot, the sister of the first dedicated AIDS ward in the UK, wrote a nursing chapter in the First edition (1987) of the textbook *ABC of AIDS* [42]. There was an ethnographic study of a New York AIDS ward between 1989 and 1991 [43], based on in-depth interviews with nurses. And contemporary training videos, research papers, and nursing textbooks provide insight into the models used, nursing philosophy and practice within HIV.

However, over the past 5–10 years, more documentaries, oral histories, and studies have been looking back at the early years of HIV care from a nursing and medical point of view. These, together with individual memoirs, provide a rich resource to better understand experiences at the time. In particular, the voice of nurses in the USA and the UK capture the tenets of nursing practice that made this period unique. What continues to strike me about these accounts is that, whether they took place in London, New York, Edinburgh, San Francisco, Brighton, or Chicago, although the stories may differ, the dominant theme is the placing of patients with HIV at the absolute centre of the care. "Patient" in this case means the "whole" person in their social, cultural, psychological, physiological, and economic context.

Before looking at what the nurses achieved, we can get a sense of what the patients—many of whom did not survive—experienced. The impact of HIV/AIDS is a story of loss. Each loss, whether it is an individual's inability to work anymore, isolation from friends or family fearing accidental disclosure, multiple bereavement or loss of function and lifestyle, has the potential to disrupt the individual's identity and place in the world. Nina H talks about the impact of these losses and why death wasn't necessarily the hardest thing to deal with:

> Patient after patient tells me that they have accepted the idea that they are going to die very
> soon. What they can't accept is losing control, or losing their independence, or losing their
> mind, or losing control of their bowels, or losing their friends who don't come to see them
> anymore. [43]

Stigma was directed at both HIV and the social groups most affected, MSM, people who inject drugs (PWID), and sex workers. It remains one of the biggest barriers in the fight against HIV, preventing people from seeking a test and accessing care and medication. Stigma in the 1980s was especially prevalent, fuelled by the popular press. It had a devastating impact on people living with AIDS who were often forced to keep their diagnosis secret. Sometimes this led to self-stigma and self-loathing. Lorna describes what the impact of stigma was on her patients and how that affected her:

> I think I was really, really saddened, in fact heartbroken, when I realised how different it
> was from other diseases, that, how bad the stigma isolated people. Isolated them to the point
> that, you think, oh my goodness, I am the only person they have talked about their deep
> personal feelings to. [44]

Rejection was common, by families, communities, partners, or friends. Many MSM living with HIV did not disclose their sexuality to their parents since there was no need while they were healthy. Sometimes parents found out about AIDS and their son's sexuality at the same time. And for some this was as, or even more, devastating than knowing their son had AIDS. Parents' reactions were either to embrace their son and his partner, or to disown their son and his partner or just his partner. Carol describes what could happen:

> They actually got the situation where the body had been left in the morgue for a year,
> because the mother would not give up access. [She wanted] the right to organise the funeral.
> The partner said, 'But I have been given the instructions by your son as to how this funeral
> will happen.' [But] it took the local vicar attached to the hospital, after months, to sit down
> and say, 'This is not doing anybody any good'. [44]

These three accounts touch on some of the issues and remind us of some of the complexities, and how the physical devastation of the illness turned people's lives upside down. Despite that, in those early days, the involvement of the community (activists and voluntary sector organisations) was unique in providing self-help and campaigning for better care, new treatments. Together with the clinicians, they put pressure on the government for effective policy and funding for HIV care and pharma companies for the release of medications [45].

In the light of the increasing numbers requiring specialist inpatient care and the prevalence of poor care on general wards NHS managers set up dedicated HIV/AIDS inpatient wards either within existing specialities or from scratch. The aim was to concentrate nursing and medical knowledge and expertise and prevent AIDS patients experiencing hostility and neglect from fearful and prejudiced healthcare staff. They sought to protect the patients' confidentiality and provide an environment that was welcoming, relaxed, and safe.

Other facilities and services were developed alongside, by charities and statutory services, to provide day care, respite, palliative and terminal care, and specialist community nursing. A large number of volunteers provided care both in the hospitals and in the community. The composition of the multidisciplinary teams established on the wards reflected the complex needs of the patients and their significant others.

1.2.1   An Applied Model of Patient-Centred Care

Cliff Morrison, a nurse, set up the world's first HIV ward in San Francisco in 1983. It was nurse led, built, and operated by nurses and volunteers. His aim was to develop a ward without the traditional doctor–nurse hierarchy, emphasising caring not curing, where patients were partners in their care, with open visiting, a focus on touch, where the concept of "family" was redefined and a patient was treated as a person with compassion and dignity [36, 46, 47]. These constituted all the elements of patient-centred, individualised care. Morrison recounts that he set the ward up essentially because no-one else wanted to [46]. He clearly saw the need for a ward that could provide both a sanctuary and care. Volunteers from the community played a big part in supporting both the nurses and the patients.

> Like the Castro [the gay cultural area of San Francisco], 5B was a judgement free zone, where patients could be themselves, love their partners and define who was family. [47]

This approach became known as the San Francisco Model. It challenged the medical model and was soon adopted by other HIV units in the USA. Meanwhile, versions of this model were developing, both consciously and spontaneously, in the UK, Europe, and Australia.

Morrison, like many HIV nurses, challenged assumptions like "next of kin," limited visiting hours, and the clinical hierarchy. As one London based nurse said, "we broke all the rules … there were no rules, it was great" [48]. This was not the arbitrary, wilful breaking of rules but part of building an alternative model of patient-centred care within a biomedical institution.

One example of this rule breaking comes up time and again in accounts from nursing staff in HIV and is illustrated by the charge nurse on the HIV Unit 371 in Chicago inducting a new nurse starter:

> We sit on the bed. You may have been taught in nursing school not to. But touching, hugging, sitting on the bed, it means so much to our patients who at one time were treated like pariahs. [49]

Touch was central to care. It enabled nurses to "let the patients know we weren't afraid of them" [43]. On my first day as ward sister of the Middlesex HIV ward, the senior medical staff expressed their concern that nurses were hugging the patients and thought this was something I should sort out. Needless to say, the nursing team demonstrated to them that touch was central to our care, as it is today (Box 1.2).

In the UK, the first purpose-built ward was opened in 1987. Care was concentrated mainly in three centres in London, St Mary's, the Middlesex, and the St Stephens and Westminster Hospitals (known now as Chelsea and Westminster) for inpatient care. By 1990 over 65% of AIDS cases in the UK were managed at these three sites [45]. This concentration of patients enabled the development of nursing expertise in all the skills required in caring for patients with HIV/AIDS, especially highly sensitive issues like confidentiality, safety, and disclosure [50]. Importantly, the medical staff recognised that care was central in the management of patients in the absence of cure.

> **Box 1.2:**
> "Up until the AIDS epidemic, we were told there was going to be a shot or a surgical treatment for just about everything. AIDS caught the medical community with its pants down. Luckily there were people who were forward thinking enough to say, 'we can't do this ourselves. My reflex mallet, my blood pressure cuff, my thermometer aren't going to do Jack shit here' For me, the ultimate message, meaning, gift, whatever of this epidemic is that there are many different ways to heal. And if you can't heal or cure, then comfort. Truly care for people" Russ Leander in Taking Turns [49]

In the UK, hands on care was delivered primarily by qualified nurses as part of the commitment to holism. It was time for experimenting and innovation. Wards established Primary or Key nursing within a team structure. During my time running the HIV wards at the Middlesex Hospital, patients were allocated a nurse and a team for the duration of their admission and subsequent admissions. The wards developed their own nursing philosophies built around a set of beliefs, values and ethics, for example:

- The right to quality care,
- The day was to be structured around the patients' needs, not a ward routine,
- The patient was a person with a life,
- Protection of patients' confidentiality,
- Care was the central role of nursing,
- Enabling patient independence,
- Partnership working,
- A non-judgemental approach,
- A commitment to multidisciplinary working.

The Nursing Process and Nursing Models, formed the foundation of nurse assessment, care planning, delivery, and evaluation. Over time the multidisciplinary structures such as ward rounds, handovers and psycho-social meetings embraced a more flattened hierarchy between doctors, nurses, counsellors, psychologists, social workers, and the patient.

The number of deaths and funerals were at times overwhelming. Formal support and supervision were available and of course just as nurses worked hard and supported each other, they also played hard. In these gruelling years, there was humour and fun but there were nurse casualties along the way due to burn out. The wards worked very closely with the HIV outpatient clinics, day care staff, respite care, and community nurses sharing the same approaches to person-centred care. The following narratives give some expression as to what this model meant in reality.

The most important lesson from this experience is that partnership working is the foundation of person-centred care. It is central to the assessment planning and evaluation process and has been central within HIV not just at an individual patient level but with the HIV community. The partnership model led to a number of changes in practice [51], for example, the requirement for informed consent for an HIV anti-body test, the implementation of "Living Wills" endorsed by the British Medical Association.

And yet it took until 2010 for the UK government to publish a white paper [51] that promoted partnership working in health and social care with the slogan "Nothing about you without you," almost 30 years after the beginning of the HIV epidemic. Eileen describes the partnership model and what it has achieved:

> This is truly a partnership model. It is organically grown through patient-healthcare professional relationships. And I think that is part of the appeal. You really get to sit alongside patients and work together. None of these remarkable achievements in HIV treatment would have happened without that partnership. [44]

Partnership depends on continuity of the relationships between nurse and patient, between doctor and patient. Continuity is valued by HIV patients and its absence particularly in primary care services is a common complaint today, having to repeat their history at each consultation. Knowing that the nurse knows your story inspires confidence and trust. Sarah describes how primary and key nursing maintains continuity:

> Each patient had a particular nurse, and there'd be a team around that nurse. So, every day you'd be given a patient, two or three patients, You had quite an intense relationship with the patients, because you spent a lot of time with them. [44]

Patients were often in hospital for long periods with frequent readmissions. The aim of the model was to enable patients to be themselves. Traditional ward rules were relaxed, partners were allowed or encouraged to stay overnight, visiting was open, inpatients were supported to safely continue normal life like going out for a meal or a coffee, celebrating a birthday or even going to Gay Pride. Nutrition was vital as the patients were generally very wasted. One of the London wards had their own chef-run kitchen providing home-cooked food.

On Broderip ward, we didn't wear uniform putting the nurse–patient relationship on a more human to human level. In the same vein, Cliff Morrison in San Francisco called himself "nursing co-ordinator" rather than "head nurse" [36]. These seemingly small gestures taken together created an environment that was less like a clinical unit and more like a home. Nicky describes her reaction to this way of working on her first day on the ward as a new member of staff:

> "I had gone from a very traditional type of nursing, as soon as you had got your handover, you'd be getting your patients up, washed, beds made, all ready for the consultant coming round and medication had to be given at a certain time. So, I was all geared up for that. And we did the handover and someone said, 'Tea and toast?' And I said, 'Yeah, who do you want me to make it for? Which bed?' And they went 'No. We now have tea and toast. We have breakfast now.' I went, 'What us the staff?' And they went, 'Yeah.' They were laughing at me because I was a bit like really? And I said, 'What about the patients?' 'Oh, they'll buzz when they're ready....' 'We get them up when they're ready to be gotten up'" [44]

All of these measures to develop non-hierarchical relationships helped to create a relaxed atmosphere. Attention was also given to the environment, introducing relaxed lighting, duvets instead of sheets and blankets, quiet spaces, art on the walls, and altering the traditional layout of the ward.

The wards were supported by volunteers some from the gay community and others affected by HIV in some way a bereaved mother, a friend, or a partner. They provided care, entertainment, practical support, complementary therapies, a listening ear, and kindness.

Finally, "going that extra mile" for patients, one nurse spoke of helping a patient move to an apartment because her family refused to help, other nurses shopped for patients on their way home from work or giving clinical care in the community at the end of a shift because no-one else would. It was tough and formal support and supervision was essential, but the day-to-day support came from the team. Anna describes how it felt:

> It was like a little mini family. And that was great. The differences here was like a warm blanket being put round you. You learnt from each other, you shared with each other; you saw people cry, colleagues cry, break down. You saw patients die. The impact of normalisation was really important, [and] that you looked out for [and] supported others. [44]

Some nurses moved from the wards to other parts of the service like research, sexual health, or the community and took this approach to care with them.

At the same time as we were busy providing patient-centred care, the political and societal values went in the opposite direction. Health services, even in the UK's publicly funded NHS, were moving down the road of commercially viable economic units and cuts in the budgets were beginning to bite. HIV services were treated as a special case and funding was ring-fenced because of the fear of the epidemic spreading into the heterosexual population. This led to resentment among our colleagues in other specialties. During this phase, HIV units were not part of the marketisation process and patients could self-refer to a unit of their choice rather than being referred by the general practitioner (GP).

1.2.2 The Impact of New Treatments on Nursing and Care Delivery

July 1996 marked a watershed for HIV treatment and care. At the XI international AIDS conference in Vancouver there were two developments that would change the face of HIV/AIDS forever: viral load testing and combination therapy, known then as HAART. Within months nurses saw dramatic changes among their patients described as the "Lazarus effect." Some patients who had been close to death literally got off their beds, and eventually were discharged home. The drug regimens were complex and burdensome with debilitating side-effects, but they had a dramatic impact on mortality.

As a result, HIV centres reduced inpatient beds by half. Whole wards closed, including the London Lighthouse inpatient unit, the nurse workforce shrank, and the focus of care shifted to outpatient departments. It was a remarkable achievement. However, it posed a new challenge to nursing. Was this the triumph of biomedicine, at last developing the "magic bullet," that would herald the renewed dominance of the medical model, relegating the importance of nursing care? And would a renewed biomedical hierarchy impact negatively on the partnership model.

The structure of an outpatient clinic was centred around the traditional doctors' consultations, with nurses supporting the doctors, the patients, and the general day-to-day management. The only difference in the HIV clinic I worked in was that the environment was more relaxed with comfy chairs and refreshments provided by volunteers. With the reduction in deaths, we saw an increase in the patient numbers and a tightening of the budget as the cost of the drugs bill increased squeezing the services. The nurses' role had narrowed to blood taking, weighing patients, supporting the busier doctors' clinics, reducing the time previously available for responding to the complex psycho-social needs of the patients.

The HIV outpatient nursing staff knew they needed to change their role to meet the holistic needs of the patient. This meant reviewing the nursing skills and structures required for a new role. Nurses were capable and well placed to provide nurse clinics such as the management of adherence to medication, triaging emergency walk-in patients and clinics where more experienced nurses managed a case load.

Despite HIV pioneering individualised care, in the UK we were late in developing advanced practice. However, in the last 10 years Advanced Nurse Practitioners in HIV are supported by Competencies and Guidelines developed by the National HIV Nurses Association (NHIVNA) and endorsed by the medical HIV organisation British HIV Association (BHIVA). It wasn't an easy journey with barriers such as financial and time constraints, lack of support from some managers and medical staff, and resistance to change. But the success has been the maintenance of a holistic partnership approach to care.

1.3   Conclusion

Today's picture of HIV looks very different from the 1980s and 1990s. HIV is now considered a manageable chronic condition, but unlike most other chronic conditions PLHIV experience stigma and discrimination. HIV disproportionately affects vulnerable and marginalised groups, including the five key populations described by UNAIDS and WHO: MSM, PWID, prisoners, sex workers, transgender people, and other vulnerable groups such as young women, adolescent girls, and indigenous people in some communities.

Important progress has been made in the last 5 years: globally, by the end of 2019 just over two-thirds of PLHIV were on treatment, still leaving 12.6 million who were not. Research has proven that if an individual has an undetectable viral load they cannot transmit HIV infection (Undetectable equals Untransmittable: U = U). Pre-Exposure Prophylaxis (PrEP) that prevents HIV infection is more widely available. We saw dramatic reductions in new diagnoses in parts of the Global North.

The world is moving closer to the UNAIDS target of 90-90-90 (90% of PLHIV are diagnosed, 90% of those diagnosed are on treatment, and 90% of those are virally suppressed).

But, as already discussed, there are fundamental flaws with a purely biomedical approach to disease such as HIV, equating "objective" indicators, such as viral load, with better health. Viral suppression is essential, but many have argued it cannot be the sole end point. HIV experts have pushed for a "fourth 90," achieving health and well-being beyond viral suppression. Clinicians have extended the fourth 90 concept to include a commitment to supporting health and well-being throughout the HIV treatment cascade from diagnosis onwards, focusing on a holistic approach to managing PLHIV [52, 53].

What have we learnt from the last 40 years of HIV nursing? First, we demonstrated that person-centred care is achievable. All the conditions were right: an engaged patient group, an active community, and, in the absence of cure, a focus on care became central. Secondly, there was a body of nursing knowledge, including nursing models, promoting a holistic approach, and philosophy of care that was non-judgemental, non-hierarchical, and committed to multidisciplinary working. The nursing teams were passionate and dedicated to making it work for the patients, their significant others, and themselves. This nursing approach influenced the way doctors worked with patients and brought the whole team closer together. They were unique times and for many, including me, the best experience of our careers.

Carol explained in a recent interview:

I did feel at the time we were living though an important era in nursing [which] would have knock-on effects. We would change nursing in every way, not just for AIDS patients. [It would influence] other things, like patients' rights to choose treatment options. And the patient-centred care really came out of the AIDS epidemic. [44]

Third, HIV nursing demonstrated that it can be flexible and adapt to the changing needs of PLHIV. The changes needed to the nursing role from the late 1990s onwards were not easily obtained but essential to retaining the partnership model of care. Had nurses not united to tread this challenging path we may have retreated once again to being a doctor's "handmaiden." Nurses bring a unique approach to advanced practice, not as a "mini-doctor" but as a "maxi-nurse." For those nurses who see the need to develop their role to better meet the complex needs of patients, but are faced with resistance and barriers, it is a long journey. But there are medical staff who support such developments and there is nursing experience, knowledge, and expertise that can be used to make those first steps.

Finally, the involvement of patients in their care, the HIV community in the shaping of clinical services and policy and providing services for PLHIV made HIV unique. Patients and the community were active from the start of the epidemic, at meetings, in the clinics, on the streets. Fighting, if necessary, for their right to be heard. This public visibility sometimes came at great cost, such as abuse from neighbours, being sacked or compromising their health for the greater good. It is a rare event nowadays to be at an HIV clinical event, or management committee without the community involvement. Buse [1] argued that, globally, the most critical aspect to the success of the HIV response has been the leadership and activism of civil society.

In the years to come, achieving health and well-being for PLHIV will require the continuance of a holistic approach which, at its heart, is the partnership between both the doctor and the nurse with the patient. Nursing brought this concept to the table as a challenge to the medical model and has successfully created HIV models of individualised patient care that are woven through the clinical services and remains central today in many parts of the world.

Key Learning Points
1. Nurses need to be aware of the social, economic, and political landscape and how it impacts on health and well-being and the values, structures, and provision of healthcare.
2. The involvement of patients and their communities in the development and provision of care and services is essential to partnership working.
3. Person-centred care is achievable and can be sustained.
4. A developed body of nursing knowledge, values, skills, and practice guidelines is essential to defining the contribution of nursing to HIV care.
5. Establishing a multidisciplinary team of equal partners is one of the foundations of developing the nursing role.

Books, Documentaries and Films of the 1980s, 1990s, and 2000s

- Oscar Moore. PWA: Looking Aids in the Face. London: Picador; 1996.
- Gideon Mendel. The Ward. Trolley Ltd., Great Britain. 2017. http://gideonmendel.com/the-ward. Accessed January 2021.
- 'How to Survive a Plague' [video]. 2012. https://vimeo.com/ondemand/howtosurviveaplague. Accessed January 2021.
- 'We Were Here' [video]. 2011. https://vimeo.com/ondemand/wewerehere. Accessed January 2021.
- 'Fire in the Blood' [video]. 2013. https://www.imdb.com/title/tt1787067/. Accessed January 2021.

References

1. Buse K, Eba P, Sigurdson J, Thomson K, Timberlake S. Leveraging HIV-related human rights achievements through a Framework Convention on Global Health. Health Hum Rights. 2013;15:96–110.
2. Kollman K, Waites MUK. Changing political opportunity, structures, policy success and continuing challenges for lesbian and gay and bisexual movements. In: Tremblay M, Paternotte D, Johnson C, editors. The Lesbian and Gay movement and the state: comparative insights into a transformed relationship. Farnham: Ashgate; 2011.

3. Varon J, Foley MS, McMillian J. Time is an ocean: the past and future of the sixties. The Sixties. 2008;1:1–7.
4. Wright J. Only your calamity: the beginnings of activism by and for people with AIDS. Am J Public Health. 2013;103:1788–98.
5. Salvage J. The politics of nursing. London: Heinemann; 2007.
6. May C, Fleming C. The professional imagination: narrative and the symbolic boundaries between medicine and nursing. J Adv Nurs. 2007;25:1094–100.
7. Samuelson H. Nurses between disease and illness. In: Holden P, editor. Anthropol. Nursing. London: Routledge; 1991. p. 190–201.
8. Benner PE, Wrubel J. The primacy of caring: stress and coping in health and illness. Menlo Park, Calif: Addison-Wesley Pub. Co; 1989.
9. Pashley G, Henry C. Carving out the nursing nineties. Nurs Times. 1990;86:45–6.
10. Gamarnikow E. The sexual division of labour: the case of nursing. In: Kuhn A, Wolpe A, editors. Feminism and materialism. London: Routledge; 1978.
11. Stein LI. The doctor-nurse game. Arch Gen Psychiatry. 1967;16:699.
12. Castledine G. Preserving nursing's identity in interdisciplinary working. Br J Nurs. 2005;14:681.
13. Cuesta C. The nursing process: from development to implementation. J Adv Nurs. 1983;8:365–71.
14. Porter S. A participant observation study of power relations between nurses and doctors in a general hospital. J Adv Nurs. 1991;16:728–35.
15. Leary A, MacLaine K. The evolution of advanced nursing practice: past, present and future. Nurs Times Line. 2019;115:18–9.
16. Sweet SJ, Norman IJ. The nurse-doctor relationship: a selective literature review. J Adv Nurs. 1995;22:165–70.
17. Schmalenberg C, Kramer M. Nurse-physician relationships in hospitals: 20,000 nurses tell their story. Crit Care Nurse. 2009;29:74–83.
18. Kuper A. Anthropology and anthropologists: the modern British school, 3rd rev. and enl. London/New York: Routledge; 1996.
19. Helman C. Culture, health, and illness, 5th ed. Hodder Arnold ; Distributed in the U.S.A. London: Oxford University Press; 1997.
20. Cassell EJ. Illness and disease. Hast Cent Rep. 1976;6:27–37.
21. Bruton J, Rai T, Day S, Ward H. Patient perspectives on the HIV continuum of care in London: a qualitative study of people diagnosed between 1986 and 2014. BMJ Open. 2018;8:e020208.
22. Brandt AM. AIDS in historical perspective: four lessons from the history of sexually transmitted diseases. Am J Public Health. 1988;78:367–71.
23. Pan D, Sze S, Minhas JS, et al. The impact of ethnicity on clinical outcomes in COVID-19: s systematic review. E Clin Med. 2020;23:100404.
24. Helman C. Suburban Shaman: a journey through medicine. Cape Town: Double Storey; 2004.
25. Fairbrother G, Chiarella M, Braithwaite J. Models of care choices in today's nursing workplace: where does team nursing sit? Aust Health Rev. 2015;39:489.
26. Merchant J. Task allocation: a case of resistance to change? Nurs Stand. 1991;5:16–8.
27. Tierney AJ. Nursing models: extant or extinct? Nursing theory and concept development or analysis. J Adv Nurs. 1998;28:77–85.
28. Draper P. The development of theory in British nursing: current position and future prospects. J Adv Nurs. 1990;15:12–5.
29. Henderson V. The Nature of Nursing. Am J Nurs. 1964;64:62.
30. Toney-Butler TJ, Thayer JM. Nursing Process. Treasure Island, FL: StatPearls Publishing; 2020. [Internet]. https://www.ncbi.nlm.nih.gov/books/NBK499937/. Accessed Jan 2021
31. Iyer PW, Taptich BJ, Bernocchi-Losey D. Nursing process and nursing diagnosis. Philadelphia: Saunders; 1986.
32. Henderson V. Basic principles of nursing care. Geneva. Geneva: International Council of Nurses; 1987.

33. Pratt RJ. HIV and AIDS: a foundation for nursing and healthcare practice, 5th ed. London: E. Arnold; 2003.
34. McCormack B. Person-centredness in gerontological nursing: an overview of the literature. J Clin Nurs. 2004;13:31–8.
35. Bennett JA. Historical overview of the HIV pandemic. In: Kirton C, editor. ANACs Core Curriculum for HIV/AIDS Nursing. Thousand Oaks: Sage; 2003.
36. Shilts R. And the band played on: politics, people, and the AIDS epidemic. New York: Penguin; 1988.
37. Rosengarten M, Imrie J, Flowers P, Davis MD, Hart G. After the euphoria: HIV medical technologies from the perspective of their prescribers. Sociol Health Illn. 2004;26:575–96.
38. Berridge V. AIDS in the UK: the making of a policy, 1981–1994. Oxford: Oxford University Press; 1996.
39. Newman C, Mao L, Canavan PG, Kidd MR, Saltman DC, Kippax SC. HIV generations? Generational discourse in interviews with Australian general practitioners and their HIV positive gay male patients. Soc Sci Med. 2010;70:1721–7.
40. Mykhalovskiy E, Rosengarten M. HIV/AIDS in its third decade: renewed critique in social and cultural analysis—an introduction. Soc Theory Health. 2009;7:187–95.
41. Hicken I, Faugier J. Establishing a nursing agenda. In: Hicken I, Faugier J, editors. AIDS HIV nursing response. London: Chapman Hall; 1996.
42. Adler MW. ABC AIDS. London: BMJ Publishing; 1993.
43. McGarrahan P. Transcending AIDS: nurses and HIV patients in New York City. Philadelphia: University of Pennsylvania Press; 1994.
44. Health Care Workers in HIV. https://www.healthcareworkersinhiv.org.uk. Accessed Jan 2021.
45. Thorlby R. Where the patient was king? A study of patient choice and its effect on five specialist HIV units in London. London: King's Fund; 2006.
46. Morrison C. "They needed to feel loved": how one nurse revolutionized patient care during the AIDS crisis. 2019. https://www.jnj.com/personal-stories/ward-5b-how-one-nurse-revolutionized-patient-care-during-the-aids-crisis. Accessed 19 Jul 2020
47. Lucas C. The San Francisco model and the nurses of Ward 5B. Lancet HIV. 2019;e819:6.
48. AIDS: Doctors and Nurses tell their Stories [video]. 2017. IMDb. https://www.imdb.com/title/tt8362448/. Accessed Jan 2021
49. Czerwiec MK. Taking turns: stories from HIV/AIDS care Unit, vol. 371. Pennsylvania: The Pennsylvania State University Press; 2017.
50. Elliott J. Nursing care. In: Adler MW, editor. ABC AIDS. London: BMJ Publishing; 1993.
51. Department of Health. Liberating the NHS. Norwich: TSO; 2010.
52. Lazarus JV, Safreed-Harmon K. Depicting a new target for the HIV response: how do you see the 'Fourth 90'? 2018. https://www.isglobal.org/en/healthisglobal/-/custom-blog-portlet/visually-depicting-a-new-target-for-the-hiv-response-how-do-you-see-the-fourth-90-/5511380/0. Accessed 19 Jul 2020
53. Safreed-Harmon K, Anderson J, Azzopardi-Muscat N, et al. Reorienting health systems to care for people with HIV beyond viral suppression. Lancet HIV. 2019;6:e869–77.

Chapter 2
Understanding and Expanding HIV Nursing Roles

Hilary Piercy

2.1 Background

Individual roles are defined by the context within which they operate and shaped by the people in those roles. They also change over time as part of the continually shifting landscape of healthcare provision, evolving and developing in response to the sociopolitical environment within they operate and the needs and expectations of those they are designed to serve. At times, they are constrained and stifled by the organisational structures within which they function and the people operating within those structures. At other times, they expand and advance, triggered by circumstances that open up new opportunities and possibilities for new ways of working. This inevitably leads to substantial variability in the way in which a role is realised. Two people who hold the same job title and might be expected to be fulfilling the same role, may in fact be working in substantially different ways and doing different things.

> **Thinking Point**
> Consider your role and how it has changed over time. What are the main factors that have influenced that change?

Capturing that role variability to provide a comprehensive and detailed account of what HIV nurses do, how they contribute to HIV care and how their contribution to care might be expanded is important. It is important for the

H. Piercy (✉)
Sheffield Hallam University, Sheffield, UK
e-mail: H.Piercy@shu.ac.uk

M. Croston, I. Hodgson (eds.), *Providing HIV Care: Lessons from the Field for Nurses and Healthcare Practitioners*,
https://doi.org/10.1007/978-3-030-71295-2_2

commissioners and providers of HIV services, tasked with responding to three major challenges. Firstly, the transformation of HIV into a manageable condition and the consequent shift in care towards chronic disease management with an emphasis on identifying and managing the comorbidities which are more prevalent in those living with HIV [1, 2]. Secondly, the demands placed on services as a result of year on year increases in the numbers accessing HIV treatment, a consequence of increasing life expectancies for those living with HIV which are now approaching those of non-HIV individuals [3] as well as continued onward transmission of infection. The increase in numbers is substantial. In the UK, the numbers receiving HIV care increased from 65,249 in 2009 to 96,142 in 2018, a 47% increase over the decade [4]. Thirdly, the challenges of caring for two distinct HIV populations; the majority who are well and have few health problems, and a minority group, including those with multiple comorbidities and those who are particularly vulnerable with psychosocial problems who have much more complex needs.

The House of Lords Select Committee report 'No vaccine no cure', identified the challenges facing HIV services of ensuring continued high-quality provision within the context of an increasingly challenging and financially constrained environment. It highlighted the urgent need for HIV services to review how care was organised and to develop models of healthcare which capitalised on the skills and expertise of their entire workforce. Recommendations included developing more innovative ways of delivering services and greater involvement of community provision [5]. Piercy et al. [6] identified three models of healthcare delivery that could be developed and collectively enable services to meet the needs of their HIV population.

1. A model that offers greater flexibility and accessibility in the way that routine HIV care is delivered.
2. A model that provides more integrated care between primary care and specialist HIV services.
3. A model that provides community-based specialist nursing care.

Activity Point
What models of healthcare operate in your service? How well do they enable you to meet the needs of the patients that you care for?

A detailed understanding of HIV nursing roles is also important for every nurse who works in HIV. It provides them with a context within which they can better understand their own role and are better able to articulate it to others. It offers them a framework against which to interrogate their role and challenges them to identify where and how they might develop and expand their role to enable them to better meet the needs of the people they care for.

2.2   Overview of the ANCHIVS Study

The ANCHIVS study was a multi-method qualitative research project involving three parts. Stage one involved semi-structured interviews with 19 representatives of key stakeholder groups: service providers, service commissioners, and service users in order to detail current provision, challenges, and opportunities for service delivery and the advanced nursing contribution. Stage two involved semi-structured interviews with a purposive sample of nurse/physician pairs from HIV services across the country to understand in detail the range of ways in which services are organised and the contribution of specialist nursing. The sampling approach ensured maximum variability across sites and included those recognised for their excellence and innovation in advanced nursing practice. A total of 42 clinicians from 21 HIV services (13% of total in England) participated in stage two. The services were situated in genitourinary medicine, infectious disease, and community services, located in metropolitan, urban, and semi-rural areas, covered high and low HIV prevalence areas, and cared for cohorts ranging from 80 to 6000.

Stage three involved a series of five case studies, involving some stage two participants and designed to provide comprehensive in-depth insight into the HIV nursing role and the service context within which it operated. Case studies were selected that individually indicated excellent and innovative advanced nursing practice and collectively provided contrasting examples of how the advanced practice role was operating in a range of different contexts and conditions. In some sites, the current role was very well established and in others it was a more recent development. They included practitioners based in hospital and community-based services and working in urban, metropolitan, and (semi) rural geographical locations and spanned areas of high and low HIV prevalence.

During site visits, data were collected from multiple sources including interviews with members of the multidisciplinary team, non-participant observation and field notes taken during clinical and managerial meetings, and documentary evidence including job description, care pathways, and service guidelines.

A framework analysis approach was used for all data analysis. This approach has a clearly defined analytic structure and is ideally suited to managing large amounts of qualitative data obtained from different sources. It involves following five data management steps to systematically sift, chart, and sort the material into key issues and themes [7]. Specific quality measures were employed to ensure the analysis benefitted from the theoretical and clinical expertise and insights of all members of the research team.

2.3   Aspects of Care Framework

The ANCHIVS study clearly established that HIV nursing is primarily a clinical role involving a range of activities through which care is delivered. The nature of those care activities and the level at which they performed varied enormously from

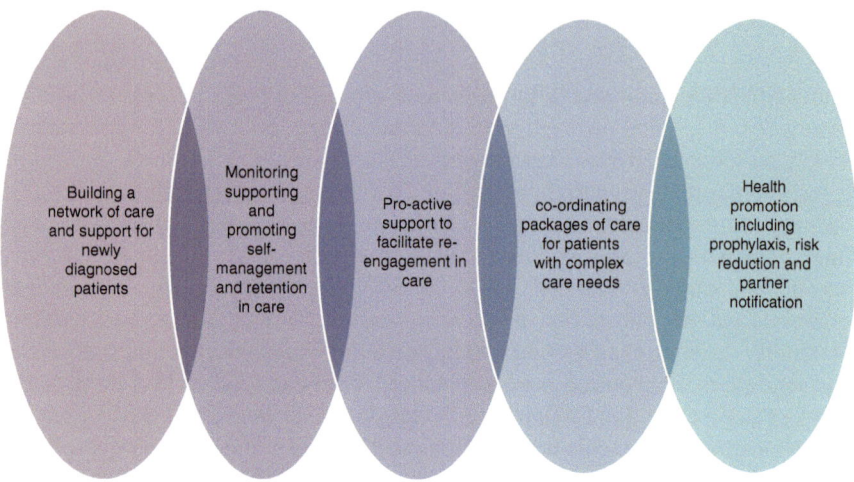

Fig. 2.1 Aspects of care framework

one service to another. The 'Aspects of Care Framework' provides an organising structure within which care activities are understood in terms of their overall purpose. Each of these is now considered in turn to understand the totality of activities involved and variability within those activities (Fig. 2.1).

2.4 Building a Network of Care for Newly Diagnosed Patients

Most of the nurses were involved with HIV patients from the point at which they were diagnosed and engaged with the service. Initial appointments were often a lengthy consultation with the specialist nurse who then served as a source of immediate and easily accessible means of ongoing contact for the patient. Nursing input in that initial period consisted of extended consultations and ongoing support. This input served three main purposes. Firstly, educational input covering aspects such as HIV prognosis and disease management including potential treatment options, secondly clinical assessment including medical history and baseline bloods on the basis of which treatment judgements were made and thirdly psychosocial assessment, support, and signposting to other agencies as required.

This early involvement was considered important for addressing psychosocial issues and allaying initial anxieties about the diagnosis and the prognosis. It also provided the basis of a long-term relationship between the patient and the service which is important for long-term retention in care.

2.5   Monitoring Supporting and Promoting Self-Management and Retention in Care

A major part of the role was directed towards supporting patients to self-manage their condition and remain fully engaged with treatment and care. This was achieved through a range of activities including periodic monitoring and review of their health status, educational input, and advice to support adherence around treatments, psychological care and support, and responding to problems and concerns.

Routine outpatient appointments provided the focus for these activities. In all services, nurses were involved in running outpatient clinics. In most services, nurse-led clinics operated and provided a substantial proportion of routine care. In areas where these clinics were well established, their scope had expanded over time such that the nurses were managing a growing cohort of patients with increasingly complex medical problems. Most of those running nurse-led clinics had qualified as non-medical prescribers. This offered clear benefits to the service in terms of the ability of the nurses to autonomously manage episodes of care which improved smooth running and efficiency of the clinics and improved the patient experience.

It was widely recognised and acknowledged that nurse consultations were particularly well suited to managing routine care because they took an explicit psychosocial perspective, adopted a holistic approach, and comprehensively covered patient concerns. One of the major stimuli for their initial introduction had been a lack of medical cover. Workforce issues continued to influence their development and expansion. Lack of an appropriate skill mix served as a major inhibitor to development. It limited the extent to which nurses were able to apply their clinical skills and expertise because they were required to spend a substantial amount of time doing jobs more appropriate for someone on a lower pay band.

In several services, nurses had been instrumental in developing clinics which were designed to expand and improve service provision in response to the specific needs of the population they cared for. For example, in a large metropolitan service, nurse-led virtual clinics had been introduced as an alternative route for those who elected to self-manage their condition with reduced direct contact with the service. In another service, based in a semi-rural low prevalence area with a large geographical footprint, a nurse-run satellite service provided clinics using community facilities to overcome problems of service access.

In addition to running clinics, nurses spent a substantial time on activities concerned with the smooth running of the service. These activities included: managing medication supplies, chasing up results, reviewing results, organising follow-up tests, repeat prescriptions, communicating with other services, and administrative tasks. Specific responsibilities were influenced by size of the service and workforce configuration.

Nurses were commonly the first point of contact with the service for all patients and dealt with a range of queries and problems. In most services, and particularly those with limited medical input over the course of the week, they were the first point of contact for unscheduled attendances. They triaged the patients and made clinical judgements that involved either dealing with the problems themselves or referring to another clinician. Additionally, they often spent a substantial proportion of time dealing with patient queries and concerns by telephone and email, contacting them with blood results and providing ongoing support related to a wide range of issues related to treatments and specific medical, psychological, or social concerns.

Most services included some community-based nursing provision for the small number of patients who required this in order to stay engaged with treatment and the service. This was most commonly provided by a hospital-based workforce on an infrequent and ad hoc basis. A small number of areas had a separate HIV community nursing workforce and offered more extensive provision. It included working with patients on short-term interventions designed to re-establish social stability. More substantially, they provided ongoing care and support for patients and their carers in their own homes or in residential care facilities. In some cases, this involved delivering all HIV treatment and care at home for those who could not engage with mainstream services.

2.6   Pro-active Support to Facilitate Re-engagement in Care

There are two sorts of reasons why people do not attend routine HIV clinic appointments: simple reasons such as forgetting an appointment, and complex reasons, where non-attendance suggests underlying problems and indicates someone may be at risk of disengaging with treatment and care. Nurses were involved in managing both and a range of related activities, to facilitate re-engagement in care.

Managing simple non-attendances involved straightforward but time-consuming administrative tasks. Responsibility for overseeing the process commonly fell to the hospital-based nurses. Inevitably this meant that when administrative support was inadequate, by default they also assumed responsibility for the tasks themselves.

Non-attendance in those with complex needs was taken as an indicator of possible disengagement from services. Considerable effort was invested in maintaining contact with these patients. The simplest approach involved the specialist nurse trying to contact patients directly, by phone or letter or indirectly through other services such as primary care. This had limited success, particularly in the larger services and those with a mobile population. A more systematic approach was to develop robust structures and processes for systematically identifying those at risk of long-term disengagement and then working proactively to build support networks involving keyworkers and outside agencies.

Where it was available, community HIV nursing provision offered the greatest likelihood of success. They were better able to make contact with patients in the community, explore their issues of concern, and work with them with the objective of re-engaging with the hospital services. They were also well integrated into community networks which enabled them to liaise effectively with other health and voluntary sector agencies.

A minority of the HIV population have highly complex needs associated with psychosocial difficulties and multiple comorbidities. Specialist nurses were commonly involved in co-ordinating care for these patients, working across settings and in partnership with a range of other agencies to establish packages of care. For hospital-based workforces, this largely involved referring into their established network of local social care services and voluntary sector organisation. For community-based teams, commissioned to manage a caseload of highly complex patients, this aspect of their role was considerably greater. Much of their time was directed towards keeping these patients engaged in treatment and care, either by working to bring them back into services or by providing those services in an outreach way. They also functioned as a care co-ordinator, working with patients and other agencies to organise and manage care packages.

Activity Point
John was diagnosed with HIV several years ago and transferred to your service 3 years ago. His attendance has recently become sporadic and he has just missed his routine review appointment. His most recent blood results indicate he has not been taking his HIV medication effectively.

Consider the points raised in this case study. How would your service respond when John misses his appointment and what role would you play in that response?

2.7   Health Promotion Including Prophylaxis, Risk Reduction, and Partner Notification

Health promotion activities included a range of specific elements: post-exposure prophylaxis (PEP), HIV testing, partner notification, risk reduction, and regular sexual health screening.

The extent to which provision and management of PEP falls within the remit of the HIV service was a matter of some contention given that it is a preventative service, for those who do not have HIV. Consequently, the extent to which HIV services were involved in PEP provision was highly variable. In some instances, PEP management had moved away entirely and in others it had been fully adopted within HIV services. Transferring it within HIV services had involved moving to nurse-led provision with responsibility for hospital trust wide responsibilities for delivery of the service.

Commonly nurses had a lead responsibility for HIV-testing activities in their service. Their testing remit varied substantially. In some instances, it was primarily concerned with testing the children of HIV-positive parents. In others it involved taking a lead role in initiatives targeted at other groups of health professionals or specific community outreach activities, working in collaboration with a range of other health and voluntary sector organisations.

Most HIV nurses had some involvement in partner notification. The extent of that involvement was largely determined by the context in which they worked and specifically the availability of health advisors. Some working in smaller services had a dual HIV nursing/Health Advisor role and thus more extensive responsibility. Others had more limited responsibilities but as they commonly had previous health advisor experience, were confident taking greater responsibility for these activities when a health adviser was not available.

In most services, nurses were largely responsible for conducting annual health reviews, either within routine follow-up appointments or as separate consultations. Sexual health screening was included, and sexual risk reduction/condom use was addressed within the context of that review.

> **Activity Point**
> Use the aspects of care framework to think about your own role and all the activities you undertake as part of your role. Does the framework provide a useful organising structure? Can you satisfactorily capture everything you do within the framework?

2.8 Developments to Improve Healthcare Delivery Models

In this section, we focus on two services which have made substantial progress towards the recommendations of the 'No vaccine, no cure' which were discussed earlier in this chapter. A brief overview of the service is provided before moving onto detailing the nurse-led initiatives they have introduced and the nursing workforce development activities that have enabled those initiatives to be introduced.

The first service is based in a major city and cares for a diverse cohort of approximately 2100 HIV patients. The nursing team is primarily hospital based. Nurse-led clinics were introduced by the lead nurse several years ago and are well established. Training and development of the five strong nursing workforce including non-medical prescribing has enabled this aspect of provision to expand considerably. Nurse-led clinics offer a comprehensive and holistic service with single consultations that cover aspects of preventative and public health as well as physical health and medication. The team capitalised on the opportunity to develop the service further when the Annual Health Review: good practice guide [8] was published and the service moved to an electronic patient record system. They amended the template for their existing electronic patient record to incorporate all the elements covered in the annual health review (AHR). This enabled them to address inconsistencies across the workforce in what was covered and to ensure that areas which were commonly overlooked, such as assessment of psychological well-being were also routinely included. Further development of the template has extended the sexual health and women's health components and improved assessment in these areas with the inclusion of a question on domestic violence and routine queries about the menopause; areas that are commonly overlooked and rarely addressed.

Introducing a robust system that ensures all clinicians are conducting a comprehensive AHR within routine appointments has enabled the team to restructure clinics and introduce substantial changes in the way that care is delivered for a substantial proportion of the cohort. The service has moved from seeing stable patients 6-monthly for routine reviews to offering one face-to-face annual review appointment and a 6-month interim review which is managed virtually by a prescribing nurse or doctor and based on patients completing a self-assessment questionnaire with support of a healthcare assistant. Streamlining and simplifying the process in this way has produced substantial benefits in terms of greater service efficiency and flexibility for patients. Extending the use of self-assessment questionnaires by introducing them into the annual review appointment will further support self-management and enable consultations to be structured around patient priorities.

The second service is a community HIV nursing service. The nursing team work alongside and in close collaboration with the main hospital-based service, caring for a caseload of approximately 70 patients with multiple psychosocial issues and highly complex care needs. The majority of their caseload do not attend mainstream HIV. To address this concern and enable these patients to remain engaged with treatment and care, they established a community clinic that enables remote management and delivery of services in the home.

Since it was introduced, the community clinic has developed substantially with expansion of provision to enable this group of patients to receive all the services that are available to those attending mainstream HIV clinics. A key element of this was to introduce a comprehensive AHR as part of the care package which enables them to identify multiple health concerns and previously undiagnosed chronic conditions. New ways of working have been developed in order to enable the health concerns that they identified to be addressed, given that this group of patients do not access healthcare and rarely access either primary care or acute services. One of these was an upskilling of the nursing workforce to address women's health issues and training is being introduced in order that the community HIV nurses can offer cervical screening at home to women for whom it is long overdue and provide long-acting contraceptive implants. Another development was driven by the need to act on the health concerns such as hypertension and hypercholesterolaemia that they identified as part of the AHR. A strengthening of relationships with primary care and other community specialist services has ensured that they can readily refer to those services so that investigation and appropriate management can be initiated. The close collaborations that have developed enable those patients to benefit from more joined up working and integrate care delivery systems.

> **Activity Point**
> Think about recent developments in your service and how you have been involved? What enabled those developments to happen and what changes in the way that services are delivered have resulted?
>   What other developments would you like to see happen in your service? What would be needed to make them possible?

2.9   Summary

In summary, this chapter has established why all HIV nurses need to have a clear sense of their own role in terms of not only what they do but also why they do it. The first part of the chapter provided a framework to help develop that understanding by drawing on the findings of the ANCHIVS study to provide a detailed and comprehensive account of HIV nursing roles in England. Those findings capture the role variability that exists between services in terms of both breadth of activities and level of clinical practice. It therefore provides a benchmark against which individuals can interrogate and better understand their own role, with a view to identifying opportunities for development and extension. This process is necessarily incremental. It occurs in parallel with and interacts in a symbiotic way with the service improvements that commonly serve as a stimulus to role development but are also dependent on that role development for their operationalisation. The two services featured in the second part of the chapter exemplify that process and the benefits it is generating.

Acknowledgments   Hilary would like to thank Justine Mellor and Elizabeth Foote for their contribution to this chapter.

References

1. De Francesco D, Wit FW, Cole JH, Kootstra NA, Winston A, Sabin CA, et al. The 'COmorBidity in relation to AIDS'(COBRA) cohort: design, methods and participant characteristics. PLoS One. 2018;13(3):e0191791.
2. Schouten J, Wit FW, Stolte IG, Kootstra NA, van der Valk M, Geerlings SE, et al. Cross-sectional comparison of the prevalence of age-associated comorbidities and their risk factors between HIV-infected and uninfected individuals: the AGEhIV cohort study. Clin Infect Dis. 2014;59(12):1787–97.
3. Nakagawa F, May M, Phillips A. Life expectancy living with HIV: recent estimates and future implications. Curr Opin Infect Dis. 2013;26(1):17–25.
4. Nash S, Desai S, Croxford S, Guerra L, Lowndes C, Connor N, et al. Progress towards ending the HIV epidemic in the United Kingdom: 2018 report. London: Public Health England; 2018.

5. House of Lords. Select committee on HIV and AIDS in the United Kingdom first report: no vaccine, no cure. HIV and AIDS in the United Kingdom. London: House of Lords; 2011.
6. Piercy H, Bell G, Hughes C, Naylor S, Bowman C. An examination of the contribution of specialist nursing to HIV service delivery. Sheffield: Sheffield Hallam University; 2015.
7. Tunnicliff SA, Piercy H, Bowman CA, Hughes C, Goyder EC. The contribution of the HIV specialist nurse to HIV care: ascoping review. J Clin Nurs. 2013;22(23–24):3349–60.
8. National HIV Nurses Association. Annual health review for people living with HIV: a good practice guide. 2018.

Chapter 3
Nurse Leadership in HIV Care

Jackie Morton

3.1 History of Nursing Leadership

We only need to look at Florence Nightingale, who transformed health care during a period of history when nursing was considered an occupation with little respect. In those days, women of Nightingale's class did not attend universities and did not pursue professional careers. Their purpose in life was to marry and bear children [1]. Heroic medicine of the day was based on infusions of arsenic, mercury, opiates, and bleeding which hastened the deaths of many more patients than it saved [2]. Nightingale believed that, by keeping patients well-fed, warm, comfortable, and above all clean, nursing could solve many problems that nineteenth century medicine could not [3]. In 1854, during the Crimean War, it is reported that Florence, to improve sanitation to the wounded soldiers, took it upon herself to remove all dirty clothing from the battlefield medical facilities that were crawling with rats and the most appalling filth. She spent her own money to purchase bandages, extra clothes, 200 scrub brushes, better food, operating tables, and other necessities for the hospital, training other nurses in her hygiene standards.

She researched and studied environmental settings that were appropriate for the gradual restoration of patient's health in the drive to understand how the external factors associated with the patient's surroundings affected their biological and physiological processes. Arguably, Florence came from a privileged background, having been privately tutored by her parents putting her in a position of leadership from her wealth. Yet she chose to focus her compassion on those less able to fight for themselves, with a steely determination and strong vision of what she wanted to achieve. Through her hands-on training of others into her techniques, she transformed nursing to become one of the most honourable professions in the country.

J. Morton (✉)
Independent Consultant, Scarborough, North Yorkshire, UK

© The Author(s), under exclusive license to Springer Nature
Switzerland AG 2021
M. Croston, I. Hodgson (eds.), *Providing HIV Care: Lessons from the Field for Nurses and Healthcare Practitioners*,
https://doi.org/10.1007/978-3-030-71295-2_3

She went on to be a leading influencer in the design and standards of hospital care adding ventilation into the ward environment, which became known as the Nightingale Ward [4]. This example highlights that transformational leadership occurs when leaders engage with their followers in pursuit of jointly held goals [5]. These rich insights from the past inform nurses of the opportunities to lead and manage change. What are the challenges for nurses to lead change in health systems of today?

3.2   The History of Nurse Leadership in the UK HIV Sector

It may be hard to believe that over 30 years ago, prejudice against young gay men with HIV produced headlines in newspapers dripping with stigma that fuelled a nation's fear against those that became infected [6].

In the UK, the famous 'tombstones' health promotion campaign, encouraging people not to 'die of ignorance of this deadly disease with no known cure', shocked British TV viewers when it appeared in 1986. This resulted in a generational fear of anyone who became infected [7]. During this time, understanding of transmission routes was limited and stigma thrived, with many patients experiencing stigmatised care from health professionals. This played out in side-rooms in the use of gloves without reason and visiting restrictions. As prejudice against this section of the population escalated, nurses, who were overwhelmed with the violence of HIV as well as the hostility of the social reactions to those with the infection, rose to challenge this global phenomenon [8]. They acted as advocates, challenged prevailing assumptions, questioned the basis of every clinical choice that mattered, and led opportunities to care for the infected and affected population [9]. Demand for out of hospital care arose from the hostility of some hospital staff, some of whom refused to treat patients with AIDS. Pioneering nurses took a leading role in the development of special wards, in partnership with peer support groups and charities led by people impacted by the virus [10].

> *"Nurses drove change through the provision of specialist advice on management and adherence to anti-retroviral medication"* [12].

Shifting the care of people living with an unpredictable and multi-pathological condition into the community resulted in hospital-based HIV nurse specialists leading the education of community nurses and the person's closest family members about the condition [11].

Implementing a model of health across the complexity of primary, secondary, community, and social care systems was not easy, yet nurses drove change through the provision of specialist advice. They emerged as leaders in complex case management, treatment management, and adherence to anti-retroviral treatment (ART).

From this leadership, a specific role emerged for the Community Nurse Specialist (CNS) supporting HIV self-care and management of a cohort of complex patients. This aimed to prevent avoidable hospital (re)admissions and speed up hospital discharge [12]. Arguably, the CNS model is well equipped to deliver a vital link between hospitals, community, and primary care [13]. But without leadership, survival of the model is difficult in an increasingly competitive economic and politically driven healthcare system. Prejudices are still rampant, and countries still display stigmatising behaviours such as imposing travel restrictions and discriminatory laws, rules, and policies that alienate and exclude people living with HIV and AIDS [14].

3.3 Leadership and Governance

According to the WHO, in 2020 there are just under 28 million nurses worldwide, with 7.3 million nurses, or about 79 nurses per 10,000 people, in the WHO European Region [15]. There is also a gender divide. Approximately 90% of all nurses are female, yet they hold only 25% of leadership positions. There is some evidence of a gender-based pay gap, as well as other forms of gender-based discrimination in the work environment [16].

The WHO recommends that the future of nursing needs strong leadership and governance. It requires nurses to hold leadership positions in government to deliver regulatory systems for monitoring nursing practice and supporting programmes that develop nurse leadership, research, and policy literacy at national and local levels [17]. Clinical governance sustains and improves high standards of patient care such as quality and safety [18]. It is the responsibility of every nurse to lead and direct the application of their own clinical practice in accordance to their professional standards. You are personally accountable for your own actions and omissions [19].

But what do we really know about leadership in healthcare services? Are leaders purely managers providing direction, alignment, and commitment within teams and organisations? Florence Nightingale had a clear vision of the type of care she expected nurses to deliver, but how did she persuade others to share her vision? When she arrived in Turkey with 38 nurses in 1854, the army doctors who worked there did not want nurses to help. After one particular battle, with many injured men arriving at the hospital [20], Florence defined the tasks of the nurses. For surgical cases, nurses' tasks were: ensuring the injured men were prepared for the doctor to give his medical opinion on what surgical intervention he recommended as treatment, supporting the doctor in the dressing of wounds and to take the doctors' recommendations on nutritional requirements of the patients. With medical conditions, tasks were dealing with bad sores, ensuring food was properly cooked and fluids were properly administered in accordance with the doctors' recommendations and to ensure the wards and the men were kept clean. This definitive model developed a culture with clear roles and functions in the supervision and delivery of clinical care [21].

Box 3.1 Leadership and Governance Indicators: Percentage of Countries with Chief Nursing Officer Position and Nursing Leadership Development Programme, by WHO Region

WHO REGION	Chief nursing officer position		Nursing leadership development programme	
	Number of countries responding/total	% yes	Number of countries responding/total	% yes
Africa	26/47	60%	28/47	64%
Americas	26/35	79%	16/35	46%
South-East Asia	6/11	60%	4/11	40%
Europe	30/53	86%	10/53	56%
Eastern Mediterranean	7/21	54%	8/21	62%
Western Pacific	20/27	74%	10/27	43%
Global	**115/194**	**71%**	**76/194**	**53%**

Source: *State of the world's nursing 2020* specific indicators, 2019. Latest available data reported by countries between 2013 and 2018

Though purely task-based nursing is not necessarily suitable for today's health systems, this example does show that effective nurse leaders are characterised as flexible, collaborative, power sharing, and employ strong personal values to promote high quality performance [22].

In a study by the World Health Organisation (WHO) covering 115 countries, 71% of respondents reported having a government chief nursing or midwifery officer position, and only 53% a nursing leadership development programme Box 3.1 [23].

From this study, the WHO report makes ten recommendations for a strengthened workforce [24]

1. Increase funding to educate and employ more nurses
2. Strengthen capacity to collect, analyse, and act on data about the health workforce
3. Monitor nurse mobility and migration and manage it responsibly and ethically
4. Educate and train nurses in the scientific, technological, and sociological skills they need to drive progress in primary health care
5. Establish leadership positions, including a government chief nursing officer, and support leadership development among young nurses
6. Ensure that nurses in primary healthcare teams work to their full potential, for example, in preventing and managing non-communicable diseases
7. Improve working conditions, including through safe staffing levels, fair salaries, and respect for rights to occupational health and safety

8. Implement gender-sensitive nursing workforce policies
9. Modernise professional nursing regulation by harmonising education and practice standards and using systems that can recognise and process nurses' credentials globally
10. Strengthen the role of nurses in care teams by bringing different sectors (health, education, immigration, finance, and labour) together with nursing stakeholders for policy dialogue and workforce planning

These recommendations highlight that nurse leadership is not just about being in a high-level government role. It is also about leading care at a local level with patients, through education. How can this be achieved in the context of HIV care?

3.4   Care Models Involving Nurse Leadership for People Living with HIV

The Royal College of Nursing recommends that all patients with long-term conditions have access to a specialist nurse. RCN: 2014

In 2014, the Royal College of Nursing UK (RCN) recommended that all patients with a long-term condition have access to a specialist nurse [25]. It has already been highlighted that having access to a CNS can be beneficial for people living with HIV for improving the quality and collaboration of care [26]. A study undertaken by the British HIV Association (BHIVA) in 2016 examined collaborative care models, or shared care, between primary, secondary, and social care. It identified that the CNS can be instrumental in meeting the needs of people living with HIV because they consider the wider determinants of health such as quality of life issues, socialisation, peer support, and psychosocial factors [27]. This study outlined that shared-care models, by definition, had an agreed protocol of responsibility between partners, facilitated by training of health professionals, appropriate and timely communication, and networks to support the co-ordination of care. The CNS leadership role in this model is an equal partner in the design and delivery of care.

Definition: 'Collaborative care' advocates a case-based approach shifting the focus of care from the health service model to a person-centred approach responsive to the individual's needs.

Person-centred care recognises that to improve people's health we must give the person more control over their own care. Whole person care recognises that care should go beyond HIV treatment, and aim to support people with the social, economic, physical, and mental health needs that are associated with the condition [28].

According to research undertaken by the UK's National Aids Trust, collaborative care is perhaps the most resource-intensive model but, in practice, may make cost savings by being preventive for people with high levels of need and deploying the most appropriate provider (e.g. a CNS instead of a senior doctor). It is the least tested of the emergent care models, but potentially the most transformative [29].

The UK's Kings Fund is a health charity that shapes health and social care policy and practice. It provides NHS leadership development to improve health and care in England. It recognises healthcare needs transformational change to deliver an entirely new model of care as opposed to incremental or small changes to the existing framework [30]. Transformation is best brought about 'from within' rather than through targets and performance management and other external stimuli [31].

As the HIV population ages, there is the potential for the HIV CNS to lead the management of health care for those with multiple health conditions [32]. HIV nurses, CNSs, or Advanced Nurse Practitioners (ANP) can guide patients through their most vulnerable and life-changing moment of an HIV diagnosis and literally, as well as metaphorically, hold the patient's hand throughout their journey [33].

Whether hospital or community based, nurses can drive change through development of specific skills, qualities, interfaces, and leadership at every level. HIV nurses have led and supported primary care testing initiatives, working with generic services in both secondary care and the community to update staff knowledge and reduce discriminatory practice [34]. This achievement has not only educated a vast range of health professionals on the management of care. It has raised the profile and leadership of HIV nurses, having been rated favourably in between the GP and HIV consultant on attitude, professional performance, and viral load control among their patient cohort [35]. The current emphasis of the Community HIV CNS role is one of the complex case managements which has been described as 'the process of planning, coordinating and reviewing the care of an individual' supporting HIV self-care and management [12].

According to a Cochrane review in 2018 nurse-led primary care services can, in certain settings and under the right circumstances, lead to similar or sometimes better patient health outcomes and higher patient satisfaction than other care delivery models. This is helped by nurses likely spending longer with their patients [36].

The following case study is one example of nurse leadership by an HIV specialist nurse.

Case Study

Meet: Geraldine, a 66-year-old woman, diagnosed and living with HIV for 10 years, viral load is undetectable and CD4 count is within normal limits of 500–1500 **per cubic millimetre of blood (cells/mm³)** *since commencing Anti-Retroviral Treatment (ART) on diagnosis.*

In November 2018, Geraldine experienced chest pain and underwent an angiogram, a special type of X-ray which uses contrast dye to examine the coronary arteries. This revealed she had a blocked Left Anterior Descending (LAD) artery across her heart resulting in the insertion of a stent, a small metal tube to unblock the artery, the procedure is called an angioplasty.

During her hospital inpatient episode, the CNS (HIV) visited Geraldine and with her permission spoke to the nurses caring for her only to find one of her newly prescribed cardiology regime could have a reaction with her ART medication. Her new regime included a daily antiplatelet drug to prevent blood clots forming in the blood, a statin to help lower 'bad' cholesterol and fats (such as LDL, triglycerides) and raise 'good' cholesterol (HDL) and a beta blocker to lower her blood pressure. The CNS took a leadership role in educating the cardiac nursing team on the Liverpool University Drug Interaction Chart, which is now a regular part of a training programme within the cardiology unit [37].

But this was not the end of the polypharmacy episode. Geraldine's blood results prior to the blocked LAD artery had shown an increasingly high cholesterol level. People living with HIV commonly have elevated cholesterol and triglycerides levels, which is caused not only by the virus itself but by the very drugs meant to treat the disease [38].

The CNS took a proactive leadership role liaising with the HIV specialist consultant and the pharmacist on the presenting causation of pharmacological side effects, resulting in the recommendation to change Geraldine's ART to a more modern and highly effective regime. Geraldine accepted the change, but 1 year later and having gained almost 9 lb in weight, Geraldine contacted the CNS HIV with concerns on the new medication.

The CNS undertook research into the new regime to find increasing evidence of weight gain as a side effect and she liaised with the HIV specialist consultant on a further change in ART for Geraldine, which she accepted. Six months later, the regime has been successful in stopping the weight gain and has not caused any other side effects or change to Geraldine's HIV status.

This case study demonstrates the unique role of the nurse. This is not only in the co-ordination of a patient care plan, but in the education and exchange of knowledge and interlinking clinical care across different care providers.

Key learning points from the case study to take away:

- Listening to the person living with HIV results in a better outcome for the individual.
- Nurses are often the primary care provider and closer to the patient than other members of the health team.
- Not all branches of nursing know about the management of people with HIV.
- Multiple health conditions can lead to polypharmacy and drug–drug interactions.
- Pharmacological side effects may exacerbate predisposing health conditions, e.g. heart disease.
- Patient history taking and a person-centred approach is essential to the long-term management of care [39].
- Sharing knowledge, skills, and expertise educates others.
- Improving patient outcomes and care provision is a partnership approach.

3.4.1 Leadership Attributes, Qualities, or Outcomes

Urban and Monarch [40] argue that there are 14 attributes or outcomes that exemplify nursing excellence. They call these the Forces of Magnetism

- Quality of leadership—nursing leaders were perceived to be knowledgeable risk takers.
- Flattened organisational structures with nursing leader serving at the executive level of the organisation and reporting to the chief executive officer.
- Management style perceived to be participative, encouraging and valuing feedback, leaders visible, accessible, and committed to communicating effectively.
- Personnel policies and programmes, participative management, and a focus on evidence-based practice, staff involved in the development of policies in general.
- Professional models of care with the responsibility and authority for the provision of patient care, accountable for their own practice, and coordinators of care.
- Quality of care—Nursing leaders are responsible for developing an environment that fostered quality of care.
- Nurses leading integration of research and evidence-based practice into clinical and operational processes.
- Nurses in leadership positions as essential consultants and resources, used as qualified experts for guidance and peer support.
- Autonomy when establishing standards, setting goals, monitoring practice, and measuring outcomes.
- Extending professional practice into the community such as discharge planning and visiting patients in nursing homes and their homes.
- Nurses incorporate teaching into all aspects of their practice.
- Aware of the importance of their image, competence, credible, valued, respected, and necessary for the survival of the hospital.
- Interdisciplinary relationships—mutual respect among disciplines.
- Professional development—emphasis on orientation, education, and career development.

Full expression of the Forces of Magnetism is required to achieve 'Magnet Designation'. It embodies a professional environment guided by a strong and visionary nursing leader who advocates and supports excellence in nursing practice. The 'Magnet Award' programme was founded in 1990 by the American Nurses Credentialing Centre (ANCC) [41]. There is increasing international support of the model in the Middle East and Asia [42]. For the UK, the RCN suggests its limited success could be the high cost of attaining the Magnet award during a time of budget constraints and other pressures.

The RCN states some of the key qualities necessary for nurses aspiring to change the face of nursing are integrity, courage, the ability to handle stress, and having a clear direction of travel [43]. By setting and monitoring goals and evaluating information, nurses can develop a shared purpose and vision to lead and engage in change, yet still be held to account for their actions. But it takes confidence to lead a team through organisational change, and this can only be achieved through training and educational programmes that support leadership development.

A key component of nursing is the value and respect of people, their individuality, rights, choices, independence, dignity, and beliefs. In today's modern health systems, a person is much more informed and in control of their health than in the time of Florence Nightingale, requiring nurse leaders to acknowledge the potential independence of the person to further plan their health. For example, pioneering advances in technology are resulting in reducing face-to-face consultations between medical teams and people living with HIV by being able to access their own personal health information through their mobile phones [44]. This Health platform enables HIV patients with stable disease to self-manage. This model of technological care has engaged many people globally to access health information and self-manage during the coronavirus (COVID-19) pandemic during 2020. Video conferencing tools offering multi-screen capabilities have connected millions of people across the world [45]. Other advantages of technology include its ability to impact hard-to-reach populations (including those who practice behaviours typically stigmatised within healthcare settings, such as injection drug users and men who have sex with men) [46]. But not all people living with HIV have access to mobile phones, tablets, netbooks, laptops, and computers. Accessing broadband in rural communities remains difficult [47]. However, in 2016, 91% of young people in the European Union made daily use of the internet, compared with 71% for the whole EU population [48]. And whilst these technological systems ensure people, hospitals, universities, schools, and other businesses can stay connected and operational, they are not without concerns. Data security and privacy of information are a significant consideration to protect individuals against cybercrime and unintentional use of personal and medical information [49].

In 2010, the WHO stated they would assist countries to strengthen their health information systems through a range of activities, including strengthening in-country capacity for improved data management, design, and implementation of integrated management information systems [50]. Research carried out by the Oxford Internet Institute shows that 71% of the UK population have sourced health information online at some time [51]. Their preliminary findings suggest access to health information through the internet may increase the individual's knowledge and recognition that they are not alone with their health condition. But there are many challenges for nurses attempting to lead change in countries where punitive and stigmatised behaviour towards people affected by HIV limit treatment options and access to health information is limited.

One example of a community group using IT solutions to provide support to people with HIV is *Teenergizer*, Ukraine. This internet group, set up by young people, aims to share information, knowledge, and experiences. In the publications section on their website, they state 'reading is power, I read the article and became stronger' [52]. Nurses working in partnership with community groups can lead a bottom-up approach in guiding patients to manage their health, where technology can complement their education on self-management of care.

There are examples of the impact of nurse leadership. The virtual elimination of the vertical transmission of HIV in the west is one, through midwives leading on educational standards and service delivery [53, 54]. Also, nurse-led drug and alcohol treatment programmes are prominent in England, supporting commissioners and specialists in HIV to redesign services [55]. Finally, in the Eastern European and Central Asia (EECA) region, where drug user registries are a primary barrier to services in some countries, nurses have linked with medical colleagues, charitable organisations and social care groups to deliver and lead excellent needle and syringe programmes (including the disposal of used syringes) and testing services [56].

Care provided for people with HIV/AIDS has changed as dramatically as its defining prognosis [9]. Pioneering nurses pushed the boundaries of care to embrace a model where the individual person living with HIV became empowered and now is seen an equal partner in planning, developing, and monitoring care [39]. Putting people and their families at the centre of decision-making is not a strange concept in the management of HIV but accepting them as experts, working alongside clinical professionals to get the best outcome is now an instrumental health component in many health systems [57]. Studies have found that key facilitators to support shared decision-making include strong leadership, changing patient and professional roles, motivated patients and professionals and appropriate infrastructure. This implies that a fundamental shift is needed in the way that both patients and professionals view their roles and, therefore, the culture and infrastructure of health services will be as important as the motivation and attitudes of patients and professionals [58]. People are more likely to stick to treatment plans and take their medicine if they feel respected, involved, and in control [59]. It motivates the person to adopt positive health behaviours that improve and help them manage their own health as described through Geraldine's care.

Finally, nurse leadership spans beyond the face-to-face interaction with patients [60]. Research into the routine use of patient-reported outcome measures (PROMs) concluded that their use in routine HIV care could afford benefits for person, clinical teams, and commissioners [61]. Benefits of using PROMs in HIV care include improved person-centredness, patient empowerment, fewer missed concerns, increased engagement with services, and informed planning of services.

3.5   Adapting Nurse Leadership for the Future

In 2020, the bicentennial of Florence Nightingale's birth, the coronavirus has shone a global spotlight on the value of nurses in the management of patient care, raising the profile of the profession and nurse leadership across health and social care systems [62]. COVID-19 required nurse leaders to adapt as care needs became more complex hour by hour [63]. There are similarities with the early days of managing the HIV virus, when there was no known cure, limited knowledge of treatment options, and worldwide fear of contagion. The difference this time is that the COVID-19 virus spreads via droplets, potentially targeting the whole population.

Even the caring professionals have succumbed. Technology has emerged as a vital part of the communication and networking process during the period of lock down to keep people safe from the coronavirus.

Technological advances in social media offer nurses expanded models of communication to target and influence healthcare service across the world. At the same time reducing face-to-face contact to make services more cost-effective. There are examples of electronic patient records projects such as the EmERGE project, run through the Brussels-based European AIDS Treatment Group and partners, which enables self-management of HIV for people with stable disease to use applications on mobile devices. It is safe, secure, and provides a 'stable person with HIV' information on their personal data held at the clinic to support self-management of their condition. It is especially useful for people not able to travel to their appointments. They have access to their hospital consultant and a link to the Liverpool Interaction Drug Chart, a UK website to empower the person with HIV when discussing medication interactions with prescribing staff [64]. The EmERGE programme interfaces directly into the hospital clinic and medical team, but not their GP. However, the individual user can show the GP their results. Currently, the HIV treating hospital team facilitates remote access to key healthcare providers across five EU countries; the UK, Spain, Croatia, Belgium, and Portugal [44].

The WHO states that the dedication of HIV activists and advocates in pushing for patient-driven care, improving access to new drugs, and expanding funding for HIV care and research, has been unparalleled in almost any other disease field [65]. But the same WHO report outlines one of the biggest challenges in the HIV response that has remained unchanged for 30 years; HIV disproportionally affects people in vulnerable populations that are often highly marginalised and stigmatised. Thus, most new HIV infections and deaths are seen where certain higher risk groups remain unaware, underserved, or neglected. About 75% of new HIV infections outside sub-Saharan Africa are in men who have sex with men, people who inject drugs, people in prisons, sex workers, or transgender people, or the sexual partners of these individuals. These are groups who are often discriminated against and excluded from health services. For example, Russia's HIV epidemic is growing. The rate of new infections is estimated to be over 250 people become infected with HIV every day. Conversely, they have achieved significant successes in the Russian Federation for vertical transmission with the government announcing in 2016 it had achieved a 98% success rate [66]. Results from the Stigma Index show that at least 20% of people living with HIV in Kyrgyzstan and 18% in Kazakhstan report being denied health services, and disclosure of HIV status by healthcare workers without consent is alarmingly common in all countries with available data [67]. In wider society, discriminatory attitudes and misconceptions about HIV were common, with at least half of adults in eight countries saying they would not buy vegetables from a shopkeeper living with HIV [67]. Community-based organisations including nursing have major roles to play in efforts to reduce stigma and discrimination towards key populations, especially people who inject drugs, sex workers, gay men, and other men who have sex with men, migrants, and prisoners. Combination prevention programmes, including harm reduction, have been implemented by city authorities in collaboration with civil society organisations, but political, legal, and technical hurdles currently block the use of PrEP in many countries of the region. Nurse leadership is essential at a local level to challenge national and local policies and address inequalities.

> *Mother to Child transmission of HIV has been virtually eliminated in the west through midwives leading on educational standards and service delivery. WHO (2014)*

With ever evolving and more complex health trends, Nkowane [68] suggested in her key note speech at the European HIV Conference in Barcelona 2016, that the roles of nurses are also dynamic and evolving with many opportunities to enhance leadership. She summarised these in five key domains:

1. **Leadership process and practice,** in creating the structures, conditions that build motivated individuals and teams, promoting participation in care and facilitating care processes.
2. **Collaborative Partnerships**—recognising the valuable contribution that others can make to the application of care, decision-making, shared knowledge and skills.
3. **Policy and regulation improvements**—identifying specific goals and objectives, target groups, specific activities to be performed and mobilising resources for professional development and education.
4. **Education and training**—Inter-professional education and training, enhancing continuous professional development.
5. **HRH management**—Driving workforce practice, competences, recruitment, and retention strategies alongside the development of performance management and information systems.

Therefore, nurse leaders of the future can look to:

- Technology to interface with people living with HIV and management of their condition.
- Spearhead and target leadership positions at government national and local levels.
- Collaborate across sectors with clarity of role and purpose.
- Seek nurse-led initiatives that focus on improved person-centred outcomes.
- Embrace and network with others with expertise on other health conditions.
- Train and educate nurses in leadership skills.
- Develop patient peer-experts in the management of the condition [69].

3.6 My Life: Personal Reflections on Leadership

Back in 1976–1988 when working as a district nurse, I was passionate about the need for person-centred. As a district nurse delivering care in the person's home, it is necessary to move beyond the boundary of the hospital and become engaged with the person's life, how they live, who they live with, their extended family members, their likes and dislikes, their frustrations and uniqueness. You are a guest in their home. They are a person and the person communicates their wants and dislikes. But once in a hospital bed the person becomes a patient, a recipient of care based on the medical model. Talcott Parsons argued that a person assuming the 'sick role' cannot fulfil the same duties as a person in good health allowing deviation from the typical behaviour of a well person legitimised by the medical model.

But a person-centred model of care keeps the person engaged and in control of their health through setting of goals jointly with clinicians. This means the person can lead and manage their conditions with their needs met as an equal partner [70]. My desire to expand leadership of person-centred care also led to my understanding of how to manage other professional groups, such as school nurses, health visitors, and nurses involved in end-of-life care, Marie-Curie nurses, and Macmillan nurses. Managing different branches of nursing enhanced my understanding of their role and function as part of the community team, and I accompanied them as they worked with their caseload of patients, attending child protection case conferences and school visits, watching and learning how and where their unique skills and knowledge benefited their work and those in their care. These informative years helped in identifying the complexity of nursing care and how different branches of the profession added their expertise to the patient's care pathway. It fuelled my thirst to learn more about bringing teams together to understand where their specific skill set added value to the person's care pathway.

This led to an ambitious programme of leadership positions in hospital and community care, managing hospital wards, medical services, pharmacy, radiology, pathology, senior doctors, and their medical teams, commissioning services with GP fund-holders, and designing performance management tools to demonstrate achievement of local and national government targets. The focus within each leadership role was on how to improve the outcome for the 'person' requiring health services. My passion took me to the top of the NHS tree, working with NHS England's decision-makers, parliamentarians, and many other health providers in England, Scotland, and Europe.

Then, in 2009, having been diagnosed with HIV and witnessing the stigma and discrimination of others, my passion to deliver person-centred care became even stronger. Driven to raise the profile of HIV and care inequalities, I joined boards of national HIV organisations, and presented at local, national, and international workshops, conferences, and working groups. I wrote articles on HIV for publication in HIV and nursing journals and sought leadership positions, at one stage becoming Chair of HIV organisations in Scotland, Europe, interim CEO of the Terrence Higgins Trust, London, and a 'Patient Public Voice' on NHS England's HIV commissioning group. But my attention remained on those men and women infected with HIV. Some had never spoken out about their condition and lived in silence, fearing what society and others would do to them once their inner secret was revealed. At one meeting, a man spoke about his diagnosis with HIV 25 years earlier to an audience of about a hundred people. I held his hand under the table as he told his story for the very first time. From his shuddering start came strength and confidence, and at the end of his session we fell into an embrace with tears streaming down both our faces. This perfect stranger had been relieved of a heavy burden he had held inside him for many years. People with HIV know resilience. They know how to hide in the shadows fearing how others will act once their story is told. HIV is a chronic disease like no other and an affected person can live in fear of how society will treat them, even in 2020.

Finally, I remember at the age of ten feeling distraught, mesmerised, and tearful as I watched, with my parents and our black and white TV, news of the assassination of John F Kennedy on 22nd November 1963. The death of this young charismatic President of the United States shocked the world, but a quote from a speech he was due to make in Dallas has stuck in my mind to this day: 'Leadership and learning are indispensable to each other' (JFK 1963) [71]. The intrinsic relationship between leadership and learning is constant. You never stop learning as a nurse. Education and learning have been the bedrock of my career. You never stop learning as a nurse and as a leader of nursing care. What I learned:

Leadership skills:

1. Identify your strengths and those of your team to make sure you are all fit for purpose.
2. Set goals that steer and guide you.
3. Be confident but not over-confident, listen and learn.
4. Everybody you meet will have a different perspective that will expand your knowledge and skills. Listen to your patients.
5. Look for opportunities to undertake training where and however it is offered to expand your education.
6. Be clear on your vision no matter how hard it may seem.
7. Examine your fitness for purpose to identify opportunities where your strengths can be built upon through training and education.
8. Sit on panels, multi-professional groups, patient forums, boards of care providers.
9. Lead educative programmes, research, and review the work of others.
10. Write articles for publishing in medical and nursing journals.
11. Speak at conferences and help individuals to speak about their stories or writing of their stories.
12. Never forget your caring and nurturing instinct. Resilience is important.

3.7 Summary

Nursing can span health and social care systems when working in partnership with other health, community, and person-centred groups. Aspiring nurse leaders need training and education on how to deliver effective management and governance at the local level. Many nurse leaders have paved the way for the profession to be recognised as an essential building block to lead and direct person-centred care and for the nurse to become the executive nurse leader of the future, working alongside inspirational people living with HIV.

Listening, and sharing personal health stories, can release a myriad of emotions for people living with HIV with a negative perception of societal acceptance. Not all countries in the world are welcoming of people living with the condition and for aspiring leaders of HIV care, there will be many challenges. Having an open mind, a vision of the desired future state of care with measurable goals of achievement linked to those who have access to and have succeeded in driving change, can aid transformational HIV nurse leaders to deliver person-centred care.

Leadership is not just about a position of hierarchy. It is the application of simple qualities; compassion, excellent communication skills; attention to detail; endurance; courage; the ability to handle stress; accountability; resilience and the ability to challenge boundaries. Person-centred values include individuality, rights, privacy, choice, independence, dignity, respect, and partnership. Technological advances aid communication to engage and learn from others and work in partnership with people living with HIV and other health conditions, community groups and linkages to research and health information. Many still have country-wide political challenges but working in partnership with advocacy groups and others in health and social care, nurses can add influence on shaping HIV care.

3.8 Learning Points: Recommendations for Nurse Leadership in HIV

1. Influence and inform service design (by sitting on executive committees, meetings, and publication of exemplary practice).
2. Lead by example. You have a unique skill set and knowledge relating to the management of HIV and other blood-borne sexual health conditions.
3. Motivate self and others, through training and education, expanding knowledge and skills.
4. Develop collaborative relationships across multiple care providers. (Leading HIV clinicians work together to ensure an effective system leadership).
5. Develop a shared purpose and vision with jointly held goals.

6. Deliver person-centred care through leadership development, learning from others to deliver hands-on training of others into new techniques working in partnership with the person living with HIV.
7. Embrace technological advances to expand knowledge, increase communication and deliver cost-effective care.
8. Develop leadership skills through training and education, publication of articles in journals and presenting at local, national, and international conferences.

3.9 Conclusions

HIV care has changed considerably since the 1980s. Nurses have played a significant part in this change through developing services in the community, away from the hospital environment. It required strong leadership and a willingness to work alongside local activists and influencers in the management of HIV care and the development of testing centres, access to anti-retroviral medication, and needle exchange programmes. But this is not happening everywhere. There are still countries without access to these services.

The World Health Organisation suggests that when countries enable nurses to take a leadership role, for example, by having a government chief nursing officer (or equivalent) and nursing leadership programmes, the regulation of nursing education and of working conditions improves [72]. But leadership is not just about a role or position. It is about being proactive in your desire to lead and manage change to improve the lives of the people you care for. Nurses are uniquely placed to work across hospital and community services to deliver person-centred services. With training, education, and technological advances, there are many opportunities to inspire and achieve exceptional models of care [73]. It requires a partnership approach with the infected and affected person living with HIV, other health, social and community teams, and local leaders able to drive change, e.g. pastors, community groups, politicians, researchers, local dignitaries, and advocates campaigning for improved access to treatment and care.

References

1. Bernard-Cohen I. Sci Am. 1984;250(3):128–37.
2. Cameron D, Jones IG. John Snow, the Broad Street pump and modern epidemiology. Int J Epidemiol. 1983;12:393–6.
3. Gill CJ, Gillian C. Nightingale in Scutari: her legacy re-examined. Clin Infect Dis. 2005;40:1799–805.
4. Onward Healthcare. Florence nightingale, the most inspirational nurse of all time, Florence's timeline of transforming nursing, Hospitals, and patient care. Onward Healthcare. https://www.onwardhealthcare.com/resources/news/florence-nightingale/. Accessed Jan 2020.

5. Page A. Keeping patients safe: transforming the work environment of nurses. Institute Of Medicine (US) Committee on the Work Environment for Nurses and Patient Safety. Washington, DC: National Academies Press; 2004.
6. Jones O. We can't go back to the deadly HIV stigma of the 1980s, The Guardian, 11 November 2015. https://www.theguardian.com/commentisfree/2015/nov/11/hiv-stigma-1980s. Accessed Jan 2021.
7. Kelly J. HIV/AIDS: why were the campaigns successful in the West? BBC News Magazine, 28 November 2011. https://www.bbc.co.uk/news/magazine-15886670. Accessed Jan 2021.
8. Bradley-Springer L. The 25th year. J Associat Nurs AIDS Care. 2012;23(1):4.
9. Johnstone F. Care-crafting and creative nursing: HIV/AIDS histories and the rise of person-centred care. 2019. https://thepolyphony.org/2019/05/01/care-crafting-and-creative-nursing-hiv-aids-histories-and-the-rise-of-person-centred-care/. Accessed Jan 2021.
10. Dickinson T, et al. Nursing a 'plague', a history of HIV & AIDS Care, 1981–1996. Research conducted 2017. London: King's College; In press.
11. Whitehead C. The specialist nurse in HIV/AIDS medicine. Fellowship Postgrad Med. 1996;72:211–3.
12. Watson S. Economic Assessment of the Community HIV Clinical Nurse Specialist. 2015; Royal College of Nursing in HIV. https://www.rcn.org.uk/clinical-topics/public-health/sexual-health/sexual-health-career-stories-and-case-studies/economic-assessment-of-the-community-hiv-clinical-nurse-specialist-role. Accessed Dec 2019.
13. Quinn D, Bowen A, Leary A. The value of the multiple sclerosis specialist nurse with respect to prevention of unnecessary emergency admission. Mult Scler. 2014;20(12):1669–70.
14. HIV Stigma and Discrimination. Avert, Global Information of HIV and AIDs. https://www.avert.org/professionals/hiv-social-issues/stigma-discrimination. Accessed Jan 2021.
15. WHO World Health Day 2020. WHO calls on governments to invest in nurses for a healthy Europe. http://www.euro.who.int/en/health-topics/Health-systems/nursing-and-midwifery/news/news/2020/4/who-calls-on-governments-to-invest-in-nurses-for-a-healthy-europe. Accessed Jan 2021.
16. World Health Organisation. State of the World's Nursing, Investing in education, jobs and leadership. Geneva: World Health Organisation. https://apps.who.int/iris/handle/10665/331677. Accessed Jan 2021.
17. Scully NJ. Leadership in nursing: the importance of recognising inherent values and attributes to secure a positive future for the profession. Collegian. 2015;22(4):439–44.
18. Royal College of Nursing (UK). Clinical Governance. https://www.rcn.org.uk/clinical-topics/clinical-governance. Accessed Jan 2021.
19. Tomblin-Murphy G, Elliott Rose A. Nursing leadership in primary health care for the achievement of Sustainable Development Goals and human resources for health global strategies. ICN policy brief. https://www.who.int/workforcealliance/knowledge/resources/ICN_PolBrief2NsgLeadershipPHC.pdf. Accessed Jan 2021.
20. The National Archives. Florence Nightingale. Why do we remember her? London: The National Archives. https://www.nationalarchives.gov.uk/education/resources/florence-nightingale/. Accessed May 2020.
21. National Health Service (NHS), NHS Improvement. The Ward Leaders Handbook. London: NHS; 2018.
22. The Kings Fund. Leadership in Health care. A summary of the Evidence Base. Faculty of Medical Leadership and Development; 2015.
23. World Health Organisation. State of the World's Nursing, Investing in education, jobs, and leadership. Geneva: WHO; 2020.
24. World Health Organisation. WHO calls on governments to invest in nurses for a healthy Europe Media Centre, Events, World Health Day, 2020. Ten recommendations for a strengthened nursing work force. Geneva: WHO; 2020. http://www.euro.who.int/en/media-centre/events/events/2020/04/world-health-day-2020/news/news/2020/04/who-calls-on-governments-to-invest-in-nurses-for-a-healthy-europe. Accessed Jan 2021.

25. Royal College of Nursing. RCN Factsheet: specialist nursing in the UK. London: RCN; 2014.
26. Bagness C, Champion B, et al. Clinical nurse specialist in early pregnancy care. London: RCN; 2017.
27. Maclellan J, et al. Shared Care: how we do it? BHIVA primary care project 2016–2017. London: British HIV Association; 2017.
28. Alderwick C. Improving and integrating HIV care. London: National AIDS Trust; 2019. https://www.nat.org.uk/blog/improving-and-integrating-hiv-care. Accessed Jan 2021.
29. National Aids Trust. Providing co-ordinated care for people living with HIV. 2020. https://www.nat.org.uk/sites/default/files/Providing%20coordinated%20care%20briefing_0.pdf. Accessed Jan 2021.
30. The Kings Fund. About us. https://www.kingsfund.org.uk/about-us. Accessed Jan 2021.
31. Dougal D, et al. Transformational change in health and care. Reports from the field. London: Kings Fund; 2018.
32. Hekkink C, et al. HIV nursing consultants: patients' preferences and experiences about the quality of care. J Clin Nurs. 2005;14:327–33.
33. Moyo TC. Making savings in HIV care delivery: are nurse led initiatives the future? Churchill Fellow Report. 2016. https://www.wcmt.org.uk/sites/default/files/report-documents/Moyo%20T%20Report%202016%20Final.pdf. Accessed Jan 2021.
34. Leber W, et al. Evaluating the impact of post-trial implementation of RHIVA nurse-led HIV screening on HIV testing, diagnosis and earlier diagnosis in general practice in London, UK. E Clin Med. 2020;19:100229. https://www.thelancet.com/journals/eclinm/article/PIIS2589-5370(19)30234-2/fulltext. Accessed Jan 2021.
35. Maclellan J, et al. Shared Care: how we do it? BHIVA primary care project 2016–17. London: British HIV Association; 2017.
36. Laurant M et al. Nurses as substitutes for doctors in primary care. Cochrane Database of Systematic Reviews. 2018. https://doi.org/10.1002/14651858.CD001271.pub3. Accessed Jan 2021.
37. HIV Drug Interactions. University of Liverpool. https://www.hiv-druginteractions.org. Accessed Jan 2021.
38. HIVinfo. Side effects of HIV medicines: HIV and high cholesterol. https://hivinfo.nih.gov/understanding-hiv/fact-sheets/hiv-and-high-cholesterol. Accessed Jan 2021.
39. Health Innovation Network. Why is person-centred care important? https://healthinnovation-network.com/resources/what-is-person-centred-care/. Accessed Jan 2021.
40. American Nurses Credentialing Centre (ANCC). Magnet model—creating a magnet culture. https://www.nursingworld.org/organizational-programs/magnet/magnet-model/. Accessed Jan 2021.
41. American Nurses Credentialing Centre (ANCC). Magnet model—creating a Magnet culture [Transformational Leadership]. https://www.nursingworld.org/organizational-programs/magnet/. Accessed Jan 2021.
42. Royal College of Nursing. The Magnet Recognition Programme. 2015. https://www.rcn.org.uk/about-us/our-influencing-work/policy-briefings/POL-0915. Accessed Jan 2021.
43. Royal College of Nursing, Leadership in Nursing. Improving patient care through quality leadership. https://www.rcn.org.uk/professional-development/professional-services/leadership-programmes. Accessed Jan 2021.
44. EmERGE Project/European AIDS Treatment Group. Creating mHealth solutions to facilitate remote access to health providers and people living with HIV. https://www.emergeproject.eu. Accessed Jan 2021.
45. BBC News. Coronavirus: zoom under increased scrutiny as popularity soars. 2020. https://www.bbc.co.uk/news/business-52115434. Accessed Jan 2021.
46. Simoni J, et al. PhD opportunities and challenges of digital technology for HIV treatment and prevention. Curr HIV/AIDS Rep. 2015;12(4):437–40.
47. Smith B, Browne CA. Today in technology: the top 10 Tech Issues for 2019. Section 8, Rural Broadband, Some progress amidst problems. https://www.linkedin.com/pulse/today-technology-top-10-tech-issues-2019-brad-smith/. Accessed Jan 2021.

48. Eurostat. Statistics explained. Being young in Europe today. Digital world. 2017. https://ec.europa.eu/eurostat/statistics-explained/index.php/Being_young_in_Europe_today_-_digital_world. Accessed Jan 2021.
49. Coventry L, Branley-Bell D. Cybersecurity in healthcare: a narrative review of trends, threats and ways forward. Maturitas. 2018. https://www.maturitas.org/article/S0378-5122(18)30165-8/fulltext. Accessed Jan 2021.
50. World Health Organisation. PMTCT strategic vision 2010–2015, Preventing mother-to-child transmission of HIV to reach the UNGASS and Millennium Development Goals Moving towards the elimination of paediatric HIV. Geneva: World Health Organisation; 2010.
51. Dutton WH, Blank G. Next generation users: the internet in Britain. Oxford internet survey; 2011. https://papers.ssrn.com/sol3/papers.cfm?abstract_id=1960655. Accessed Jan 2021.
52. Teenergizer. https://teenergizer.org/en/articles/. Accessed Jan 2021.
53. BHIVA. The management of HIV in pregnancy and post-partum. London: British HIV Association, 2019. https://www.bhiva.org/pregnancy-guidelines. Accessed Jan 2021.
54. World Health Organisation. HIV/AIDS Epidemic Europe/Mother to Child Transmission. Geneva: World Health Organisation; 2014. https://www.euro.who.int/en/health-topics/communicable-diseases/hivaids/news/news/2014/07/hivaids-epidemic-in-europe-mother-to-child-transmission. Accessed Jan 2021.
55. Public Health England. The role of nurses in alcohol and drug treatment services, a resource for commissioners, providers and clinicians. London: Public Health England; 2014. p. 6–8. https://assets.publishing.service.gov.uk/government/uploads/system/uploads/attachment_data/file/652963/Role_of_nurses_in_alcohol_and_drug_services.pdf. Accessed Jan 2021.
56. World Health Organisation. WHO calls for urgent action to accelerate HIV response in Eastern Europe and central Asia. Geneva: World Health Organisation; 2018. https://www.euro.who.int/en/health-topics/communicable-diseases/hivaids/news/news/2018/7/who-calls-for-urgent-action-to-accelerate-hiv-response-in-eastern-europe-and-central-asia. Accessed Jan 2021.
57. Ashby ME, Dowding C. Hospice care and patients' pain: communication between patients, relatives, nurses and doctors. Int J Pall Care Nurse. 2001;7(2):58.
58. Da Silva D. A review of evidence considering whether shared decision making is worthwhile. Evidence: Helping people share decisions. Health Foundation. 2012. https://www.health.org.uk/publications/helping-people-share-decision-making. Accessed Jan 2021.
59. NHS England. Involving people in their own health and care: statutory guidance for clinical commissioning groups and NHS England. https://www.england.nhs.uk/wp-content/uploads/2017/04/ppp-involving-people-health-care-guidance.pdf. Accessed Jan 2021.
60. Dowsett SM, Saul JL, Butow PN, Dunn SM, Boyer MJ, Findlow R, Dunsmore J. Communication styles in the cancer consultation: preferences for a patient-centred approach. Psycho-Oncology. 2000;9(2):147–56.
61. Harding R, Bristowe K, et al. Towards person-centred care for people living with HIV: what core outcomes matter, and how might we assess them? A cross-national multi-centre qualitative study with key stakeholders. HIV Med. 2019;20:8.
62. Catton H. World's nurses are 'stepping up' to COVID-19 crisis. Nursing Times. 2020. https://www.nursingtimes.net/news/leadership-news/worlds-nurses-are-stepping-up-to-covid-19-crisis-says-icn-chief-02-04-2020/. Accessed Jan 2021.
63. Bailey S, West M. Covid-19: Blog: why compassionate leadership matters in a crisis. 2020. https://www.kingsfund.org.uk/blog/2020/03/covid-19-crisis-compassionate-leadership. Accessed Jan 2021.
64. Liverpool HIV Drug Interactions. Liverpool University, Interaction checker. https://www.hiv-druginteractions.org/checker. Accessed Jan 2021.
65. World Health Organisation. HIV/AIDS fact sheet. https://www.who.int/news-room/fact-sheets/detail/hiv-aids. Accessed Jan 2021.
66. Clark F. World report: gaps remain in Russia's response to HIV/AIDS. Lancet. 2016;388:857–8.
67. UNAIDS. Global AIDS Update 2018. https://www.unaids.org/sites/default/files/media_asset/miles-to-go_en.pdf. Accessed Jan 2021.

68. Nkowane AM. Transforming nursing, enhancing nurse clinical leadership in the HIV testing and treatment. Barcelona, Spain: European Nursing Conference; 2016. https://www.iapac.org/ EHNC/presentations/EHNC2016-keynote-nkowane2.pdf. Accessed Jan 2021.
69. Positively UK. Peer mentor training programme. https://positivelyuk.org/peer-mentor-training/ project-100-peer-mentors/. Accessed Jan 2021.
70. Health Innovation Network. What is person-centred care? https://healthinnovationnetwork. com/system/ckeditor_assets/attachments/41/what_is_person-centred_care_and_why_is_it_ important.pdf. Accessed Jan 2021.
71. Spencer B. Leadership and learning are indispensable to each other. 2015. https://blog. teamsatchel.com/leadership-and-learning-are-indispensable-to-each-other-j.f.k.   Accessed Jan 2021.
72. World Health Organisation. A Capacity Building Manual, Roles and responsibilities of Government Chief Nursing and Midwifery Officers. WHO. 2015:15–6. (ISBN 978 92 41509473).
73. Piercy H, et al. How does specialist nursing contribute to HIV service delivery across England? Int J STD AIDS. 2017;28(8):808–13.

Chapter 4
HIV is a Small Word with a Big Impact: Psychosocial Interventions to Support Children, Young People, and Families with HIV

Tomás Campbell

4.1 Introduction

In Europe, there are declining numbers of children born with HIV which is a testament to the success of antiretroviral medication interventions, and These advances have prevented approximately 1.4 million children from acquiring HIV since 2000 [1] and reduced the global incidence of HIV among children by 50% since 2010 [2]. The elimination of MTCT is now an achievable goal and core to the strategy to stop new infections [3].

However, at a global level, HIV/AIDS continues to take a heavy toll on families and children. Currently, the bulk of the families in which there is HIV live in sub-Saharan Africa [4], where there is still much work to be undertaken with regard to implementing proven MTCT interventions. Of the approximately 36.7 million people currently living with HIV globally [5], the largest proportion are now of child-bearing age. This presents challenges with regard to both effectively interrupting onward transmission of HIV and supporting young HIV+ parents to cope effectively with the new challenges of parenthood while managing their own health status.

Children have been affected in other ways and HIV-negative children often face complex challenges associated with parental HIV. During the first 30 years of HIV epidemic, approximately 17 million children have lost one or both parents to HIV disease [6]. Millions more children are living with HIV-infected parents/caregivers and the number has grown over the past few decades [4]. Similar to young people with HIV, this group of uninfected children have now grown up and are now of child-bearing age themselves.

T. Campbell (✉)
Cogito Psychological Services, London, UK

© The Author(s), under exclusive license to Springer Nature Switzerland AG 2021
M. Croston, I. Hodgson (eds.), *Providing HIV Care: Lessons from the Field for Nurses and Healthcare Practitioners*,
https://doi.org/10.1007/978-3-030-71295-2_4

HIV presented many challenges to the affected families at the time and, nearly four decades later, many of the complex set of social, medical, psychological, and emotional challenges remain in the context of this highly stigmatized disease.

4.2   The Presence of HIV Disrupts Normal Family Functioning

HIV can be considered to be a disease that alters the normal life functioning of individuals and families, as its diagnosis and management present individual family members, both HIV positive and negative, and the family as a whole, with unwanted and unwelcome challenges [7].

As HIV may affect several family members simultaneously, each person affected will be faced with difficulties and dilemmas that require them to make often tough decisions about treatment, how to discuss the diagnosis with others, how to seek support and what to expect and how to prepare for the future. Challenges include the personal medical management of HIV but also the consideration of treatment for others, coping with daily and life-long adherence to antiretroviral therapy and the management of possible side-effects to antiretroviral therapy. For families, there are always issues with regard to explaining and discussing the diagnosis with schools. Further challenges include the psychological issues associated with positive status (e.g., coming to terms with HIV, management of HIV-related mental health difficulties), social issues (e.g., housing, employment), and social issues (e.g., the effects of HIV-related stigma, discussion with family members, friends, and sexual partners about the presence of HIV) [8].

From a child developmental perspective, the presence of HIV infection may have negative influence directly on neurodevelopmental, psychological, and psychosocial outcomes. This can occur both directly through the impact of infection on physical and neurocognitive development, and indirectly through increased risks at the family and community level [9]. Children who are HIV+ face life-long risk of related illnesses and are more likely to experience cognitive and motor development delays, stigma, trauma, and low mood [10].

From a family and community perspective, HIV can negatively affect the ways in which families cope with challenges, the ways in which they communicate and the effects on their mental health. As the family structure is usually the context in which children, adolescents, and young people are cared for and grow up in, the quality of parental coping capacity is important in determining how HIV-related issues are dealt with in the family but can be placed under huge strain as a result of the presence of HIV [11].

Parental HIV-related illness and the psychological impact of living with the disease may greatly affect their ability to adequately care for their children, placing stress on both the parent(s) and child(ren) [12]. Evidence has suggested that children living with HIV, or living in families affected by HIV, are vulnerable to emotional and behavioural difficulties including psychological distress [12, 13], disrupted school attendance [14] and increased rates of psychological and behavioural issues [15]. Adolescents with HIV-positive parents are likely to be more vulnerable to higher sexual risks, increased alcohol, drug use, and mental health problems [16, 17].

There are probably many factors that affect how children and young people cope in a family in which there is HIV. The presence of family conflict has been suggested as a significant risk factor for increased psychological and social difficulties among young people [18]. Disruptions to familiar, effective, and supportive family routines have been reported to be associated with poorer social and psychological functioning in young people [18]. The presence of multiple family stressors has also been suggested to negatively affect all family members. In a review of London-based family clinic attendees, most families were headed by a single parent. Multiple other stressors were present including parental death due to HIV, high levels of mental health issues in parents and high levels of other social problems [19]. The presence of such factors strains the coping abilities of parents, children, and young people.

On the contrary, the presence and maintenance of effective family routines have been associated with lower rates of aggression, anxiety, depression, binge drinking, and behavioural disorders in HIV-affected adolescents [20]. Supportive adult–child relationships have been reported to be protective against the development of social and psychological issues in children and young people [21]. Changes to routines can be changed drastically by a family member's illness that in turn negatively affects individual family roles and responsibilities [22].

Discussion Points
What social factors distinguishes HIV from other diseases?
Why does can the presence of HIV disrupt normal family functioning?
What are the links between disrupted family life and the emergence of psychological and social difficulties?

4.3   The Family is the Point of Intersection of HIV, Coping, and Well-Being

For parents, children, and young people with HIV, the family is the point of intersection between HIV infection and parental coping and child and family well-being. In high-prevalence environments, transmission occurs mainly in the family, between mothers and children and between sexual partners [23]. The family is the basic unit of care for children and young people and is the single greatest influence on a child's health and well-being. The consideration of the health, psychological, and social needs of all the members of the family affected by HIV is not a new idea, but it has been extremely difficult to implement as an approach in most parts of the world and particularly where HIV has been most prevalent.

Clinical services that integrate health and social support for both adults and children are probably the most effective way of ensuring good clinical and psychosocial outcomes for HIV-positive children [24] and several family-focused HIV clinics have been established in the UK and elsewhere in Europe that provide coordinated multidisciplinary medical, psychological, nursing, and social care for all HIV-positive members of the family [25].

Family-focused care can be difficult to define as there is no generally accepted definition of what constitutes a 'family', what appropriate treatment or interventions should be and how they should be delivered. However, any group of people who depend on each other for care, support, and comfort should be considered to be a family. Traditionally, family-focused approaches have tended to focus on mothers and children for many reasons: they are easier to access as a population via child health and immunization clinics, mothers' gender and social roles emphasize that child-care and rearing is a female responsibility and fathers have historically been very absent from child-focused health settings compounding the difficulty of delivering health interventions to them and considering how the presence of HIV has affected them. However, there is a growing awareness that males and fathers should be more involved and that new strategies need to be developed and implemented to achieve this aim [26].

Models of care that support effective family functioning have been demonstrated to be effective in supporting good outcomes for children including better psychosocial functioning in children [27] and have been demonstrated to assist parents in making decisions about disclosure of HIV status, planning for children's long-term adjustment to HIV [28], and the development of long-term coping skills to cope with HIV infection [29].

The core concepts of family-centred care for children and young people can be described as [24]:

1. Families are the constant in the lives of children (and adults) while interventions are intermittent and generally short lived and contact with services might be infrequent and brief.
2. Families must be variously and inclusively defined.
3. Family-centred approaches are those that are comprehensive and integrated.
4. Love and care within families, when recognized and reinforced, promote improved coping and wellness among children and adults.

A family-focused approach has been demonstrated to be effective for recruiting HIV-positive women into treatment and consequently reduced mother to child transmission, supported adherence, and improved paediatric adherence to antiretroviral medication [30]. There is some evidence that providing group-based interventions for parents aimed at strengthening skills regarding issues such as disclosure can be effective [29].

Supportive group interventions utilizing cognitive-behavioural theory and psycho-education have also been demonstrated to be effective in enhancing mood and coping behaviours and reducing negative affect [31]. However, family-focused programmes have been less successful in recruiting males and fathers into treatment and care and programmes and have reported mixed success regarding supporting disclosure of HIV status between females and their male partners. Finally, studies have also shown that HIV-positive adults in care did not consistently and routinely refer their children to the same treatment centre or programme where they themselves were receiving treatment [30].

> **Discussion Points**
> *Do you think that integrated medical, social and psychological care is an effective model to address HIV?*
> *Why is it difficult to include fathers and males in family-focussed interventions?*
> *What underlying principles do you consider to be important in the design and implementation of HIV services and interventions?*
> *Why is it important to maintain a focus on the family when it comes to HIV treatment and care?*

4.4 HIV Stigma: What Is It?

Goffman [32] provided a seminal conceptualization of health-related stigma in which he considered it to be 'an attribute that is deeply discrediting' and one which 'reduces the bearer from a whole and usual person to a tainted, discounted one." The mechanism for this process is a societal one by which difference (that which is undesirable) is identified and located in an individual or group.

Subsequent conceptualizations have attempted to explain the mechanisms by which the experience of stigma is created and how it affects the cognitions and behaviours of both those who enact stigmatizing behaviours and attitudes and those who are affected by stigma. In this model, stigma is created when four distinct but related components converge:

1. Differences among people are articulated and labelled as being bad/evil/immoral/dangerous.
2. Dominant cultural beliefs link labelled persons to undesirable characteristics (or negative stereotypes).
3. Labelled persons are placed in distinct categories that facilitate the separation of 'us' from 'them'.
4. Labelled persons experience status loss and discrimination that leads to unequal outcomes (e.g., health, economic, social).

HIV stigma can also be considered as a layered experience [33]. This idea refers to HIV being particularly prevalent in certain groups (gay men, drug users, Black Africans) or associated with particular sexual behaviours (oral sex, anal sex, or other sexual practices that might be considered to be "kinky" or fetish) or social behaviours that are stigmatized (addiction, selling sex). In this way, HIV stigma also becomes attached to other 'traits or behaviours that are undesirable' and may deepen the experience of stigma [34].

In this way, the interaction of personal characteristics that may already have stigma attached to them (e.g., young age, female gender, Black ethnic origin, African ancestry) and HIV disease provides a context in which the contribution and importance of any one factor becomes blurred and stigma is experienced at many levels.

Discussion Points
Why do you think HIV has so much stigma attached to it?
  Can you think of examples of how stigma might affect care and treatment?
  What are ways to reduce the effects of stigma in clinical services?
  What approaches would you take to address issues of stigma in your own clinical practice?

4.5   HIV and the Family: The Effects of Stigma on Care, Treatment, and Functioning

The effects of HIV stigma are complex and mostly negative in the lives of HIV-positive people. Stigma may be experienced at an individual level, but stigmatizing behaviours and attitudes can become embedded at organizational and societal levels affecting the ways in which HIV testing and treatment interventions are delivered.

HIV stigma can also be a barrier to accessing health care and its effects discourage HIV people from the outset, placing many at risk for poor medical outcomes if they are HIV+ [34]. There is substantial evidence that people with HIV who experience stigma have poorer social support, poorer mental health [35] and poorer adherence to antiretroviral therapy [36].

With regard to young people specifically, evidence suggests that higher levels of stigma in HIV-positive young women in particular was associated with poorer adherence to antiretroviral medication [37]. Higher levels of stigma may also negatively affect adherence to antiretroviral therapy in young adults living with HIV [38]. However, in their systematic review and meta-analysis of published studies regarding adherence patterns to antiretroviral therapy for adolescents and young adults living with HIV, Kim et al. [38] reported wide variations in patterns worldwide. Adherence was reported to be highest in Africa and Asia and lowest in Europe and North America. While this meta-analysis did not control for the effect of stigma, this study suggests that membership of a marginalized group is associated with poorer adherence and the mediating factor may be the effects of stigma.

Discussion Points

How does the effect of HIV stigma pose a barrier to accessing HIV testing and treatment?

What do you consider to be the effects of stigma on the lived experience of people with HIV?

What are the psychological and psychosocial interactions between HIV and adherence to antiretroviral therapy?

4.6 What Are Examples of Family-Focused Interventions?

Intervention types are varied but all share the aim of reducing psychological distress (depression, anxiety, behavioural problems, drug and alcohol use), and improving individual and family coping skills. Some have included both parents and children, others have focused on parents only and still others have focused on children/young people only. There have also been a range of intervention types that have included psychological interventions (e.g., support groups, psychological debriefing), support programmes (e.g., home visiting or play groups), and social programmes (e.g., cash transfer programmes, material assistance, skills building programmes) [19, 39, 40].

4.6.1 Intergenerational Interventions

Family-centred psychosocial interventions have been implemented in several countries, mostly in sub-Saharan Africa where the burden of HIV is highest. Bell, Gibbons, & McKay (2008) [41] described a family group-based intervention in South Africa which included both caregiver and child. The intervention was randomized into the study arm and a control arm which included usual clinical care. The intervention was delivered over 10 weekends and focused on reducing youth HIV risk-behaviours by the strengthening of family relationships, targeting negative peer influences through enhancing social problem-solving and peer-negotiation skills for youths. On evaluation, there was no differences between the study and intervention groups for psychosocial outcomes. In the intervention group, there was improved HIV-transmission knowledge and lower stigmatizing attitudes towards people with HIV.

In a randomized control study, families attended a six-session intervention delivered to HIV affected family groups in China [42]. Families also attended community events. The intervention focused on improving the family's capacity to develop new skills to address the impact of living with HIV. Adult family members attended separate sessions, followed by joint activities with children, and the cohort also attended three community events as a family group. Mixed results were reported, with no differences in psychological measures of self-esteem or problem behaviours between groups. There was improved perceived parental care at 6 months in the intervention group compared to controls.

In an American randomized control trial, mothers and their children (aged between 6 and 20 years) met in a twice-weekly group-based cognitive-behaviour therapy intervention over a 16-week period. Mothers in the intervention arm met concurrently in their own groups for some sessions and attended groups with their children at other times [43].

The intervention aimed to improve mothers' physical and psychological health, maintain effective parenting when unwell, address HIV-related stressors, and reduce HIV-transmission behaviours. Participants were followed up 18 months after the end of the intervention. For adolescents, the intervention goals were to: (1) improve family relationships; (2) reduce mental health symptoms; (3) reduce multiple problem behaviours (e.g., drug use, criminal acts, school problems, teenage pregnancy); and (4) increase school retention. Results indicated that for most outcomes, mothers did not significantly differ between the intervention and control condition over time. However, compared to mothers in the control condition, the women in the intervention arm were significantly more likely to monitor their own CD4 cell counts and their children were more likely to decrease alcohol and drug use.

In a related study of the same group of mothers, women in the study arm showed several indications of the stress of living with HIV including lower rates of employment and more financial hardship in comparison with HIV-negative mothers [43]. These results may have been in part due to HIV-related illnesses. However, an additional factor was that more HIV-positive than HIV-negative mothers were head of a single parent household that may have resulted in a smaller household income, while the number of children in the households were similar between the study and control group. Additionally, mothers with HIV reported more emotional distress (declining over time) and lifetime and current substance use than women in the control group.

There were also differences between the two groups around issues of family relationships. Mothers with HIV reported higher levels of family cohesion at baseline, but those gains were lost over time. They also reported lower conflict reasoning and less physical violence than the control group at baseline. However, over time, HIV+ mothers reported increased levels of conflict and lowered levels of physical violence, social interactions, and engagement than HIV-negative women.

In a study conducted in South Africa, HIV+ mothers and children in a participated in randomized trial aimed at the promotion of resilience of young children with HIV-positive mothers [44]. The intervention was delivered over 24 weekly sessions, with over half of the sessions held with caregivers and children separately and the rest held together. The focus of the sessions was to improve the well-being of the mother and child, family relationships, and to provide information about HIV. The intervention group children showed a significant improvement in externalizing behaviours, communication and daily living skills, and no difference in internalizing behaviour and emotional intelligence between groups. On the other hand, children in the intervention group reported significantly higher levels of anxiety. Boys tended to gain greater benefit from the intervention than did girls.

In a further American study, 62 HIV+ mothers and their children participated in four 75-min group sessions. Enrolled mother/child pairs were interviewed at baseline and 3-, 6-, and 12-month follow-ups [45]. The intervention aimed to improve parenting practices (e.g., increase parent–child communication and parental monitoring), improve mental and physical self-care skills, reduce child mental health indicators (e.g., behavioural problems, poor self-concept and poor coping), and improve family functioning. The intervention was based on the IMB model (information, motivation, and behavioural skills model [46]). Interventions based on this model should focus on imparting relevant information, increase personal motivation and social support, and train skills to promote self-efficacy in performing targeted behaviours. For maternal outcomes, findings suggested the intervention improved parenting efficacy (better parental monitoring and involvement with children) and maternal mental health. Improved mental health in the intervention group was also reported. With regard to child outcomes, the strongest findings were evident for coping behaviours in the intervention group, with additional beneficial effects on child depression and self-concept. Results also indicated that parental–child relationships improved with regard to better communication.

In summary, results of group-based psychological interventions that include HIV+ parents (usually mothers) and their children indicate generally positive effects for parents living with HIV, their children, or both. Positive outcomes have been demonstrated in the improvement of parent–child communication, improved parental self-care, and increased positive coping behaviours and emotional outcomes for children.

However, we also need to consider some of the methodological constraints of the studies reported here [47]. Small sample sizes and short follow-up periods mean that longer term intervention effects are unknown. High rates of participant attrition may bias outcomes and some studies (usually American) lacked complete racial/ethnic diversity. The cognitive-behaviour therapy approach on which many studies were based might not be the most appropriate given that the studies focused on changing parent–child communication patterns. A more family-based and ecological framework may be necessary for the development and evaluation of effective future intergenerational interventions, as most of the studies included in this review utilize group-based programming in their intervention methodology.

In summary, there is some evidence available that family focused interventions improve health and well-being outcomes for affected young people and their families. However, many interventions are not evaluated effectively and if they are evaluated, results often do not reaching the evidence base [40].

Discussion Points

If you had to design a family-based intervention, what lessons from the studies reported above would you consider?

What do you consider to be the most important components of effective coping in families with HIV?

What are the ways mechanisms to improve coping in families with HIV?

4.6.2   Parent/Caregiver Only Interventions

In a study conducted in [48] Kenya, Thurman, Jarabi, and Rice (2012) evaluated an ongoing support group programme for parents and caregivers of HIV+ orphans and vulnerable children. The intervention was delivered on a weekly basis in 3-hour sessions. Caregivers attended groups of up to 25 participants facilitated by trained counsellors. The topics covered were participant led and included issues of HIV prevention, life skills, children's rights, and the effects of HIV stigma. Evaluation of the intervention reported that support-group members considered that the behaviour of children in their care improved and that behavioural difficulties had reduced. Caregivers reported less social marginalization, better family functioning and more positive feelings towards the children.

Interventions to improve parental coping abilities have been reported [49]. In a group intervention informed by social action theory [50], HIV-positive African parents raising their children in a British cultural context attended a 6-week intervention run during the school summer holidays. The intervention focused on improving functioning in three psychological domains: responses to internal affective states that influence the self-regulation process, the self-regulation capabilities of the individual and the external environmental context. Within this model, interventions are aimed at increasing coping skills, improving communication skills between parents, children, other family members and new sexual partners, and psycho-education about child and adolescent development. Enhancing parental confidence and skills in relation to coping with HIV was a focus for each session, including topics such as: exploring fears of and approaches to the disclosure of parental HIV status and of HIV-positive children's status; promoting ongoing conversations about HIV within the family rather than a one-off discussion of diagnosis; enhancing children's resilience in the face of HIV-related stigma; dealing with parental fears of adolescence within the context of HIV.

The evaluation of the effectiveness of this intervention [49] indicated that participants reported an increase in confidence or knowledge with regard to talking to their children about their own HIV status, and their children's HIV status (for those who had HIV-positive children). Parents also reported feeling more confident talking to HIV-negative children about HIV. However, despite expressing more confidence with HIV-related discussion, there was also a drop in confidence to help their families cope with HIV and participants agreed more strongly at evaluation than at baseline that it was more difficult to raise children in London than in Africa.

Overall, the authors concluded that interventions provided to young people had potential for improving cognitive, psychosocial, and reducing risk behaviours (alcohol and drug use, sexual risk taking). Interventions that transferred cash and had therapeutic components had the highest effect sizes. However, therapeutic approaches had positive effects on fewer outcomes and demonstrated some negative effects. Successful components of other types of intervention were identified, including cash grants, mentorship, and family therapy.

However, there are some methodological issues to be considered with regard to all the studies. Many interventions are not based on randomized control trials (RCT) and so do not get published limiting the amount of published evidence available. Conversely, randomized control trials are time limited, are easier to implement and evaluate than already functioning parental support interventions but do not neces-sarily reflect how services can deliver interventions in the real world. Lastly, results from RCTs cannot always be easily implemented into healthcare programmes.

Discussion Points
What are the advantages/disadvantages of interventions focused only improv-ing coping in parents with HIV?
What important issues emerge from the research discussed above?

4.6.3   Child/Young Person Only Interventions

Structured interventions have been directed at children or adolescents specifically. A group-based intervention in Tanzania was delivered weekly over 28 weeks after school or on weekends to young people who were orphaned through HIV. It focused on increasing self- and collective-efficacy through public education and community mobilization. The authors found a positive impact on different types of self-efficacy, but no difference in academic efficacy or peer resistance [51].

Soccer was used as an intervention tool in the WhizzKids programme in South Africa. A HIV-prevention intervention was delivered in eight sessions over 12-weeks to large groups of orphaned and vulnerable young people [52]. Attendees were local school children (aged 10–18) who participated in structured discussions before soc-cer training which aimed to change attitudes towards HIV and to improve self-efficacy to make healthy choices, including the uptake of HIV testing and sexual health services. Intervention participants had a significantly lower likelihood of engaging in drug and alcohol use than the comparison group and lower reported HIV stigma.

School-based interventions have shown some success. Mueller, Alie, Jonas, Brown, and Sherr, 2011 [53] reported on the results of an art-based intervention with children orphaned by HIV or vulnerable to HIV. The intervention aimed to increase self-esteem, self-efficacy, and psychological well-being and was delivered during class over 6 months and participants received 50 or more sessions. Results were mixed; children in the intervention arm had significantly better self-efficacy than comparisons on evaluation. However, key outcomes of levels of self-esteem, depression, and behavioural problems remained the same as the control arm.

In Uganda, another school-based group intervention delivered to groups of chil-dren only, in the form of exercise (e.g., a game or play) over a period of 10 weeks [54]. The intervention focused on sharing experiences of being an orphan and the development of coping strategies to deal with these issues. Intervention children had significantly lower anxiety, depression, and anger than controls, but similar levels of self-esteem.

In the UK, the 'Looking Forward Day' programme was developed [49] to support young HIV+ people aged between 10 and 18 years. The intervention ran over a 10-year period and was delivered four times yearly during school holidays. Each session was a whole day event which aimed to empower participants about a range of topics, including antiretroviral therapy, experiences of being told about the diagnosis, how HIV is managed within families, sharing difficult experiences, discussion of HIV with sexual and romantic partners, and improving communication with healthcare providers. The approach was underpinned by a Narrative Therapy approach [55] in which psychological problems are considered to occur when the dominant narratives people have about themselves are pathologizing and unhelpful, and people begin to feel and think that they as individuals are a problem. The approach focuses on emphasizing and strengthening skills and giving experiences of being valued as individuals and developing communication and resilience skills. The evaluation suggested that the events were effective addressing issues that young people could not ask elsewhere. Optimism for the future improved, as did confidence in healthcare consultations.

An economic intervention tested on two different occasions in Uganda which was aimed at school age children orphaned or vulnerable because of HIV [56]. In the first study, the intervention group received usual care for orphaned children (counselling and education supplies). Additionally, a comprehensive microfinance intervention consisting of matched savings accounts, financial management classes, and an adult mentor for children was implemented over 10–12 months. Children in the intervention group had significantly better self-esteem and lower depression compared to controls at follow-up. In the second study, the same intervention was delivered, but with the addition of ten workshops focused on starting family-based income generating activities. Children in the treatment group reported significantly lower levels of hopelessness than control children as well as significantly higher scores of self-concept [57].

The evaluation of a week-long residential camp for young people with HIV (aged 16–19 years) in the UK aimed at enhancing well-being and improving HIV-related outcomes has been described by Evangeli, Lut, and Ely, 2019 [58]. At evaluation, results suggested improvements in both participants' HIV knowledge and attitudes and feelings towards discussing their HIV status with others which was maintained at 6-month follow-up. There were also improvements in antiretroviral adherence beliefs and self-perception from baseline to 6-month follow-up. The authors concluded that these beneficial changes might also mediate and promote changes in other areas of difficulty including adherence to antiretroviral therapy to reduce onward transmission of HIV.

Finally, in another study from South Africa, Sherr, Akubovich, Cluver, Skeen, Hensels, Macedo, and Tomlinson (2016) [59] compared outcomes for children attending community-based HIV programmes and those who were not, drawing data from two comparable studies. The community-based programmes differed with regard to their interventions including income generation/supplementation, emotional support, child development education, medical provision, or emergency support. The authors found that children engaged with community-based programmes were less likely to experience domestic violence, suicidal ideation, depression, stigma, peer problems, and conduct problems, and more likely to display prosocial behaviour. However, there was no difference between the groups in perceived parental praise/regard or post-traumatic stress symptoms.

In conclusion, there has been a welcome increase in the number of psychological and psychosocial randomized control trials undertaken with HIV+ children and young people which are gold standard for intervention evaluation and provide the best evidence for the effectiveness of any intervention [60]. However, such trials are usually developed specifically for research purposes only and do not have to fit into the realities of delivering care and treatment in complex and often messy real-world situations. While an intervention might be beneficial within the context of a tightly controlled trial context, it might not be easy or possible to deliver the intervention in existing healthcare contexts. In contrast, it is more difficult to evaluate the effectiveness of community-based programmes, where study methodology often needs to fit into the reality of how programmes are delivered.

Discussion Points
Do you think that outcomes such as lowered levels of depression and anxiety are the appropriate outcomes to focus on?
    Can you think of other outcomes that could be more important?
    What are the challenges of outcome measurement with children and young people?

4.7 Can the Most Effective Components of Support Programmes Be Identified?

In the preceding sections, I have presented outcomes of interventions aimed at improving parental and child coping skills to deal with the effects of HIV in their lives. What approaches, components, or interventions can be identified from these studies that are the most effective and most likely to significant increase ability to cope with the psychological effects of HIV?

Firstly, interventions that are run over a longer period of time are more likely to be effective than those that are time-limited. There are many reasons for this: it is easier to run and deliver time-limited interventions as they require fewer resources in terms of effort, planning, and staff management than longer-term interventions, so they are attractive to both organizations and staff who wish to improve functioning for people who benefit from their interventions. Evaluation of such time-limited interventions is also easier as there is a planned framework from the outset for the delivery of the programme and its evaluation. Usually, such interventions deliver only the components of the study design in contrast with long-term programmes that have multiple interventions and more complex service delivery structures. However, while acknowledging that longer-term interventions are both more difficult to deliver and evaluate, they seem to be more beneficial for participants. People's lives change, new challenges emerge and, especially with regard to families, children grow up, and their needs change. It is important that families are able to access interventions when they require them in order to meet the challenges of effective coping with HIV.

Secondly, it is important not to be too ambitious in terms of what can be delivered. Complicated interventions are more likely not to be sustainable in the real-world contexts due to staff changes, pressures on services, and funding issues. Focusing on more simple interventions probably ensures that they are more likely to be able to withstand the pressures of the healthcare context (constant change, new goals and targets, required savings). The most important component of any effective programme is the quality of the staff relationships between staff and programme beneficiaries. It is probably the single most important driver for change and underpins every successful intervention but it is rarely, if ever, evaluated within a randomized control trial framework. Positive, warm, and empowering relationships are at the core of effective interventions and the longer these relationships can be sustained, the more benefit recipients of care will likely derive.

Thirdly, interventions based on a theoretical model, approach, or framework are more likely to deliver a consistent approach which will be beneficial to participants. The underlying framework also helps guide what can and should be evaluated. However, this is easier said than done as organizations that which deliver health care are always under pressure with regard to funding, time, and resources, and it can be very difficult to take the time to consider the evaluation process. Few if any of the interventions described here addressed the impact of stigma in any meaningful way, yet stigma is a huge barrier to the uptake and maintenance of HIV treatment and care and is a factor that underpins poor mental health, poorer coping, increased use of alcohol and drugs, and poorer medical outcomes. It is surprising that in the fourth decade of HIV treatment that effective ways of addressing stigma using techniques derived from cognitive–behavioural therapy have not been a core feature of every intervention.

Lastly, the components of any successful programme are likely to be those that provide a warm and nurturing framework within which people can share HIV-related experiences in a context that is not stigmatizing and valuing of their contributions. Such a framework will allow skills transfer to occur in natural ways as people will naturally exchange ideas and experiences of how they dealt with different problems, challenges, and difficult times. Adults are more likely to benefit from this kind of approach and children and young people probably require something that is more specific. Interventions directed at young people are probably most effective when delivered through 'doing' activities, e.g., the doing of art, football, drama rather than expecting them to speaking openly and easily about difficult experiences. The sharing of experiences is an essential part of adolescent life and is the mechanism through which we have all explored identity, possibilities, dreams, and ambitions. However, it probably occurs more naturally when young people have had other shared experiences of play, sport, etc. by which trust and familiarity has been established and where there are safe boundaries to facilitate sharing.

4.8 Conclusion

There has been an increased and welcome focus on strategies to strengthen families' capacity to respond most effectively to the challenges of HIV. Advocates for a family-focused approach point to a number of reasons for this perspective: firstly, HIV infections frequently occur within the family context via sexual relationships, pregnancy, delivery, and breastfeeding. Secondly, the family is the unit in which most HIV-positive children and young people are raised and the one best placed to meet their needs—both developmentally and medically. Lastly, all members of the family (both positive and negative) are affected by the social consequences of HIV, including stigmatization, social exclusion, and discrimination. Perinatally infected HIV-positive young people are developing into adulthood and are now having children of their own and we are seeing a new generation of people and families in which there is HIV.

In this chapter, I have discussed that HIV is a family issue that requires both individual and family responses. Effective parental coping factors are very important, not only because parents need to look after themselves in order to be able to take care of those dependent on them, but also because through their own HIV-related behaviours, parents provide a model to children and young people of more effective and less effective ways of managing the disease. It is not surprising that parents who cope better and who manage the HIV stressors in their lives are better able to assist their children to mitigate the negative psychological and psychosocial effects of HIV in their lives. Conversely, children and young people who are exposed to poor parental coping will find it harder to develop effective HIV coping strategies themselves. Within this complicated context, a multi-disciplinary and multi-factorial approach is key. Early identification of families in which there are coping difficulties is essential as interventions are more likely to be successful if addressed in a timely way.

As we are now in the fourth decade of the disease, we need to ensure that families and young people are equipped as well as possible with psychological and emotional tools to manage this infection in the long term. However, it is unlikely that one off interventions will be effective in facilitating the development of effective coping strategies. If psychological interventions are to be of maximum efficacy, they need to be interwoven into the provision of medical and social care for young people and their families. There is no doubt that this is a challenge. Healthcare teams delivering HIV care in the developed world have disproportionate access to such resources and young people in resource poor settings (which is where the majority of young people with HIV live) are much less likely to be able to access sophisticated psychological interventions. However, much of the work that needs to be undertaken does not require sophisticated technology or highly trained staff. It could be argued that what is necessary is a paradigm shift for those who provide the medical care. Being aware of the likely issues that arise at different points of the life span and what are effective interventions to address the common issues that are underpinned by stigma are likely to be successful. I suggest that it is through a stance of curiosity about the ways in which HIV is managed in the lives of both individuals and their families that allows for different and transforming conversations to occur.

References

1. UNAIDS. On the fast-track to an AIDS-free generation. Geneva: UNAIDS; 2016.
2. UNAIDS. Global plan towards the elimination of new HIV infections among children by 2015 and keeping their mothers alive. Geneva: UNAIDS; 2011.
3. United Nations General Assembly. Political declaration on HIV and AIDS: on the fast track to accelerating the fight against HIV and to ending the AIDS epidemic by 2030. New York: United Nations; 2016.
4. Short SE, Goldberg RE. Children living with HIV-infected adults: estimates for 23 countries in sub-Saharan Africa. PLoS One. 2015;10(11):e0142580. https://doi.org/10.1371/journal.pone.0142580.
5. UNAIDS. Global AIDS update 2016. Geneva: UNAIDS; 2016.
6. United Nations International Children's Emergency Fund (UNICEF). UNICEF data: monitoring the situation of children and women, current status R progress. New York: UNICEF; 2018. https://data.unicef.org/topic/hivaids/protection-care-and-support-for-children-affected-by-hiv-andaids/. (Updated January 2018; Accessed 17 Nov 2020).
7. Davey MP, Duncan TM, Foster J, Milton K. Keeping the family in focus at an HIV/AIDS pediatric clinic. Fam Syst Health. 2008;26(3):350–5.
8. Wilkins R, Campbell T, Beer H. Preparing HIV-positive young people for the challenges of adult life: a group-work approach. AIDS Hepat Dig. 2007;119:1–4.
9. Stein A, Pearson RM, Goodman SH, Rapa E, Rahman A, McCallum M, Pariante CM. Effects of perinatal mental disorders on the fetus and child. Lancet. 2014;384(9956):1800–19.
10. Vreeman RC, Scanlon ML, McHenry MS, Nyandiko WM. The physical and psychological effects of HIV infection and its treatment on perinatally HIV-infected children. J Int AIDS Soc. 2015;18:20258.
11. Richter L, Sherr L. Strengthening families: a key recommendation of the Joint Learning Initiative on Children and AIDS (JLICA). AIDS Care. 2009;21(1):1–2.
12. Chi P, Li X. Impact of parental HIV/AIDS on children's psychological well-being: a systematic review of global literature. AIDS Behav. 2013;17(7):2554–74.
13. Sherr L, Mueller J. Where is the evidence base? Mental health issues surrounding bereavement and HIV in children. J Publ Ment Health. 2009;7(4):31–9.
14. Sherr L, Cluver LD, Betancourt TS, Kellerman SE, Richter LM, Desmond C. Evidence of impact: health, psychological and social effects of adult HIV on children. AIDS. 2014;28:S251–9.
15. Lee SJ, Detels R, Rotheram-Borus MJ, Duan N, Lord L. Depression and social support among HIV-affected adolescents. AIDS Patient Care STDs. 2007;21(6):409–17.
16. Murphy DA, Herbeck DM, Marelich WD, Schuster MA. Predictors of sexual behavior among early and middle adolescents affected by maternal HIV. Int J Sex Health. 2010;22(3):195–204. https://doi.org/10.1080/19317611003800614.

17. Murphy DA, Roberts KJ, Herbeck DM. Adolescent response to having an HIV-infected mother. AIDS Care. 2013;25(6):715–20. https://doi.org/10.1080/09540121.2013.769495.
18. Li L, Comulada WS, Lan CW, Lin C, Xiao Y, Ji G. Behavioral problems reported by adolescents and parents from HIV affected families in China. J Child Fam Stud. 2018;27(2):365–73. https://doi.org/10.1007/s10826-017-0906-2.
19. Campbell T, Griffiths J, Beer H, Tungana J, Bostock V, Parrett N. A group approach to facilitate family-focused coping with HIV+ African parents in London. Clin Psychol Forum. 2011;220:31–6.
20. Murphy DA, Marelich WD, Herbeck DM, Payne DL. Family routines and parental monitoring as protective factors among early and middle adolescents affected by maternal HIV/AIDS. Child Dev. 2009;80(6):1676–91.
21. Zolkoski SM, Bullock LM. Resilience in children and youth: a review. Child Youth Serv Rev. 2012;34(12):2295–303.
22. Crespo C, Santos S, Canavarro MC, Kielpikowski M, Pryor J, Féres-Carneiro T. Family routines and rituals in the context of chronic conditions: a review. Int J Psychol. 2013;48(5):729–46.
23. Dunkle KL, Stephenson R, Karita E, Chomba E, Kayitenkore K, Vwalika C, Allen S. New heterosexually transmitted HIV infections in married or cohabiting couples in urban Zambia and Rwanda: an analysis of survey and clinical data. Lancet. 2008;371(9631):2183–91.
24. Richter LM, Sherr L, Adato M, Belsey M, Chandan U, Desmond C, Madhavan S. Strengthening families to support children affected by HIV and AIDS. AIDS Care. 2009;21(supp 1):3–12.
25. Miah J, Campbell T, Fakoya A, Poulton M. Providing psychological care to families living with HIV in London's East End. AIDS Hepat Dig. 2003;95:1–2.
26. Hosegood V, Madhavan S. Data availability on men's involvement in families in sub-Saharan Africa to inform family-centred programmes for children affected by HIV and AIDS. J Int AIDS Soc. 2010;13(Suppl 2):S5. https://doi.org/10.1186/1758-2652-13-S2-S5. (need the end page of this ref)
27. Nostlinger C, Bartoli G, Gordillo V. Children and adolescents living with HIV positive parents: emotional and behavioural problems. Vulnerab Child Youth Stud. 2006;1(1):29–43.
28. Rotheram-Borus MJ, Lee MB, Murphy DA, Futterman D, Duan N, Birnbaum J. The teens linked to care consortium efficacy of a preventive interventions for youths living with HIV. Am J Public Health. 2001;91:400–5.
29. Nyandiya-Bundy S, Gatsi R, Machokoto S, Beta N, Montaño D, Kasprzyk D. TALC TO PIP: the adaptation of TALC for Zimbabwe. Gaborone, Botswana: AIDS Impact Conference; 2009.
30. Leeper SC, Montague BT, Friedman JF, Flanigan TP. Lessons learned from family-centred models of treatment for children living with HIV: current approaches and future directions. J Int AIDS Soc. 2010;13(Suppl 2):S3. https://doi.org/10.1186/1758-2652-13-S2-S3. (need the end page of this ref)
31. Chesney MA, Chambers DB, Taylor JM, Johnson LM, Folkman S. Coping effectiveness training for men living with HIV: results from a randomized clinical trial testing a group-based intervention. Psychosom Med. 2003;65(6):1038–46.
32. Goffman E. Stigma: notes on the management of spoiled identity. New York: Simon and Schuster; 2009.
33. Swendeman D, Rotheram-Borus MJ, Comulada S, Weiss R, Ramos ME. Predictors of HIV-related stigma among young people living with HIV. Health Psychol. 2006;25(4):501.
34. Campbell T. The seemingly intractable problem of HIV-related stigma. In: Croston M, Rutter S, editors. Psychological perspectives in HIV care: an inter-professional approach. London: Routledge; 2020.
35. Logie C, Gadalla TM. Meta-analysis of health and demographic correlates of stigma toward people living with HIV. AIDS Care. 2009;21(6):742–53.
36. Dlamini PS, Wantland D, Makoae LN, Chirwa M, Kohi TW, Greeff M, Holzemer WL. HIV stigma and missed medications in HIV-positive people in five African countries. AIDS Patient Care STDS. 2009;23(5):377–87.

37. Martinez J, Harper G, Carleton RA, Hosek S, Bojan K, Glum G, Ellen J. The impact of stigma on medication adherence among HIV-positive adolescent and young adult females and the moderating effects of coping and satisfaction with health care. AIDS Patient Care STDS. 2012;26(2):108–15.
38. Kim S-H, Gerver SM, Fidler S, Ward H. Adherence to antiretroviral therapy in adolescents living with HIV: systematic review and meta-analysis. AIDS. 2014;28(13):1945–56.
39. Campbell T, Griffiths J. "I can still be happy, I can still get my life again": psychological interventions with children, young people and families living with HIV in the United Kingdom. In: Liamputtong P, editor. Children, Young people and living with HIV/AIDS: a cross-cultural perspective. Dordrecht, Netherlands: Springer; 2016.
40. King E, De Silva M, Stein A, Patel V. Interventions for improving the psychosocial well-being of children affected by HIV and AIDS. Cochrane Database Syst Rev. 2009;2:CD006733. https://doi.org/10.1002/14651858.CD006733.pub2.
41. Bell CC, Gibbons RT, McKay MM. Building protective factors to offset sexually risky behaviors among black youths: a randomized control trial. J Natl Med Assoc. 2008;100(8):936–44.
42. Li L, Liang LJ, Ji G, Wu J, Xiao Y. Effect of a family intervention on psychological outcomes of children affected by parental HIV. AIDS Behav. 2014;18(11):2051–8.
43. Rotheram-Borus MJ, Rice E, Comulada WS, Best K, Li L. Comparisons of HIV-affected and non-HIV-affected families over time. Vulnerab Child Youth Stud. 2012;7(4):299–314. https://doi.org/10.1080/17450128.2012.713532.
44. Eloff I, Finestone M, Makin JD, Boeving-Allen A, Visser M, Ebersöhn L, Ferreira R, Sikkema KJ, Briggs-Gowan MJ, Forsyth BW. A randomized clinical trial of an intervention to promote resilience in young children of HIV-positive mothers in South Africa. AIDS (London, England). 2014;3(3):S347–57. https://doi.org/10.1097/QAD.0000000000000335.
45. Murphy DA, Armistead L, Payne DL, Marelich WD, Herbeck DM. Pilot trial of a parenting and self-care intervention for HIV-positive mothers: the IMAGE program. AIDS Care. 2017;29(1):40–8. https://doi.org/10.1080/09540121.2016.1204416.
46. Fisher JD, Fisher WA. Changing AIDS risk behaviour. Psychol Bull. 1992;111:455–74.
47. Han HR, Floyd O, Kim K, Cudjoe J, Warren N, Seal S, Sharps P. Intergenerational interventions for people living with HIV and their families: a systematic review. AIDS Behav. 2019;23(1):21–36. https://doi.org/10.1007/s10461-018-2223-1.
48. Thurman TR, Jarabi B, Rice J. Caring for the caregiver: evaluation of support groups for guardians of orphans and vulnerable children in Kenya. AIDS Care. 2012;24(7):811–9.
49. Campbell T, Beer H, Wilkins R. The looking forward day: an evaluation of group work with HIV+ young people in London. Clin Psychol Forum. 2010;205:26–30.
50. Gore-Felton C, Rotheram-Borus MJ, Weinhardt LS, Kelly JA, Lightfoot M, Kirschenbaum SB. The healthy living project: an individually tailored, multidimensional intervention for HIV-infected persons. AIDS Educ Prev. 2005;17(Suppl A):21–39.
51. Carlson M, Brennan RT, Earls F. Enhancing adolescent self-efficacy and collective efficacy through public engagement around HIV/AIDS competence: a multilevel, cluster randomized-controlled trial. Soc Sci Med. 2012;75(6):1078–87.
52. Balfour L, Farrar T, McGilvray M, Wilson D, Tasca GA, Spaans JN, Cameron WD. HIV prevention in action on the football field: the WhizzKids United program in South Africa. AIDS Behav. 2013;17(6):2045–52.
53. Mueller J, Alie C, Jonas B, Brown E, Sherr L. A quasi-experimental evaluation of a community-based art therapy intervention exploring the psychosocial health of children affected by HIV in South Africa. Tropical Med Int Health. 2011;16(1):57–66.
54. Kumakech E, Cantor-Graae E, Maling S, Bajunirwe F. Peer-group support intervention improves the psychosocial well-being of AIDS orphans: cluster randomized trial. Soc Sci Med. 2009;68(6):1038–43.
55. White M. Narrative practice and exotic lives: resurrecting diversity in everyday life. Adelaide: Dulwich Centre Publications; 2004.

56. Ssewamala FM, Neilands TB, Waldfogel J, Ismayilova L. The impact of a comprehensive microfinance intervention on depression levels of AIDS-orphaned children in Uganda. J Adolesc Health. 2012;50(4):346–52.
57. Ssewamala FM, Karimli L, Torsten N, Wang JSH, Han CK, Ilic V, Nabunya P. Applying a family-level economic strengthening intervention to improve education and health-related outcomes of school-going AIDS-orphaned children: lessons from a randomized experiment in Southern Uganda. Prev Sci. 2016;17(1):134–43.
58. Evangeli M, Lut I, Ely A. A longitudinal evaluation of an intensive residential intervention (camp) for 12–16-year olds living with HIV in the UK: evidence of psychological change maintained at six-month follow-up. AIDS Care. 2019;31(1):85–9.
59. Sherr L, Yakubovich AR, Cluver LD, Skeen S, Hensels IS, Macedo A, Tomlinson M. How effective is help on the doorstep? A longitudinal study of the impact of community-based organisation support on child behaviour and mental health. PLoS One. 2016;11(3):e0151305.
60. Skeen SA, Sherr L, Croome N, Gandhi N, Roberts KJ, Macedo A, Tomlinson M. Interventions to improve psychosocial well-being for children affected by HIV and AIDS: a systematic review. Vulnerab Child Youth Stud. 2017;12(2):91–116.

Chapter 5
Advancing the Role of the Nurse: Sexual Health for People Living with HIV

Matthew Grundy-Bowers

5.1 Defining Sexual Health

Sexual health is broader than the 'physical' of sexually transmitted infections (STIs) or contraception [1, 2], as it encompasses many things including unintended pregnancy and abortion, infertility, sexually transmitted cancers, and sexual dysfunction. As such, it is influenced by a wide range of factors including behaviour, attitude, society, biology, genetics [2], and importantly politics [1]. Furthermore, as highlighted by Starr and Anderson (2016: 7) [1] *'operates on multiple levels—individual, relational, familial, and community'*. While not a formal definition, the World Health Organisation statement on sexual health has provided an enduring overview:

> A state of physical, emotional, mental and social well-being related to sexuality; not merely the absence of disease, dysfunction or infirmity. Sexual health requires a positive and respectful approach to sexuality and sexual relationships, as well as the possibility of having pleasurable and safe sexual experiences, free of coercion, discrimination and violence. For sexual health to be attained and maintained, the sexual rights of all persons must be protected, respected and fulfilled
>
> (WHO, 2002) [2]

M. Grundy-Bowers (✉)
Imperial College NHS Trust, London, UK
e-mail: matthew.grundybowers@nhs.net

5.1.1 Reflection Point

Take some time to consider what sexual health means to you? What are the stories/images/messages about sex you have receive from your culture?

- How do these relate to gender?
- To relationships?
- To sexual knowledge and contraceptive use?
- To responsibility?
- How have these changed over time?

5.1.2 Sexual Health and People Living with HIV

Given the intersecting breadth and levels of sexual health, it is useful to consider how sexual health affects people living with HIV. PLWH are disproportionally affected by STIs [3], particularly gay, bisexual, and other men who have sex with men (GBMSM) [4]. Compared to their HIV-negative counterparts, women living with HIV (WLWHIV) are significantly less likely to use prescribed contraception such as long-acting reversable contraception (LARC) or short-acting hormonal methods [5] and have high levels of unintended pregnancy [6]. In addition, sexual dysfunction is common among both HIV-positive men and women [7, 8]. Furthermore, a significant number of HIV-positive GBMSM engage in sexualised drug use also known as 'chemsex', a portion of which also engage in sexualised injection drug use (IDU) or 'slamming' [9]. All of which can negatively impact on the health and well-being of people living with HIV.

5.1.3 Impact of Poor Sexual Health

The effects of poor sexual health can detrimentally impact people living with HIV physical, emotional, and psychological well-being. For instance, although the management of the majority of STIs are the same as for those who do not have HIV [10], there are nuanced differences, especially in the relationship between STIs and HIV which are both complex and bidirectional [11]. An example of this can be seen in the epidemiological synergy between Herpes Simplex Virus (HSV) a common STI in people living with HIV [12]. Having HSV-2 not only increases the risk of acquiring HIV [13], but also activates HIV viral replication [12]. PLWH may experience extensive, prolonged, repeated, or severe episodes of genital herpes and resistance to HSV treatment is more common [14] and the initiation of HIV anti-retroviral treatment can temporarily increase HSV viral shedding [15]. Both HSV and HIV are also associated with stigma and shame [13, 15], which can increase isolation and depression, and be linked to risk behaviours [10] leading people living with HIV to avoid forming new sexual relationships or, if they are in a relationship avoid having sex [16].

5.1.4 The Role of the ACP (HIV)

Given the significant impact of poor sexual health on people living with HIV, it would be useful to examine the pivotal role of the ACP (HIV) in relation to sexual health. NHIVNA (2013) [17] suggest that ACPs should demonstrate an understanding of the issues relating to the sexual health needs of people living with HIV, especially in relation to:

- Cultural and belief issues.
- Confidentiality.
- Routine screening.
- Women's and men's health issues.
- Preconception advice.
- Health promotion.

Even those with little or no sexual health experience have transferable skills (e.g., advanced communication), knowledge (e.g., the impact of stigma on health and well-being, behaviour change interventions), and behaviours (e.g., empathy and being non-judgemental) which they can build upon. These can be used to create a safe, non-judgemental relationship with their patients, supporting them where necessary with advice, signposting, and behaviour change interventions. In addition, ACPs can (with appropriate training) undertake detailed sexual health histories and risk assessments, develop action plans and make onward referrals, working with key statutory and non-statutory providers, especially around risk reduction [10, 17].

5.1.5 Activity

Spend 5 min finding the answers to these questions:

- Where could I find further information, training with regard to sexual health within my area?
- What national websites could I access for more information to support my learning.

5.1.6 STIs

This next section provides an overview of the common sexually transmitted infections. It is essential however, that ACP refer to the most recent versions of the national guidelines for the management of STIs which can be found on the British Association for Sexual Health & HIV (BASHH) website. This is especially pertinent in relation to treatments, as these change in light of resistance patterns. In 2020, there was a 5% increase in STIs, disproportionately affecting young people, GBMSM, and people from BME backgrounds [18].

5.1.7   Gonorrhoea

Gonorrhoea (*Neisseria gonorrhoeae*) is a bacterial infection, which is highly infectious. It is transmitted through direct contact of the discharge from one mucus membrane to the other (normally sexual contact, but can be passed vertically), and the incubation period is 2–5 days [19]. Symptoms depend on the site of infection, in penile urethral infections it causes a purulent discharge and dysuria, while infection of the endocervix it causes a change in vaginal discharge, and lower abdominal pain [20]. Infection in the rectum it is often asymptomatic, but can cause discharge and discomfort/pain, and pharyngeal infection occasionally causes a sore throat, but is generally asymptomatic [19]. Diagnosis is made in three ways: (1) a swab or first catch urine sample which is tested using nucleic acid amplification tests (NAATs); (2) a swab which is cultured; or (3) via Gram's stain microscopy [20].

The management is the same for HIV-positive and HIV-negative patients [20]. All patients with a positive NAATs test or Gram's stain microscopy should also have cultures taken before they are treated. Treatment is normally with a cephalosporin, or spectinomycin for those with a penicillin allergy [20]. Patients should be advised to avoid sexual contact for 7 days after treatment (and until 7 days after any sexual partner has been treated) and should have a test-of-cure to ensure the infection is resolved [20]. Partner notification of all partners in the 2 weeks prior to the onset of symptoms, and 3 months in asymptomatic patients is required [20, 21]. Complications include disseminated gonorrhoea, pelvic inflammatory disease (PID), epididymo-orchitis (EO), and conjunctivitis [19].

5.2   Chlamydia and Lymphogranuloma Venereum (LGV)

Chlamydia (*Chlamydia trachomatis*) is a common bacterial infection, serotypes D-K cause genital infection, while types L1–3 cause LGV [19]. It is transmitted primarily through condomless penetrative sex (although can be passed vertically) and the incubation period is between 7 and 21 days [22]. Most individuals with chlamydia are asymptomatic (especially infections in the pharynx and rectum), infections in the penile urethra can cause discharge and dysuria, infections in the endocervix can cause increased vaginal discharge, post-coital and intermenstrual bleeding, lower abdominal pain, and dyspareunia. Infection in the rectum can cause discharge and discomfort/pain, while infections in the eye can cause conjunctivitis [19]. LGV is generally an infection associated with HIV-positive GBMSM and causes rectal discharge, discomfort/pain, tenesmus, and diarrhoea/altered bowel habit [23]. Diagnosis is made using a swab or first catch urine sample which is tested using nucleic acid amplification tests (NAATs), in HIV-positive GBMSM rectal swabs (especially in symptomatic patients) should be tested for LGV if their initial chlamydia test is positive [22].

The management is generally the same for HIV-positive and HIV-negative patients. Treatment is normally with a tetracycline or macrolide [22]. HIV-positive patients with rectal infection should be tested for Lymphogranuloma Venereum (LGV), in the absence of testing should be treated empirically for LGV (normally 3 weeks) [22]. Patients should be advised to avoid sexual contact until they have completed their treatment (at least 7 days if given a shorter treatment) and until 7 days after any sexual partner has been treated [22]. Patients do not routinely require a test-of-cure, unless they are pregnant, have rectal infection, continue to be symptomatic, or if there are issues of compliance [22, 24]. Partner notification of male patients with urethral symptom of all partners in the 4 weeks prior to the onset of symptoms, and 6 months in all other cases is required [22]. Complications include PID, EO, sexually acquired reactive arthritis (SARA), ectopic pregnancy, tubal infertility, and perihepatitis [19].

5.2.1 Syphilis

Syphilis (*Treponema pallidum*) is a bacterial infection, which is common among GBMSM, especially those living with HIV [18]. It is transmitted through direct contact with a lesion (such as a sore or rash) or vertically [19]. The incubation period is 9–90 days (normally 21 days), with symptoms depending on the stage of the disease [19].

5.2.2 Primary Syphilis

Primary infection typically causes a single, painless, indurated ulcer (chancre) at the site of entry (normally ano-genital) which resolve after 3–8 weeks, and lymphadenopathy [19]. In PLWH, there may be multiple ulcers, which last longer (into the secondary stage), and are deeper and painful [25].

5.2.3 Secondary Syphilis

Secondary syphilis occurs in approximately one-fourth of untreated patients which occurs 3 months after the initial symptoms [19]. Typically, patients have a macular/popular rash, the rash is normally on the trunk, but can also be found on the soles of the feet and palm of the hands [19]. In addition, patients can have patchy hair loss, mucosal ulceration in the mouth (snail track ulceration), and wart-like lesions of the perineum and anus (*condylomata lata*) which are highly infectious [25]. More serious symptoms include neurological symptoms, hearing loss/tinnitus, and uveitis [19].

5.2.4 Latent Syphilis

The symptoms of secondary syphilis would normally resolve after 3/12, and they would then enter a period of latency, where they are asymptomatic [19]. This latency is divided between early (up to 2 years) and late (after 2 years) [25].

5.2.5 Late Latent Syphilis (Tertiary)

Late or tertiary disease occurs between 20 and 40 years after initial infection in approximated one-third of untreated patients [25]. Symptoms include necrosis of the skin and bone (*gummatous syphilis*), dilatation and regurgitation of the aorta (*cardiovascular syphilis*), and stroke, general paresis, and tabes dorsalis (*neurological syphilis*) [19].

Diagnosis is made on clinical history, examination, and laboratory investigations. Lesions can be sampled for dark field microscopy or multiplex PCR testing [25]. Blood tests 'Serological tests for Syphilis' (STS) are divided into specific screening tests:

- Treponemal enzyme immunoassay (EIA) or Treponema pallidum particle agglutination assay (TPPA)/Treponema pallidum haemagglutination assay (TPHA).

  Non-specific which are undertake if the initial screen test is positive:

- Venereal Diseases Research Laboratory (VDRL) or rapid plasma regain (RPR) and are also used to monitor treatment effect.

Confirmatory testing should be performed on patients with a positive result as false negatives and positive tests can occur, and these results can be difficult to interpret so senior advice is essential, especially when reinfection is suspected [25].

Management is similar for people living with HIV and those without HIV; however, HIV-patients presenting with neurological symptoms should be investigated for neurosyphilis examination of Cerebrospinal Fluid (CSF) [25]. Treatment is normally penicillin injections or oral doxycycline, with longer treatment in late syphilis. Some of the treatments are unlicensed, so this should be clearly documented in the patient's records, and reactions to treatment can occur so this should be clearly explained to patients [25]. Patients should avoid sex for the duration of treatment (and until any lesions have healed). Patients should have extended follow-up serology (minimum 12 months), especially if non-penicillin treatments are administered [25]. Partner notification should be 3 months prior to initial symptoms in primary syphilis, extended to 2 years in secondary syphilis [25].

5.2.6 Genital Warts

Genital warts are caused by the human papilloma virus (HPV), typically genotypes 6 and 11 which are classed as low-risk types which can cause ano-genital warts, and high-risk genotypes such as 16 and 18 can cause pre-cancerous skin changes and lesions [19]. Transmission is through skin-to-skin contact of the ano-genital tract; however, genital HPV can also be detected in the oral cavity [26]. The incubation periods range from 3 weeks to 8 months but can be much longer and symptom are lesions which occur in the ano-genital area (penis, meatus, vulva, vagina, cervix, perianal, anus, rectum) which can be single or multiple [19]. Diagnosis is made on clinical examination; however, biopsies may be required where lesions are persistent, or for unusual looking skin/lesions to exclude intraepithelial neoplasia [26].

Management for people living with HIV is the same as HIV-negative individuals and depends on the type, distribution and number of warts, and the patient's preference. Treatments include topical applications and physical ablation; it should be noted that some treatments are contraindicated in pregnancy [26]. Partner notification may be of benefit for current partner (to exclude undiagnosed infection) but is not required for previous partners [26]. People living with HIV may experience more persistent infection or more likely to have recurrent episodes [19].

5.2.7 Herpes Simplex Virus

Herpes is a common viral infection which is caused by the herpes simplex virus (types 1 or 2) and transmitted through skin-to-skin contact, normally ano-genital to ano-genital, or oral to ano-genital (although other sites can be affected) [19]. The incubation period is 2 days to 2 weeks, however only one-third of individuals will develop symptoms at acquisition [12]. Symptoms include painful blisters which lead to ulceration, dysuria, discharge, fever, myalgia, and symptoms of proctitis (which is more common in HIV-positive GBMSM). Symptoms can be significantly more aggressive and frequent in people living with HIV (especially those not on treatment) and lead to systemic complications (e.g., neurological disease, fulminant hepatitis, disseminated infection, and pneumonia) [12]. Diagnosis is made on clinical observation and confirmed on HSV NAAT swabs taken from the lesion [12].

Management depends on whether this is an initial or recurrent episode. Salt water bathing, over the counter analgesia, topical analgesia, and antiviral medication if initiated within 5 days of the start of symptoms (unless there are new or persistent lesions), while serve infections may require IV antiviral therapy [12]. As recurrences are self-limiting, the patient can self-manage with SWB, petroleum jelly, topical analgesia, and OTC analgesia, or can be treated with oral antiviral medication taken episodically or suppressively [12]. Patients should avoid sexual contact for the duration of symptoms, and partner notification can be useful [12]. As the diagnosis of herpes can be very distressing, patients may require extra support. Detailed information should be provided to the patient about the infection, recurrences, self-management, and treatment [12]. In addition, the risk of transmission, condom use, and disclosure should also be discussed and documented [12]. Complications can include superinfection of lesions, autonomic neuropathy, and aseptic meningitis [19].

5.2.8 Reflection Point

With regard to sexually transmitted infections consider what health promotion advise you would give to someone who has received a diagnosis of one of the above infections.

5.2.9 Contraception

Having considered the common STIs, this next section now provides an overview of the main contraceptive methods for women living with HIV. For women living with HIV planning and preventing pregnancy is very important for women without HIV (see Chap. 5 for more information about women's health) [10]. Most methods of contraception can be used by women living with HIV although special consideration is required if the women is on treatment; this includes potential pill burdens [10]. Long-acting reversable contraception (LARC) should be discussed with women, as these provide more effective, long-term contraception.

As with the previous section, it is important to refer to the most up-to-date national guidelines, which can be found on the Faculty of Sexual and Reproductive Healthcare (FSRH) website. In addition to the guidelines, the website has the UK medical eligibility criteria for contraceptive use known as the UKMEC. Developed by the FSRH clinical effectiveness unit (CEU) the UKMEC provides an evidence-based guide for clinicians for which contraceptives can be prescribed safely for their patients, based on their medical conditions (Table 5.1).

Table 5.1 Definition of UKMEC categories (adapted from FSRH 2016:2 [27])

UKMEC	Category 1	Category 2	Category 3[a]	Category 4
Definition of category	A condition for which there is no restriction for the use of the method	A condition where the advantages of using the method generally outweigh the theoretical or proven risks	A condition where the theoretical or proven risks usually outweigh the advantages of using the method	A condition which represents an unacceptable health risk if the method is used

[a]The provision of a method requires expert clinical judgement and/or referral to a specialist contraceptive provider since use of the method is not usually recommended unless other more appropriate methods are not available or not acceptable

Contraceptives can be broken down into 'hormonal' and 'non-hormonal' methods.

5.2.10 Non-hormonal Methods

5.2.10.1 Barrier Methods

Barrier methods provide a barrier between the ejaculate and cervico-vaginal secretions and include the male and female condoms, diaphragms, and cervical caps. Diaphragms and cervical caps are a UKMEC 3 for women living with HIV (the risk of use outweighs the benefit), therefore will not be discussed [27]. Condoms if used correctly are between 98% (male condom) and 95% (female condom) effective are only used at the time of sex non-hormonal, easily available, and have no side effects (for most) [28]. Condoms also have the additional benefit of offing protection against STIs and be used with sex toys, especially if they are shared between partners [28]. They also come in latex and non-latex varieties, and a range of sizes, colours, flavours, thicknesses, and textures (e.g., ribbed, dotted).

Caution is required to prevent condom breakages and slippages, such as sharp objects (e.g., finger nails), sex lasting longer the 30 min, and ill-fitting condoms (slippages); however, the thickness of the condom doesn't affect condom breakages [28]. Additional lubrication (not nonoxynol-9 as this irritates the genital epithelium, increasing the risk of lesions) can prevent breakages, however may be associated with slippages [29]. In addition, oil-based lubricants should be avoided with latex condoms as this may damage them, and caution should be used if the patient is using/prescribed vaginal/topical preparations as these can also damage latex condoms [29]. Condoms should be replaced if the sex lasts longer the 30 min or if moving from the anus to the vagina [28].

5.2.10.2 Intrauterine Device

The intrauterine device (IUD) also known as the 'coil' is a highly effective, non-hormonal, long-acting contraceptive method. It is a small, T-shaped plastic device with copper on the body and arms, which depending on the device lasts for 5–10 years [29]. As well as being an LARC, the IUD is also the most effective emergency contraceptive method [30]. The mode of action is the copper is toxic to sperm and ovum, and the subsequent change in copper content of the cervical mucus, prevents sperm penetration, while an inflammatory action has an anti-implantation effect [29].

Following insertion, the device is effective immediately, and if used as EC, can be then used as an ongoing method [30]. As well as being non-hormonal, and long-acting other benefits of the IUD include reduced risk of endometrial and cervical cancer [31]. One of the drawbacks of the method is that it requires a procedure, which is invasive and can be uncomfortable. Other side effects and complications include longer and more painful periods, the risk of ectopic pregnancy (reduced risk overall, however if the woman does fall pregnancy 50:50 of ectopic pregnancy), expulsion (1:20), perforation (2:1000, higher if breastfeeding), and infection [31].

5.2.11 Hormonal Methods

5.2.11.1 Progestogen

Hormonal methods all contain a synthetic form of progesterone (progestogen), which is a steroid hormone is released by the ovaries and influences the menstrual cycle and pregnancy [29]. The two main modes of action for progestogens are thickening the cervical mucus to form a 'plug' at the endocervix which prevents the sperm from penetrating the uterus (and thus reaching the ovum), or suppressing ovulation (to varying effect) [29]. Other effects include changes to the endometrium which prevent implantation and slowing of the ovum from the ovaries by reducing the activity of the cilia in the fallopian tubes. Common side effects associated with progestogens are skin changes, changes in mood, decreased libido, breast tenderness, headache, nausea, and irregular bleeding/amenorrhoea [29]. The main risk associated with progestogens are ovarian cysts; however, these will often be resolved without treatments, and the link between progestogens and breast cancer is still being researched but is thought to be low [32].

Progestogens can be delivered in several ways:

Short-acting contraception

- Oral (progestogen-only pill): self-administered daily, 99% effective (if taken correctly) [32].

  Long-acting reversable contraception

- Intramuscularly (Depo-Provera): administer every 13 weeks, 99% effective [33].
- Subcutaneously (Sanya Press): self-administered every 13 weeks, 99% effective [34].
- Subdermal (Nexplanon): inserted 3 yearly, 99% effective [35].
- Intrauterine (intrauterine system or IUS): inserted 3–5 yearly [31] 99% effective [31].

5.2.12 Oestrogen

Some hormonal methods also contain a synthetic form of oestrogen (estrogen), which like progesterone is a steroid hormone released from the ovaries and influences the menstrual cycle [29]. Contraceptively, oestrogen works with progestogen to suppress ovulation [29]. Common side effects of oestrogen are oedema, weight gain, premenstrual stress, and nausea [36]. There are several risks associated with oestrogen including deep vein thrombosis, pulmonary embolus, cerebrovascular accident, and increase the risk of breast and cervical cancer [36].

Estrogens (in combination with progestogens) can be delivered in several ways: Short-acting contraception

- Oral (combined oral pill): self-administered, daily for 21, with a 7-day break* [36].
- Transdermal (combined transdermal patch (CTP)): self-administered, renewed each week for 3 weeks, then 7-day break* [36].
- Vaginal (combined vaginal ring (CVR)): left in place continuously 21 days, then 7-day break* [36].

*Tailored regimens include: extended use (tricycling) for 9 weeks (3 × 21 tablets, 9 patches, or 3 rings), flexible extended use (continuous until breakthrough bleed occurs), or continuous use, and shortened hormone-free intervals (4 days) [36].

5.2.13   Emergency Contraception

Emergency contraception (EC) is used to reduce the risk of conception where there has been condomless sex, or a contraceptive failure such as a condom break, or missed pill [29]. EC comes in two forms; oral levonorgestrel (LNG-EC) or ulipristal (UPA-EC) and the IUD (discussed previously). Intrauterine devices (IUDs) are not only the most effective method of emergency contraception [30] can be used with all ART regimens [10]. The mode of action of oral methods delay ovulation; this means that oral methods are only effective prior to ovulation. Whereas the IUD has both pre- and post-fertilisation modes of action work by delaying preventing fertilisation or preventing implantation, which means that it can be used post-ovulatory [30].

Although known colloquially as 'the morning after pill' oral EC can be taken up to 72 h (levonorgestrel) or 120 h (ulipristal), and the IUD can be inserted up to 120 h after condomless sex, or within 120 h of the earliest estimated date of ovulation [29]. The most effective EC is the IUD, while ulipristal is more effective than levonorgestrel [30]. In women who are overweight (>70 kgs/BMI > 26) oral EC is potentially less effective and should be offered IUD-EC. If IUD-EC is not appropriate/acceptable, then they should be offered UPA-EC or a double dose of LNG-EC (3 mg instead of 1.5 mg) [30].

5.3   Drug–Drug Interactions

5.3.1   Interactions

It is important to assess not only ARTs, but also other medications that the women may be on, for example, antibiotics, anti-epileptics, or antidepressants as these too can interact [30]. Some methods such as injectable contraceptive (e.g., depo-provera, sanya press) and the intrauterine systems (e.g., Mirena, Levosert) can be used with all ART regimens, however because generally hormonal methods are metabolised via cytochrome P450, ARTs which induce or inhibit this may produce drug–drug interactions [10]. Also, as of some of the contraceptives might need to be used outside of their product licence this should be discussed and documented in their notes [10].

This is also true for emergency contraception, drug–drug interactions with some ARTs mean that Upristal should be avoided with enzyme inducers such as efavirenz, while levonorgestrel can be used with a double dose, although its effectiveness is unknown [10]. In addition, UPA-EC is a progesterone receptor modulator, which means it may be less effective if progestogen is taken 7 days prior or 5-days after administration. In this situation women should be offered LNG-EC or IUD-EC [30]. As discussed previously IUDs can be used with all ART regimens [10].

5.3.2   Sexual Dysfunction

An individual's sexual functioning changes over time, however, sexual dysfunction (SD) is common in the general population around 50% of men [37], and 40–50% of women will experience SD in their lifetime [38]. As with other chronic health conditions, HIV is associated with impaired sexual functioning [16] and is common in patients receiving ARTs (in particular PI) [39]. Furthermore, conditions which are also associated with SD (such as mental health issues and substance use) are also more common in people living with HIV [16], as is stigma [40]. The impact of HIV on sexual functioning: Considerations for clinicians. Psychotherapy. This means that over half of people living with HIV will experience SD [41]. SD has a significant impact on quality of life [41], relationships, and forming relationships. Furthermore, SD can also be a marker for other health conditions such as diabetes and cardiovascular disease, as well as being linked to lower adherence to treatment. [41].

5.3.3   Female Sexual Dysfunction

There are a range of SD conditions which affect women. The most common is dyspareunia (painful intercourse) with an estimate three-fourth of women experiencing this in the lifetime [42]. There are a range of potential causes including psychological problems or stress, history of non-consensual sex, dermatosis, or gynaecological conditions.

Hypoactive sexual desire disorder (HSDD) or low sexual desire affects around 40% of women in their lifetime [43]. There are a large number of possible causes for LSD including medications, recreational drugs, medical condictiones (such as hypertension), life changes (pregnancy, care commitments), surgery (breast or genital tract), hormonal changes (e.g., during menopause), and other SD such as dyspareunia.

Anorgasmia (difficulty in reaching orgasm or sexual climax) affects at least 20% of women and can be primary (never having reached orgasm), secondary (previously reaching orgasm, then not being able to), situational (happening in certain sexual encounters or with particular partners), or general [44, 45]. Physical causes include medical problems, medications or substance use, psychological causes include performance anxiety, stress, cultural/religious beliefs; however, other causes include relationship issues such as unresolved conflict, lack of connection, breaches in trust. These conditions are however are often intertwined, for example, a lack of desire, arousal, or both can lead to dyspareunia.

5.3.4 Male Sexual Dysfunction

Erectile dysfunction is one of the most common (and probably most well-known) SD in men affecting up to 75% at some point in their life [46]. It can be the sign of underlying organic disease such as hypertension, diabetes, benign prostatic hyperplasia, and ischemic heart disease [46]. Causes of ED can be physical such as neurological disease, atherosclerosis, hepatic disease, and substance use, while psychological causes include performance anxiety, altered body image (e.g., lipoatrophy), relationship issues, and stress.

Ejaculatory issues such as premature ejaculation are also common, affecting between 20% and 30% of men [47] and similar to anorgasmia in women can be lifelong (always had), acquired (previously having no problems, then occurring), or variable (happening in particular situations or with some partners) [48]. Causes can be organic (e.g., neurological, vascular disease, pelvic injury, or surgery) or psychogenic (e.g., anxiety/stress, poor body image, performance anxiety).

Hypoactive sexual desire disorder is also common in men, with around 15% of men reporting HSDD [49]. Again, like other SD has a range of potential causes including other sexual problems (e.g., ED), medications (e.g., antidepressants, antihypertensives, analgesics), recreational drugs (including alcohol), medical conditions (diabetes, coronary artery disease, hypertension), previous genital surgery, lifestyle changes, relationship issues, and body building.

5.3.5 Management

Following identification/disclosure of SD reassurance should be given that it is common and can in most cases be treated [50]. The ACP should explore the patient's expectations and desire for treatment and make an onward referral for further specialist investigation and treatment as per local pathways. SD can have a physiological and/or psychological basis, and these factors can be interlinked. The type and cause of the SD will influence the treatment options, and multiple interventions may be required. Common treatments include sexual education, counselling (both individual and couples), lifestyle changes (such as exercise [including pelvic floor], weight loss, smoking cessation, reduction in drugs and alcohol), relationship changes (e.g., protected time for intimacy, improved communication), and interventions to manage stress [50]. In addition to these, there are also pharmacological and surgical interventions. The management of SD can however take time, and some of the interventions may not be acceptable for some patients. For example, some interventions require the patient to masturbate, which can be unacceptable for some patients of faith, while others involve talking therapies, which some patient may not wish to engage in.

5.3.6   Sexualised Drug Use

Sexualised drug use (SDU), 'chemsex', or 'Party and Play' (PnP) is using particular recreational drugs prior to, or during sex [51, 52]. These substances are used as a social lubricant to enhance sex and maximise sexual experiences, as a self-treatment for negative affective states or to escape from reality, or for their disinhibitory effect [53–56]. SDU is associated with increased risk of STI, addiction, and mental health issues [57]. It is estimated that around 30% of HIV-positive GBMSM engage in SDU and around 10% engage in sexualised injection drug use (SIDU) [58].

5.3.7   Drugs Associated with SDU

Individuals have used drugs with sex for millennia [51], however within the context of GBMSM and SDU the substances taken have evolved since the 1990s [59]. While almost any drug can be used in the context of sex, the drugs specifically associated with SDU are crystal methamphetamine ('crystal', 'tina'), gamma-Hydroxybutyric acid ('GHB')/gamma-butyrolactone ('GBL'), and methylmethcathinone ('mephedrone') [51]. The substances can be taken via nasal insufflation 'snorting' (mephedrone, crystal), orally 'bomb' (mephedrone, GHB/GBL), smoked (crystal), injection 'slamming' (crystal, mephedrone), or rectally 'bootybump' (crystal, mephedrone, GHB/GBL).

Polypharmacy is common as these substances are often taken in combination to achieve the desired effects which include increased euphoria, increased libido, being sexually adventurous, increased confidence, and able to have sex over a long duration [57]. In addition to taking the drugs associated with SDU, individuals may also take other substances either before (e.g., alcohol or the more traditional 'party drugs' such as 3,4-methylenedioxymethamphetamine [MDMA/ecstasy] and cocaine), during (e.g., alkyl nitrite or sildenafil), or after to help with the 'come down' (e.g., alcohol, cannabis, MDMA, or prescription drugs such as Alprazolam [Zanax]).

SDU or chemsex sessions can be characterised by their duration with sessions lasting for days. They can be between two partners or more (threesome, foursomes, group sex), with partners remaining at the same organised event, or with partners coming and going over a weekend. Location-based dating apps such as 'Grindr' are often used to seek out potential partners. The drugs are often used in a facilitative way to enable the type of sex that individuals want, which is why SDU is often associated with more adventurous sexual practices such as the use of sex toys, fisting, bondage, domination, and sado-masochism.

While some patients report no problems associated with their SDU, it can have a significant impact on health and well-being. Physically, it can cause weight, oral, cardiovascular, hepatic, renal issues, injection site problems such as phlebitis. In addition, GHB/GBL in particular causes serious physical problems such as collapse as the therapeutic range is narrow and the medication builds up over time, and it also can cause convulsions if stopped abruptly. Overdose, especially associated with GHB/GBL can also lead to collapse and death [60]. Mentally, drugs such as crystal and GHB/GBL are highly addictive. More distressingly, one of the common side effects of crystal is that paranoia and psychosis, which is compounded by with lack of sleep.

Furthermore, SDU doesn't just affect the individuals who partake, it can have a much wider psychosocial impact. For example, SDU can affect relationships with family and friends as individuals become withdrawn, or put participating in chemsex over other commitments [59]. There are financial implications too, buying drugs can be expensive [61], and poor performance or absenteeism from work because of SDU can lead to termination of employment [59]. Another issue within the SDU context is that intoxication can create a blurred line in relation to consent [62], and some individuals intentionally overdose their partners in order to sexually assault them.

Supporting patients engaging in SDU requires the practitioners to non-judgemental, as patients will often feel stigmatised by their behaviours. Individuals, especially those who are injecting drugs (slamming), do not fit into existing drug services. It is important to remember that patients have to be in a space where they are ready to change, if they are not, interventions are unlikely to be effective. Behaviour change intervention such as motivational interviewing can be effective in supporting patients; however, relapses are common. Some patients, especially those using GHB/GBL may require formal detoxification with an experienced professional to help patients titrate off GHB/GBL.

5.3.8 Service Provision Models

For successful integration of sexual health within the HIV clinical setting, ACPs also need to contribute strategically by leading cultural change and the development, implementation, and monitoring of local pathways for SRH care provision for

PLWH [17] that facilitates access and management of HIV-positive patients presenting with sexual health issues:

- Sexual health screening.
- Immunisation.
- Contraception.
- Assisted conception.
- Cervical screening [17].

Where ever possible service development should involve key stakeholders, including patients [17]. Sexual health is a rapidly changing speciality, and a key responsibility of an ACP is to develop consistent policies and standards. It is therefore of paramount importance for them to keep abreast with current trends, clinical guidance, research, and policy [17]. The first place to start is having a good understanding of the various legal, policy, and government initiatives that influence current sexual healthcare provision for people living with HIV. For example, people living with HIV need appropriate services to ensure their sexual and reproductive health [63], so in the UK the BHIVA standards (2017) [10] recommend that HIV out-patients services should provide the following related sexual health care:

- *Facilities for partner notification.*
- *GU/sexual health screening and services.*
- *Access to contraception and preconception care.*

(BHIVA, 2017:5 [10])

Promoting and protecting sexual health for people living with HIV is not just talking about condoms and safer sex but incorporates a range of strategies. These include:

- Sexual health histories and risk assessment review at all routine appointments [10],
- Hepatitis A & B vaccinations [64, 65],
- And where appropriate HPV vaccination [65, 66],
- Asymptomatic STI screening (including hepatitis and syphilis) annually if partner change since previous visit, every 3 months for higher risk patients (MSM and frequent partner change, substance use, especially injection drug use, commercial sex workers, those engaging in 'chemsex', young people, and those with chaotic lifestyles [67],
- Annual cervical cytology [10, 67],
- Although unproven annual anal cytology [65].

In addition to the above, discussions about safer drug use; conception and contraception; diagnosis and treatment of sexual dysfunction and access to PEPSE and PrEP for sexual partners [10]. There are a number of ways that SRH can be provided within the HIV clinical setting, wherever possible this should be with minimal input as much as possible to have single points of access [10, 17]. This next section will explore some of the ways that this can be achieved.

5.3.9 Asymptomatic STI Screening

All clinical staff working in HIV services should encourage and promote regular health checks and screening as appropriate. Patients should be offered a full sexual health assessment at diagnoses (if not already had one), then a review of their sexual histories at every routine visit, and offered an annual sexual health screen (if partner change since previous visit) which should be documented in their notes [10]. And ACPs should proactively discuss sexual health with their patients (and where ever possible encourage the incorporation of discussions about sexual health issues into the routine provision of HIV nursing service, undertake sexual health risk assessment as part of routine assessment of patients with HIV [17]. They should also demonstrate an awareness of HIV and STI transmission risk and the resources available (free condoms, leaflets, PrEP, PEPSE advice to patients) as they have an integral role in promoting a positive attitude to issues around sex and patients' sexual and reproductive health [17].

In addition, ACP have an important role in supporting junior staff to be able to assist in the assessment of patients, for example, in taking a full sexual history, blood-borne virus risk assessment, asymptomatic STI screening, cervical cytology, and support patients to maintain healthy lifestyles, including around drugs and alcohol [17].

5.3.10 Swab and Urine Tests

Routinely, investigations for *neisseria gonorrhoeae* and *chlamydia trachomatis* in asymptomatic patients are self-taken vulvo-vaginal swabs in women, first catch urine samples in men, and self-taken rectal and pharyngeal swabs in those reporting anal/oral sex Nucleic Acid Amplification Tests (NAATs) [68]. When conducting these investigations, it is essential to give advice around the relevant window periods [68] 2 weeks for both *neisseria gonorrhoeae* and *chlamydia trachomatis* [20, 22] and retesting (if necessary).

More recently, most areas in the country have options for asymptomatic STI screening, including blood tests via free online services. Patients diagnosed with an STI are contacted by the service by one of their clinical staff, who makes an assessment of the patient and either signposts them to clinical services or arranges treatment which is delivered to the patient in the post, or a prescription at a local pharmacy.

5.3.11 Blood Tests and Vaccinations

Routinely all patients should be screened initially on diagnosis and have ongoing blood tests for syphilis, hepatitis A, B, and C immunity status at their initial assessment, then annually [67]. As co-infection with hepatitis C is of concern for some patient populations already infected with HIV, more frequent hepatitis C testing (both antibody and PCR testing) may in indicated in those individuals considered at higher risk [68]. Hepatitis C is more infectious than HIV and can be passed on through injecting drug use (of particularly concern given the popularity of injecting methamphetamine (known as 'slamin' or 'getting to the poinT'). [69] Some MSM have caught hepatitis C through traumatic anal sex such as fisting (inserting the hand into the vagina or rectum), sharing lube so they become the vehicle of transmission/or not washing hands and/or changing gloves/washing toys between partners, as well as condomless anal sex, so discussion of all risks should form the sexual bi-annual sexual health assessments [64, 70].

In addition to screening, vaccination plays a key role in protecting health. All people living with HIV identified as being at risk of hepatitis A (MSM, IDUs, haemophiliacs, individuals with special needs) and as not having immunity should be offered vaccinations for hepatitis A [65]. Hepatitis A vaccination consists of two doses administered at least 6 months part for patients with a CD4 count greater than 350 cells/μL, and three doses (administered 0, 1, and 6 months) for those with a CD4 count of less than 350 cells/μL [65]. Further boosters should be offered every 10 years [65].

All people living with HIV identified as not having immunity should be offered vaccinations for hepatitis B [65]. Hepatitis B vaccination consists of four doses (administered 0, 1, 2, and 6 months) with immunity status checks of the hepatitis B 4–8 weeks post vaccination [10]. Subsequent titre checks should be performed 2–4 yearly in individuals with an HBsAb response greater than 100 μ/mL and a CD4 count greater than 350 cells/μL, annual checks should be performed in other patients. Where HBsAb level are below 100 μ/mL, booster doses or repeat courses of vaccinations should be offered depending on their history [67].

As men and women living with HIV are at greater risk of acquiring Human Papilloma Virus (HPV), having persistent HPV infection, and HPV-related disease such as intraepithelial dysplasia and malignancy (HPV) vaccination is recommended for HIV-positive men and women under 26 years old [65], MSM up to the age of 45 years old [66], and is suggested for unvaccinated women up to 40-years old [65]. It consists of three doses which is administered 0, 1–3, and 6 months [65] and does not require booster doses.

5.3.12 Symptomatic Patients

It is beyond the scope of this chapter to discuss each of the STIs in detail and most STIs are generally managed the same for people living with HIV as those without [10]. Refer to local and national guidelines such as BASHH for more details on how to recognise, diagnose, investigate, and treat sexually transmitted infections and related conditions [10]. Some infections are seen more frequently in men who have sex with men (MSM) especially those with HIV such as lymphogranuloma venereum (LGV) or syphilis [23, 25] and STIs should be considered in the differential diagnosis of skin conditions and proctitis [10]. People living with HIV may have exacerbated presentations of infections such as syphilis, ano-genital warts, or herpes [12, 25, 26].

5.3.13 Managing Symptomatic Patients

There are a number of ways that symptomatic patients can be managed, and it will be dependent on individual services. In integrated HIV and SRH services, people living with HIV can be fast tracked to the SRH service. In services without a general sexual health service, liaise with local SRH providers to gain experience and understanding of local referral pathways [12] to ensure smooth access as required. Alternatively, where services are not co-located, patients should be signposted to the appropriate local sexual health service.

Some services have dedicated sexual health pathways embedded within their HIV service. These pathways can be delivered by experienced ACPs (SRH) for STI management and contraception. The ACPs complete the whole episode of care including history, examination, microscopy, diagnosis, treatment, and follow-up.

Diagnosis and treatment of the STI however, are only part of the story, as risk taking is common with some MSM (see risk-taking section). ANPs also need to use effective communication skills to explore patient's individual attitudes, beliefs, and motivations towards behavioural changes to improve their sexual health, and one-to-one skills building support such as negotiating safer sex [17, 71]. Having staff who are training in motivational interviewing or other brief intervention techniques is therefore essential, and clear pathways for more intensive interventions if required [71].

5.3.14 Case Study

One of your patients has come into clinic and informs you that they have been informed that their partner has been diagnosed with a sexually transmitted infection. Your patient is concerned that they might also have an infection. During the consultation your patient confides in you that they have lost interest in sex but have been forced to have sex with their partner on several occasions.

- What thoughts, beliefs, and values come to mind with this situation?
- What support might your patient need?
- Based on the information within this chapter what might you want to consider when providing support to your patient?

5.4   Conclusion

This chapter has provided a foundation in sexual health for ACPs to work with their patients to improve and maintain their sexual health. It has explored some of the key issues facing people living with HIV including STIs, sexual function, contraception, and sexualised drug use, before concluding with some models of service provision. It has discussed how by working in partnership with patients and the MDT, HIV nurses can promote and improving the sexual health of their patients. It is however, this is only a brief introduction to sexual health, and to acknowledge that there are many other important aspects of sexual health which could not be covered due the constraints of the chapter such as sex and sexuality, abortion, infertility, and sexual assault. It should also be acknowledged that the confines of the chapter prevent detailed and contemporary guidance of the specific clinical management, and further information should be sought from the relevant national guidelines.

It is essential that ACPs working in HIV to continue to develop their knowledge, skills, and behaviours relating to sexual health in order to provide the best care for their patients. And for those with a specialist interest there are opportunities to develop more advanced and specialist skills in particular areas such as women's health or sexual dysfunction. There are a range of ways that this can be achieved, for example, reading around the various aspects of sexual health (e.g., national guidelines or journals), perhaps focusing on areas where there may be a knowledge deficit or interest in a particular topic. Alternatively, development may centre around areas which are particularly pertinent to the patient cohort or requirements for service delivery. Other approaches to development may include working with experienced practices in sexual health or arranging clinical attachments or placement with sexual health services. Finally, there are more formal programmes of learning such as those provide by higher education institutions or professional organisations.

References

1. Starrs AM, Anderson R. Definitions and debates: sexual health and sexual rights. Brown J World Aff. 2015;22:7.
2. World Health Organisation. Defining Sexual Health. 2002. http://www.who.int/reproductive-health/topics/gender_rights/sexual_health/en/. Accessed 1 Oct 2020.
3. Lucar J, Hart R, Rayeed N, Terzian A, Weintrob A, Siegel M, Parenti DM, Squires LE, Williams R, Castel AD, Benator DA. Sexually transmitted infections among HIV-infected individuals in the district of Columbia and estimated HIV transmission risk: data from the DC cohort. Open Forum Infect Dis. 2018;5(2):ofy017, US: Oxford University Press.
4. Public Health England. Sexually transmitted infections and screening for chlamydia in England. London, UK: Public Health England; 2019.
5. Haddad LB, Monsour M, Tepper NK, Whiteman MK, Kourtis AP, Jamieson DJ. Trends in contraceptive use according to HIV status among privately insured women in the United States. Am J Obstet Gynecol. 2017;217(6):676–e1.

6. Loutfy MR, Raboud JM, Wong J, Yudin MH, Diong C, Blitz SL, Margolese SL, Hart TA, Ogilvie G, Masinde K, Tharao WE. High prevalence of unintended pregnancies in HIV-positive women of reproductive age in Ontario, Canada: a retrospective study. HIV Med. 2012;13(2):107–17.
7. Santi D, Brigante G, Zona S, Guaraldi G, Rochira V. Male sexual dysfunction and HIV—a clinical perspective. Nat Rev Urol. 2014;112:99–109.
8. Agaba PA, Meloni ST, Sule HM, Agaba EI, Idoko JA, Kanki PJ. Sexual dysfunction and its determinants among women infected with HIV. Int J Gynecol Obstet. 2017;137(3):301–8.
9. González-Baeza A, Dolengevich-Segal H, Pérez-Valero I, Cabello A, Téllez MJ, Sanz J, Pérez-Latorre L, Bernardino JI, Troya J, De La Fuente S, Bisbal O. Sexualized drug use (Chemsex) is associated with high-risk sexual behaviors and sexually transmitted infections in HIV-positive men who have sex with men: data from the U-SEX GESIDA 9416 study. AIDS Patient Care STDs. 2018;32(3):112–8.
10. British HIV Association. BHIVA/BASHH/FSRH guidelines for the sexual & reproductive health. 2017. https://www.bhiva.org/file/zryuNVwnXcxMC/SRH-guidelines-for-consultation-2017.pdf. Accessed 03 Oct 2020.
11. Chun HM, Carpenter RJ, Macalino GE, Crum-Cianflone NF. The role of sexually transmitted infections in HIV-1 progression: a comprehensive review of the literature. J Sex Transmit Dis. 2013;20:13.
12. Patel R, Green J, Clarke E, Seneviratne K, Abbt N, Evans C, Bickford J, Nicholson M, O'Farrell N, Barton S, FitzGerald M. UK national guideline for the management of anogenital herpes. Int J STD AIDS. 2015;26(11):763–76. https://www.bashhguidelines.org/media/1019/hsv_2014-ijstda.pdf. Accessed 03 Oct 2020.
13. Looker KJ, Elmes JA, Gottlieb SL, Schiffer JT, Vickerman P, Turner KM, Boily MC. Effect of HSV-2 infection on subsequent HIV acquisition: an updated systematic review and meta-analysis. Lancet Infect Dis. 2017;17(12):1303–16.
14. British HIV Association. British HIV Association guidelines on the use of vaccines. 2015. https://www.bhiva.org/file/NriBJHDVKGwzZ/2015-Vaccination-Guidelines.pdf. Accessed 03 Oct 2020.
15. Ford ES, Magaret AS, Spak CW, Selke S, Kuntz S, Corey L, Wald A. Increase in HSV shedding at initiation of antiretroviral therapy and decrease in shedding over time on antiretroviral therapy in HIV and HSV-2 infected persons. AIDS. 2018;32(17):2525–31.
16. Wilson T, Jean-Louis G, Schwarts R, Golub E, Cohen M, Maki P, Greenblatt R, Massad S, Robinson E, Goparaju L, Lindau S. HIV infection and women's sexual function. J Acquire Immun Def Syndr. 2010;54(4):360–7.
17. National HIV Nurses Association. National HIV nursing competencies. London: Mediscript; 2013. https://www.nhivna.org/ebooks/ebook/index.html. Accessed 03 Oct 2020.
18. Public Health England. Sexually transmitted infections and screening for chlamydia in England, 2019. London, UK: Public Health England; 2020.
19. Holmes KK, Sparling PF, Stamm WE, Piot P, Wasserheit JN, Corey L, Cohen MS, Watts DH. Sexually Transmitted Diseases. 4th edition. 2007. New York: The McGraw-Hill Companies; 2008.
20. Fifer H, Saunders J, Soni S, Sadiq ST, FitzGerald M. 2018 UK national guideline for the management of infection with Neisseria gonorrhoeae. Int J STD AIDS. 2020;31(1):4–15.
21. Society of Sexual Health Advisors. Guidance on Partner Notification. 2015. https://ssha.info/wp-content/uploads/ssha-guidance-on-partner-notification-aug-2015.pdf. Accessed 03 Oct 2020.
22. White J, O'Farrell N, Daniels D. UK National Guideline for the management of lymphogranuloma venereum: Clinical Effectiveness Group of the British Association for Sexual Health and HIV (CEG/BASHH) Guideline development group. Int J STD AIDS. 2013;24(8):593–601.
23. White J, O'Farrell N, Daniels D. UK National Guideline for the management of lymphogranuloma venereum: clinical effectiveness group of the British Association for Sexual Health and HIV (CEG/BASHH) Guideline development group. Int J STD AIDS. 2013;248:593–601.

24. Dragovic B, Nwokolo N, BASHH clinical effectiveness group: update on the treatment of Chlamydia trachomatis (CT) infection. 2018. https://www.bashhguidelines.org/media/1191/update-on-the-treatment-of-chlamydia-trachomatis-infection-final-16-9-18.pdf. Accessed 03 Oct 2020.
25. Kingston M, French P, Higgins S, McQuillan O, Sukthankar A, Stott C, McBrien B, Tipple C, Turner A, Sullivan AK. Syphilis guidelines revision group UK national guidelines on the management of syphilis 2015. Int J STD AIDS. 2016;27(6):421–46. https://www.bashhguidelines.org/media/1148/uk-syphilis-guidelines-2015.pdf. Accessed 03 Oct 2020.
26. Gilson R, Nathan M, Sonnex C, Lazaro N, Keirs T. UK national guidelines on the management of anogenital warts 2015. Br Associat Sexual Health HIV. 2015;2015:1–24.
27. Faculty of Sexual and Reproductive Healthcare. UK Medical eligibility criteria for contraceptive use (UKMEC 2016) Amended September 2019. 2016. https://www.fsrh.org/standards-and-guidance/documents/ukmec-2016/fsrh-ukmec-full-book-2019.pdf. Accessed 03 Oct 2020.
28. Faculty of Sexual and Reproductive Healthcare. Barrier Methods for Contraception and STI Prevention (amended October 2015). 2012. file:///C:/Users/Admin/Downloads/ceuguidance-barriermethodscontraceptionsdi%20(2).pdf. Accessed 03 Oct 2020.
29. Guillebaud J, MacGregor A. Contraception: Your questions answered. 7th ed. Edinburgh: Elsevier; 2017.
30. Faculty of Sexual and Reproductive Healthcare. Emergency Contraception (amended December 2019). 2017. file:///C:/Users/Admin/Downloads/fsrh-guideline-intrauterine-contraception-sep-2019%20(2).pdf. Accessed 03 Oct 2020
31. Faculty of Sexual and Reproductive Healthcare. Intrauterine Contraception (amended September 2019). 2015. file:///C:/Users/Admin/Downloads/fsrh-guideline-intrauterine-contraception-sep-2019%20(2).pdf. Accessed 03 Oct 2020.
32. Faculty of Sexual and Reproductive Healthcare. Progestogen-only Pills (amended April 2020). 2015. file:///C:/Users/Admin/Downloads/fsrh-guideline-intrauterine-contraception-sep-2019%20(2).pdf. Accessed 03 Oct 2020.
33. Faculty of Sexual and Reproductive Healthcare. Progestogen-only Injectable Contraception (amended June 2020). 2014. file:///C:/Users/Admin/Downloads/cec-ceu-guidance-implants-feb-2014%20(1).pdf. Accessed 03 Oct 2020.
34. Faculty of Sexual and Reproductive Healthcare. CEU statement of self-administration of Sayana Press. 2015. file:///C:/Users/Admin/Downloads/ceustatementsayanaselfadmin%20(1).pdf. Accessed 03 Oct 2020.
35. Faculty of Sexual and Reproductive Healthcare. Progestogen-only Implants. 2014. file:///C:/Users/Admin/Downloads/cec-ceu-guidance-implants-feb-2014%20(1).pdf. Accessed 03 Oct 2020.
36. Faculty of Sexual and Reproductive Healthcare. Combined oral contraception (amended July 2019). 2019. file:///C:/Users/Admin/Downloads/fsrh-guideline-combined-hormonal-contraception-july-2019%20(2).pdf. Accessed 03 Oct 2020.
37. Chen L, Shi GR, Huang DD, Li Y, Ma CC, Shi M, Su BX, Shi GJ. Male sexual dysfunction: a review of literature on its pathological mechanisms, potential risk factors, and herbal drug intervention. Biomed Pharmacother. 2019;112:108585.
38. Nappi RE, Cucinella L, Martella S, Rossi M, Tiranini L, Martini E. Female sexual dysfunction (FSD): prevalence and impact on quality of life (QoL). Maturitas. 2016;94:87–91.
39. Monero-Perez O, Escoin C, Serna-Candel, Pico A, Alfayate R, Merino E, Reus S, Boix V, Sanchez-Paya, Portilla. J Risk factors for sexual and erectile dysfunction in HIV-infect men: the role of protease inhibitors. AIDS. 2010;24(2):255–64.
40. Baker BD, Lea EJ, Lavakumar M. The impact of HIV on sexual functioning: considerations for clinicians. Psychotherapy. 2020;57(1):75–82.
41. Huntingdon B, Muscat DM, de Wit J, Duracinsky M, Juraskova I. Factors associated with general sexual functioning and sexual satisfaction among people living with HIV: a systematic review. J Sex Res. 2020;57(7):824–35.

42. Harlow BL, Kunitz CG, Nguyen RH, Rydell SA, Turner RM, MacLehose RF. Prevalence of symptoms consistent with a diagnosis of vulvodynia: population-based estimates from 2 geographic regions. Am J Obstet Gynecol. 2014;210(1):40–e1.
43. Clayton AH, Kingsberg SA, Goldstein I. Evaluation and management of hypoactive sexual desire disorder. Sexual Med. 2018;6(2):59–74.
44. Wolpe RE, Zomkowski K, Silva FP, Queiroz APA, Sperandio FF. Prevalence of female sexual dysfunction in Brazil: a systematic review. Eur J Obstet Gynecol Reprod Biol. 2017;211:26–32.
45. Karatas OF, Gumus II, Bayrak O, Yildirim ME, Badem H. A novel method to treat primary anorgasmia: vestibuloplasty: a case report. Int J Womens Health Wellness. 2016;2:011.
46. Kessler A, Sollie S, Challacombe B, Briggs K, Van Hemelrijck M. The global prevalence of erectile dysfunction: a review. BJU Int. 2019;124(4):587–99.
47. Gillman N, Gillman M. Premature ejaculation: aetiology and treatment strategies. Med Sci. 2019;7(11):102.
48. Saitz TR, Serefoglu EC. The epidemiology of premature ejaculation. Transl Androl Urol. 2016;5(4):409.
49. Rubio-Aurioles E, Bivalacqua TJ. Standard operational procedures for low sexual desire in men. J Sex Med. 2013;10(1):94–107.
50. Hackett G, Kirby M, Wylie K, Heald A, Ossei-Gerning N, Edwards D, Muneer A. British Society for Sexual Medicine guidelines on the management of erectile dysfunction in men—2017. J Sex Med. 2018;15(4):430–57.
51. Stuart D. Chemsex: origins of the word, a history of the phenomenon and a respect to the culture. Drugs Alcohol Today. 2019;19(1):3–10.
52. Edmundson C, Heinsbroek E, Glass R, Hope V, Mohammed H, White M, Desai M. Sexualised drug use in the United Kingdom (UK): a review of the literature. Int J Drug Policy. 2018;55:131–48.
53. Halkitis PN, Siconolfi D, Fumerton M, Barlup K. Facilitators of barebacking among emergent adult gay and bisexual men: Implications for HIV prevention. J LGBT Health Res. 2008;4(1):11–26.
54. Adams J, Neville S. Men who have sex with men account for nonuse of condoms. Qual Health Res. 2009;19(12):1669–77.
55. Natale AP. Denver MSM sociostructural factors: preliminary findings of perceived HIV risk. J HIV/AIDS Soc Service. 2009;8(1):35–56.
56. O'Byrne P, Holmes D. Drug use as boundary play: a qualitative exploration of gay circuit parties. Subst Use Misuse. 2011;46(12):1510–22.
57. Evers YJ, Hoebe CJPA, Dukers-Muijrers NHTM, Kampman CJG, Kuizenga-Wessel S, Shilue D, Bakker NCM, Schamp SMAA, Van Buel H, Van Der Meijden WCJPM, Van Liere GAFS. Sexual, addiction and mental health care needs among men who have sex with men practicing chemsex-a cross-sectional study in the Netherlands. Prev Med Rep. 2020;2020:101074.
58. Pufall EL, Kall M, Shahmanesh M, Nardone A, Gilson R, Delpech V, Ward H, Hart G, Anderson J, Azad Y, Positive Voices Study Group. Sexualized drug use ('chemsex') and high-risk sexual behaviours in HIV-positive men who have sex with men. HIV Med. 2018;19(4):261–70.
59. Bourne A, Reid D, Hickson F, Torres-Rueda S, Weatherburn P. Illicit drug use in sexual settings ('chemsex') and HIV/STI transmission risk behaviour among gay men in South London: findings from a qualitative study. Sex Transm Infect. 2015;91(8):564–8.
60. Corkery JM, Loi B, Claridge H, Goodair C, Schifano F. Deaths in the lesbian, gay, bisexual and transgender United Kingdom communities associated with GHB and precursors. Curr Drug Metab. 2018;19(13):1086–99.
61. Flores-Aranda J, Goyette M, Aubut V, Blanchette M, Pronovost F. Let's talk about chemsex and pleasure: the missing link in chemsex services. Drug Alcohol Today. 2019;19(3):45.
62. Morris S. Yes, has no meaning if you can't say no: consent and crime in the chemsex context. Drug Alcohol Today. 2019;19:1.

63. World Health Organisation. Advancing the sexual and reproductive health and human rights of people living with HIV: a guidance package. Amsterdam: The Global Network of People Living with HIV/AIDS; 2009.
64. British HIV Association. British HIV Association guidelines for the management of hepatitis viruses in adults infected with HIV 2013. 2013. https://www.bhiva.org/file/TcrCoXjAGRaHb/HepatitisGuidelines2013.pdf. Accessed 18 June 2020.
65. British HIV Association. British HIV Association guidelines for HIV-associated malignancies 2014. 2014. https://www.bhiva.org/file/qUSRLDwncBEYp/MalignancyGuidelines2014.pdf. Accessed 18 June 2020.
66. National Health Service. Who should have the HPV vaccine? NHS website. 2019. https://www.nhs.uk/conditions/vaccinations/who-should-have-hpv-cervical-cancer-cervarix-gardasil-vaccine/. Accessed 18 June 2020
67. British HIV Association. BHIVA guidelines for the routine investigation and monitoring of adult HIV-1-positive individuals (2019 interim update). 2019. https://www.bhiva.org/file/DqZbRxfzlYtLg/Monitoring-Guidelines.pdf. Accessed 18 June 2020
68. British Association for Sexual Health & HIV. Standards for the management of sexually transmitted infections. 2019. https://www.bashh.org/about-bashh/publications/standards-for-the-mngement-of-stis/. Accessed 16 June 2020
69. Hibbert MP, Brett CE, Porcellato LA, Hope VD. Psychosocial and sexual characteristics associated with sexualised drug use and chemsex among men who have sex with men (MSM) in the UK. Sex Transm Infect. 2019;95(5):342–50.
70. Turner J, Rider A, Imrie J, Copas A, Edwards S, Dodds J, Stephens J. Behavioural predictors of subsequent hepatitis C diagnosis in a UK clinic sample of HIV positive men who have sex with men. Sex Transm Infect. 2006;82(4):298–300.
71. Clutterbuck DJ, Flowers P, Barber T, Wilson H, Nelson M, Hedge B, Kapp S, Fakoya A, Sullivan AK. UK national guideline on safer sex advice. Int J STD AIDS. 2012;23(6):381–8.

Chapter 6
Nurses in HIV Care in Eastern Europe: Past, Present, and Future

Anna Maria Żakowicz

6.1 Introduction

The challenges in HIV epidemic in the Eastern European region are related to the course of epidemic itself and how the healthcare system reacted to and managed to address the needs of affected populations. The chapter describes the beginning of HIV epidemic and current situation in the region. As one of the challenges is related to organisation of health care and role of the nurses the text considers the approaches of task shifting and nurse engagement in HIV care more deeply. Interventions from Kazakhstan, Kyrgyzstan, Tajikistan and Siberia, Russia related to nurse engagement in HIV treatment delivery, home care for HIV clients, support with retention and return to care are discussed. Additionally, a study on nurses' engagement in linkage to care in Ukraine is described.

The best practices and research on nursing interventions in Easter Europe are scarce; therefore, the author interviewed a team working in a *Test&Treat Clinic* in Odessa, Ukraine: the chief doctor, chief nurse, and nurse tester. The team strives to implement people-centred care approach in practice, with the aim to support and serve the community of people who live with HIV in Odessa. The *Test&Treat Clinic* team practices teamwork using notions of task shifting, joint decision-taking and interchangeability. In practice, they refer to the values of respect and care for their clients in their everyday work. They share their experience of quality improvement both for the client and clinic staff and building clients' trust in the facility which supports clients' retention and promotes better treatment outcomes.

A. M. Żakowicz (✉)
AIDS Healthcare Foundation (AHF), Amsterdam, The Netherlands
e-mail: anna.zakowicz@aidshealth.org

© The Author(s), under exclusive license to Springer Nature
Switzerland AG 2021
M. Croston, I. Hodgson (eds.), *Providing HIV Care: Lessons from the Field
for Nurses and Healthcare Practitioners*,
https://doi.org/10.1007/978-3-030-71295-2_6

The chapter includes recommendations for nursing practice for the Eastern European region based on the previous work related to nurse engagement, the WHO's Europe strategy, and case study based on interviews with staff working at the *Test&Treat Clinic*.

6.2 Role of Nurses in Public Health in the Region: Historical Outlook

The start of public health care available to all people, including those living in rural areas in Russia dates to 1861 when serfdom was abolished and *zemstvo* or elected local self-governing councils were established. *Zemstvo* oversaw rural health care and hospitals which were built in bigger villages. Back then on average one physician oversaw between 25,000 and 30,000 people who lived within one geographic district [1]. Along the district health care, municipal care, factory care, and private care were available to the citizens. The structure and the governance were quite complex, not able to address emergency situations during epidemics of typhus, cholera, typhoid fever, and smallpox which were ravaging the country at the turn of the century. Total mortality was between 25 and 30 people per 1000 and life expectancy was approximately 40 years [2].

Following the October Revolution of 1917, the Soviet health service was established by creating a People's Healthcare Commissariat, a governing body overseeing all healthcare services and commissioned to provide free medical care to the population. It was led at the establishment level by Dr. N. Semashko [2]. The 'Semashko model' of health care, as it became known, was a highly centralised, central government-controlled model of care with state-owned facilities managed at the local and regional level. The goals of the model were: unification of care, guaranteed free care for citizens and focus on preventive care. Primary care was provided at outpatient clinics, called polyclinics by specialists such as internists, paediatricians, obstetricians, and others. Hospitals played an important role in the system [2, 3].

The differences between Semashko model and the UK's NHS lie in the level of government regulations, which are much stronger in the former. The latter allows the private sector to provide some services and private health insurance. The entry point to health care is outpatient care in Semashko model and family doctors and community services in NHS. Additionally, the Soviet approach focuses extensively on occupational health [3]. After the Second World War when communist regimes were instituted in the countries of Central and Eastern Europe the Semashko approach was used for the transformation of health care although some features of the national health care were retained in the countries. The Central-Asian republics of former USSR were introducing the model more fully [3].

In the Semashko model, primary care was solely based on doctor physicians (DPs) [4]. In rural areas when there was no access to DPs, physician assistants known as *feldchers* played an important role. These included *feldchers* and *feldcher midwives*. Feldchers are personnel who finished middle medical school education and, as well as assisting physicians, in the physician's absence could work to a certain level independently. The role was therefore either complementary or as a substitute. Middle medical workers, a level of professional between doctors and non-professional workers of polyclinics or hospitals, included both feldchers and nurses, with the nurses being much bigger in number [5]. The nurses, 'sisters of mercy', were low in the hierarchy with less professional prestige and were not able to exercise any medical professional autonomy [6]. In Russia, the nurse was perceived as a technical support to the doctor [7].

Following the dissolution of the USSR in December 1991, Russia and former Soviet Union republics needed to look for efficient and cost-effective approaches. The population was ageing; there was an increase of chronic diseases, new diseases such as HIV, and increasing care costs. The new approaches included home care, development of hospices, and strengthening the focus on preventive care and improving the general health of the population. The role of the nurses to address medical, psycho-social needs of the population, family planning, and providing accessible care in rural areas were important directions to consider [7]. However, structural, organisational, and educational challenges needed to be addressed. The challenges included doctors with functions that could be performed by well-trained nurses, decreasing the role of nurses as a support to doctors and performing technical tasks, low motivation to become a nurse due to low social status and prestige of the profession, lack of well-qualified human resources such as chief nurses and senior nurses that would be trained in the organisation of health, management, leadership, medical supply management, and limited possibilities of professional growth within the nursing profession [7].

6.3 HIV Epidemic in Eastern Europe

The first cases of HIV in the USSR were diagnosed in 1986 among foreign students from African countries, followed by outbreaks among children in hospitals caused by poor infection control including limited sterilisation facilities and a shortage of single use disposable syringes [8]. In the following year, more cases were reported, majority of cases coming from continental Africa and living in the USSR, followed by citizens in certain key risk groups: men who have sex with men (MSM), sex workers, and people who inject drugs [8]. The first case of AIDS among Soviet citizens was officially registered in 1987 [9]. New regulations introduced mandatory HIV testing for foreign nationals, and all pregnant women to be screened for HIV [8, 9]. In the late 1980s, there was no clarity of the extent of the HIV epidemic, no willingness to work with people from key populations, and shortage of single use disposable instruments [9]. Since 1995, the region of Eastern Europe has been experiencing a rapid increase of HIV infections [10] and the increase continues in 2020 [11].

Currently, the region of Eastern Europe and Central Asia is disproportionally affected by HIV where the epidemic continues to grow [11]. In 2018, there was an estimated 1.7 million people who lived with HIV in the region [12]. In 2019, there were just 63% [52–71%] of people who live with HIV who received lifesaving antiretroviral treatment and 41% [34–46%] of those who live with HIV who were virally suppressed [11]. There is a need to address a gap in services that would prevent new HIV infections, deliver targeted testing interventions for affected populations, services that would link positive clients to care [11], ensure rapid start of HIV treatment and support clients in being retained in care. Additionally, EuroSIDA cohort highlights higher rates of AIDS-related mortality among patients from Eastern Europe with those who died being younger and with lower CD4 count at the time of death [13]. TB:HIV study group in EuroCoord emphasises major challenges connected with the management of TB in HIV-positive patients related to high pill burden, toxicities, high rate of MDR-TB, HCV co-infection, and drug use [14].

More recently, there has been a stronger focus on nurse engagement in HIV care. In 2013, WHO included in their Consolidated Guidelines on the Use of Antiretroviral Drugs for Treating and Preventing HIV infection guidance on operations and service delivery in HIV care. An attempt was made to move towards task shifting and delivery of services at different locations, such as STI clinics, TB, and OST sites [15]. Task shifting, which "involves rational redistribution of tasks among healthcare workforce teams" [15] recommended nurses, midwives, and non-physician clinicians to initiate first-line ART, maintain ART, and dispense ART between regular clinical visits [15].

Following the WHO recommendations, there were a few attempts to bring task shifting to the level of national discussions and implementation on the ground in Eastern European region. In 2018, a home-based nurse-led adherence support intervention SUPPORT4HEALTH (S4H) was launched by ICAP, a global health programme at Columbia University, at nine sites in Kazakhstan, Kyrgyzstan, and Tajikistan with the aim to improve retention and adherence to HIV treatment. The intervention included higher percentage of people in the intervention group to start ART, restart ART, and become virally suppressed. In the S4H group, there was no significant difference in VL suppressions related to drug use or between women and men [16].

Similar work was done in Krasnoyarsk, Siberia, by the NGO 'We Against AIDS' with support of the AIDS Healthcare Foundation (AHF) Russia. The programme started in 2015 and focused on home-based physician's assistants-led interventions, with the aim to re-engage people in HIV care, start and restart ART, and support with retention in HIV care. Between 2016 and 2019, 4375 people were targeted by the intervention, 3138 (72%) returned to HIV care, 2099 (67%) people restarted and continue ART and 1289 were virally suppressed for 1 year [17].

Additionally, a nurse-led intervention focusing on linkage to care, a Modified Antiretroviral Treatment Access Study (MARTAS), which was conducted in Ukraine between 2015 and 2019 showed efficacy in linkage to care [18] and feasibility and acceptability of the intervention, which included up to six sessions with a nurse, addressing stigma, fear of HIV status, and referral to other services depending on clients' needs [19].

6.4 Nurses' Experience in Test&Treat Clinic in Odessa

In October 2017, Ukraine launched healthcare reform which started at primary healthcare level. The reform related to HIV care aimed to move HIV patients to primary care level. In December 2017, AIDS Healthcare Foundation (AHF) in collaboration with Odessa Regional Centre for Socially Significant Diseases opened *Test&Treat Clinic*, a service based on primary health care for people who live with HIV which coordinates different services within the clinic with possibility of referrals to other specialists. AHF is a global non-profit organisation established in the USA in 1987, which through its regional and country offices delivers HIV prevention, testing and medical interventions within their own programmes and in collaboration with governmental and non-governmental institutions with the goal to bring cutting-edge medicine to the clients regardless of their ability to pay.

In December 2018, *Test&Treat Clinic* became a separate legal entity, received medical licence in primary health care and continues to work in collaboration with the Odessa Regional Centre. The clinic is unique in the Easter-European region as it aims to build people-centred models of care for people who live with HIV and people in high risk groups, which include integration, rapid treatment initiation, support to the clients along the continuum of care, user-driven care and co-production of care [20]. The HIV care at the primary care setting is based on greater engagement of nursing cadres and task shifting within the current legal framework of Ukraine [21–25].

The clinic embraces people-centred care approaches by integration of services, simplification of procedures, reduction of waiting time through appointment system, task shifting, and introduction of clear patient pathways for patients without and with symptoms of progressive HIV infection and TB, mental health screening and referral to care, family planning, and GP services [23–25]. The services are provided free from stigma, at a friendly and attractive setting in central location in Odessa. The clinic introduced consultations until 19:00 with prolonged hours of work and on Saturdays. All services are free, there is no out-of-pocket payment.

The clinic organises StART Clubs in a face-to-face and online format, the initiative to re-engage in HIV care and support with starting and restarting HIV treatment. The clinic encourages clients of the clinic to meaningfully engage in its life by participation in Patient Advisory Group (PAG) [20].

The clinic provides rapid HIV, HCV, HBV, and syphilis testing, information and counselling, HIV treatment and care, laboratory monitoring, OIs and HIV-associated diseases diagnostics, treatment and prevention. Gynaecological services and reproductive health, TB screening and diagnosis, TB prevention, mental health care: screening, diagnosis, and referral to treatment and CVD risk screening and prevention are a part of integrated approach. The clinic focuses on preventive care, provides condoms, post-exposure prophylaxis (PEP), pre-exposure prophylaxis (PrEP), and support for sero-different couples [20, 26].

The team consists of a chief doctor who is a gynaecologist, GP, chief nurse, nurse, receptionist and clinic navigator, social worker and peer tester [27]. Psychiatrist consultations happen once a week in the clinic. The clinic work is based on the principle of task shifting and efficient exchange of responsibilities. Trained in infectious diseases general care specialist such as family doctor and gynaecologist manage ART for the patients. Additionally, a nurse can dispense ART for stable patients and supervise them. Senior nurse is additionally responsible for medical supply management [21–25].

For 1 August 2020, there were 1299 HIV-positive clients receiving care in the clinic, 1195 (97%) were on ART and 1142 (95.6%) achieved undetectable viral load (<1000 RNA/mL) [28]. Cohort analysis among patients from the clinic shows that out of 535 people who started ART in August 2018, 494 (92.3%) are retained in care and remain on HIV treatment [28].

6.4.1   Case Studies

In September 2020, the author had informal conversations with the staff of *Test& Treat Clinic*: a chief doctor, chief nurse, and nurse. Due to COVID19, the conversations were done via a virtual platform. The conversations focused on the role of nurses in the clinic: organisation of work, the role of the nurse, task shifting and task sharing, prestige of the profession, motivation to work, and education and training. The author would like to thank the clinic's team for sharing their views and openness in sharing their experience.

6.4.1.1   Organisation of Work

The purpose of the work in the clinic is to maximally identify HIV cases through testing, engage and retain patients in care. When a new client comes to the clinic, they are met by the receptionist who is a junior nurse and a social worker. Testing procedure is done by a nurse in the testing room and she establishes good report with the client. Results of the test are communicated by the nurse along with post-test counselling. The nurse is at the front line and supports the client with the emotional side if the test is positive. Then the client meets a doctor and after having received an ART prescription from the doctor, they come back to the nurse to receive additional information related to treatment and care. The doctor always informs the nurse on the results of appointment and what is needed to be done after the appointment.

The team looks into different ways of delivery ART to patients. The clinic provides treatment and prevention of OIs and all examinations for free. It helps a lot with retention. The clinic focuses also on preventive care. There is a group of clients who are in high risk of acquiring HIV who became clients of the clinic. They receive HIV/HBV/HCV/syphilis combination tests, condoms in the needed number and other prevention interventions. These clients are invited to the clinic for testing once in 3 months. There is a PrEP programme for about 20 clients. PEP is also available; the clinic receives approximately one client for PEP each week.

There is an appointments system, with no lines and waiting time for the clients, due to that it is possible to keep efficiency of the patient flow and confidentiality.

The appointments are scheduled in convenient for the client time and can be rescheduled if needed. On the other hand, the clients can receive counselling without waiting in line and phone requests are answered immediately. If a person misses an appointment, it is followed by the receptionist and the new appointment is scheduled. The team keeps registry of patients who have challenges with retention or adherence. The team connects with them more often, and as they know their life style, they can predict when they can miss the visit or need more attention.

The clinic introduced patients' pathways to differentiate between HIV patients without symptoms of progressive HIV infection, HIV patients with symptoms of progressive HIV infection and patients with positive screening for TB infection. Consecutive visits and specified time frame of the visits is described within responsibilities clearly defined by each function. The team highlights that having patients' pathway is very helpful for workflow and convenience. *Test&Treat Clinic* is the only HIV clinic in the city open on Saturdays, which is also convenient to the clients.

The team mentioned they were able to build good communication and interaction between each other. The team meetings happen every week where they discuss current issues, complicated cases, and plans for the next week. The challenges are solved quickly as good communication and trustful atmosphere are present. As the team works on implementation of task shifting and task sharing, they can easily replace each other when needed or in case of emergency. They feel confident as a team. They were able to build trustful and friendly relations with their patients, who are open and share their challenges and concerns during consultations.

During COVID19 quarantine, the clinic team kept continuous contact with patients and delivered medicines. They were monitoring the clients remotely and for complicated cases they had appointments in the clinic. They had PPEs and disinfectants in sufficient amount. Their main purpose during this time was to keep the continuity of treatment and avoid disruptions and breaks. People at risk to discontinue HIV treatment were especially in focus during this period.

As people were not able to come for visits, the team delivered medicines by post. They were able to keep their distribution schedule. Clients received their ARVs for 3–6 months. The contact with clients was kept with phone counselling, especially if they had some symptoms. Some patients were able to visit the clinic and all services were provided to them.

> It is great that we have enough time for each patient due to appointments system.
>
> We communicate a lot during work because we have complicated cases, and we need to follow up closely the procedures. Each week we have team meeting to discuss the most critical situations of the week and how to settle some issues. We feel like hosts in this clinic and we feel the responsibility for it. We communicate almost 24 h because in the evening we plan the actions for the next days based on the results of the previous day.
>
> I had a client who came for testing. He had appointment but he had to wait 5 min and fill in the questionnaires. At the same time the other patient came to doctor's appointment. They met at the reception desk and I realised that they knew each other but were shocked to meet in this place. Without saying anything to each other, together with receptionist we reacted immediately and showed the situation as if they both came just for testing and had never been in the clinic before. We also try to support couples and people who are not ready to open their status to their partners. We try to set up individual approaches to each client.

6.4.1.2   Increasing the Role of the Nurse

In *Test&Treat Clinic,* the nurses perform primary screening. If the patient is stable, a planned visit with a doctor is scheduled and if there any urgent issues an earlier visit to a doctor is arranged. The medicines are dispensed by a nurse to stable patients who continue to receive the same ART regiment. For stable patients, ART can be dispensed for 3–6 months. Such an approach gives more time to doctor for complicated cases and patients who need more attention. Senior nurse additionally manages logistics of ART and medical supplies, including financial administration.

The nurses can replace each other, they can dispense ART, provide counselling and other procedures, including talking and counselling by phone and reporting within electronic medical information system (MIS). Nurses provide counselling on ART, PEP, and PrEP, how they should be taken, interpret results of basic blood tests, and advise on the necessity to come to doctor. The nurses can answer majority of the questions and the decision related to initiation and treatment choice is done by doctors. Receptionist coordinates requests to refer patients to other medical facilities, explains how the testing is done, and takes care of administrative issues.

Each patient has a register where doctors and nurses can see all the notes from the doctors and other nurses about previous visits and tests, it helps with addressing the needs of individual patients. The nurses shared that at *Test&Treat Clinic* they have more interactions within the team and more communication and involvement in the work with patients. They do not only do the procedures, but really interact with the clients. They often need to address the needs of people who tested positive, take care of their emotional state, and explain HIV treatment and importance of retention.

The nurses and the doctor referred to Ukrainian legislation which needs to be updated to include these new roles of the nurses. All of them stressed that stable clients with good conditions do not need doctors' examination and nurse can take care of them, but as per the procedure in any other clinic, each time the patient comes to clinic he should be seen by the doctor. When talking about the nurses' role in the health system in general, they mention that a nurse is completely subordinated to doctors and dependent on doctors as per legislation. They pointed to a very strict hierarchy, which might not be efficient. They felt it would be advisable that doctors can share some duties with the nurse.

> Nurses should interact more with the patients, provide more counselling and work on psychological state of the patients, be in contact all the time to make them feel comfortable and confident. It is important to have good interaction with the doctors and the team as well. Shifting duties is also very much helpful. We have very good communication, we have team meetings where we exchange opinions, discuss work issues and cases, all decisions are taken together.
>
> If we have stable patients or if somebody comes without appointment I speak with such patients. I distribute ART to stable patients and interpret results of basic tests to them. It saves time for doctors and patients as I do not go into detailed examination unless I see that patient's condition is not good.

6.4.1.3   Prestige and Motivation to Work

The team values possibility to work in a clinic that implements new approaches and that they work on their implementation together. They recognise the differences between governmental structures and *Test&Treat Clinic* related to conditions and services for the patients and for the staff. They highlight openness and communication as important factors for them.

The team says that they have learned a lot together, they gained new experiences and changed their approaches in providing services. When they analyse the data, they see that they achieved good results, the patients are registered in care soon after they are diagnosed, they try to prescribe ART as soon as possible and at the end 2020 they were the only clinic in Ukraine meeting 90-90-90 threshold. They recognise that it could have been done because they have effective teamwork and good experience in adjusting services to the needs of the patients. They are proud of their achievements.

They mentioned having received additional trainings on testing and ART, they have started implementing new programmes for patients such as PrEP and Hep C treatment. Each day they try to upgrade and think of new approaches. However, they still have a lot of paperwork and registers to fill in including electronic data to medical information system.

> *I feel confident, I feel support and back up.*
>
> *If to compare to my previous job, I should say that the difference is big as Test&Treat Clinic demonstrates European approach in everything, which is not possible in governmental structures.*
>
> *I am proud of my nurses, they are highly qualified, they can even advise me; we interact [with one another] and we all know how to accept comments and criticism from colleagues, and we are spiritually united. I see that community and patients feel the difference and get more and more adherent to our clinic, but we still have space for development as a clinic and as staff.*

6.4.1.4   Education and Training

Nurses in Ukraine graduate from medical college, and every 5 years they have trainings to confirm their qualifications and grade. They mention that *Test&Treat Clinic* provides more opportunities to learn and grow professionally, they have more trainings and webinars for professional development and learn about innovations in medical area.

They state that it would be advisable to have less bureaucracy and more learning and development activities, including learning from international experience and best world practices. Exchanging the experience on domestic and international level would be beneficial for the team. They share that in the clinic the model works, the interventions that were implemented allow on smooth processes for the clients and the staff and they would like to share their practice with other sites. They also highlight the need to keep good communication and continue experience sharing between AHF sites.

I also have a dream to apply for bachelor's degree and later for master's degree in health care.

Learning Points

- The change was possible to happen with a vision, commitment, and strong belief that structural changes are possible even within challenging circumstances.
- Building relationships with national authorities including education about the model, its advantages, expected results for the public health benefit and regular communication were essential to ensure sustainability of the model.
- Implementation of innovative approaches required persistence from the management and continued support and clear communication with the staff.
- For the innovation to become common practice, it needed to benefit both the patients and the staff.
- Long-term strategy and detailed action planning was crucial for the structural interventions to take place.
- Clarity about tasks and responsibilities for each team member helped to create positive attitude to change.
- Motivated and engaged team was key to success as they are the ones to implement the change.
- Ownership of the change process and its results by all the staff helped with the success and a wish for the future to improve even further.

6.5   Recommendations

Health 2020. A European policy framework and strategy for twenty-first century, adopted by 53 European countries at the 2012 Regional Committee for Europe, prioritises areas of investment in health, tackling communicable and non-communicable diseases, strengthening people-centred systems and creating resilient communities [29]. The common goal is to provide health and well-being for populations in equitable manner while strengthening sustainable health systems [29]. These goals cannot be achieved without rethinking the healthcare structure and investment in human resources in health to build competent workforce.

The groundwork is to build legal and regulatory framework to meaningfully include nursing cadres into care provision. The roles and functions of doctors, nurses, physician's assistants need to be rethought and reshaped. Legal changes need to be followed by organisation of education which also needs to be supported by legal acts.

The change in regulatory framework will allow on upgrading procedures in facilities. Nurses can take a lot of functions, and they are ready for this shift. HIV care, where there are groups of stable patients and those who need more attention, provides a strong grounding for such a change. The change is feasible and can be organised by teamwork, communication, and using clear patient pathways.

This structural shift also has a potential to benefit everyone: a doctor with more time for more difficult cases and time for education, a nurse with increased role and possibility to take clinical decisions, which as an effect could impact motivation, a patient with better care, more efficient use of time and no need for formal appointments and finally the governments and health budgets with better use of human resources for health.

Proper remuneration of frontline work and a culture of career development is crucial to attract new cadres and promote staff retention. Refreshing knowledge, closer educational links between institutions nationally and internationally could help to exchange experience, ideas and best practices, build competence, and support better provision of quality of care.

Nurses in Eastern Europe are ready for this change. The frameworks and road maps leading to policy change are also well defined. It takes the first bold step to make the shift towards a healthier society. The historical foundation of public health in the Eastern Europe is based on equity. Enabling the nursing workforce to increase their contribution has a potential to lead the region towards more universal, equitable, sustainable, and quality public health.

References

1. Lichterman B. From Prussia to Russia: Russian critics of "Aerztliche Ethik". J Med Ethics Hist Med. 2019;12:19. https://doi.org/10.18502/jmehm.v12i19.2201.
2. Reshetnikov V, Ekkert NE, Capasso L, et al. The history of public health in Russia. Med Hist. 2019;3(1):16–24.
3. Marrée J, Groenevegen PP. Back to Bismarck; Eastern European Health Care Systems in Transition. ISBN 1 85972 617 8. 1997. p. 7–12.
4. Sheiman I, Shishkin S, Shevsky V. The evolving Semashko model of primary health care: the case of the Russian Federation. Risk Manag Healthc Policy. 2018;11:209–20. https://doi.org/10.2147/RMHP.S168399.
5. Storey P. The Soviet Feldsher as Physician's Assistant. US Department of Health, Education and Welfare. DHEW Publications No. (NIH) 72-58. 1972. p. 3–8.
6. Grant S. Introduction. In: Grant S, editor. Russian and Soviet health care from an international perspective. Cham: Palgrave Macmillan; 2017. https://doi.org/10.1007/978-3-319-44171-9_1.
7. Perfilieva G, Perfilieva Galina Michailovna, Sestricheskie delo v Rossii.Nursing in Russia. Moscow. 1995. http://medical-diss.com/docreader/386607/a?#?page=1 Accessed 16 Sept 2020.
8. Medvedev Z. Evolution of AIDS policy in the Soviet Union. Br Med J. 1900;300:890–1. https://www.bmj.com/content/bmj/300/6728/860.full.pdf. Accessed 21 Sept 2020.
9. Medvedev Z. Evolution of AIDS policy in the Soviet Union. Br Med J. 1900;300:932–4. https://www.bmj.com/content/bmj/300/6729/932.full.pdf. Accessed 21 Sept 2020.
10. UNAIDS. Global Report: UNAIDS report on the global AIDS epidemic. 2010. https://www.unaids.org/globalreport/documents/20101123_GlobalReport_full_en.pdf. Accessed 20 Sept 2020.
11. UNAIDS Seize the moment. Tackling entrenched inequalities to end epidemic. 2020. https://aids2020.unaids.org/chapter/region-profiles. Accessed 21 Sept 2020.
12. UNAIDS. UNAIDS Data 2019. 2019. https://www.unaids.org/sites/default/files/media_asset/2019-UNAIDS-data_en.pdf. Accessed 24 Oct 2020.

13. Reekie J, Kowalska JD, Karpov I, et al. Regional differences in AIDS and non-AIDS related mortality in HIV-positive individuals across Europe and Argentina: The EuroSIDA Study. PLoS One. 2012;7(7):e41673. https://doi.org/10.1371/journal.pone.0041673.

14. Efsen AM, Schultze A, Post FA. Major challenges in clinical management of TB/HIV coinfected patients in Eastern Europe compared with Western Europe and Latin America. TB: HIV Study Group in EuroCoord. PMID: 26716686 PMCID: PMC4696866 DOI: 10.1371/journal. pone.0145380. https://pubmed.ncbi.nlm.nih.gov/26716686/.

15. Consolidated Guidelines on the Use of Antiretroviral Drugs for Treating and Preventing HIV Infection. Recommendations for Public Health Approach. June 2013. https://apps.who.int/iris/ bitstream/handle/10665/85321/9789241505727_eng.pdf?sequence=1.

16. Deryabina A, Ivakin V, Kuddusova Y. High rates of Viral load suppression among patients participating in a home-based, nurse-led ART adherence support interventions in Kazakhstan, Kyrgyzstan and Tadjikistan. https://programme.ias2019.org//PAGMaterial/eposters/605.pdf. Accessed 19 Sept 2020.

17. Kandlen K, Chuykov A, Boiko A et al. Comprehensive retention to care model: results of the pilot in Krasnoyarsk, Russia 2016 to 2019. https://onlinelibrary.wiley.com/doi/full/10.1002/ jia2.25616. Accessed 24 Oct 2020.

18. Neduzhko O, Postnov O, Sereda Y, et al. Modified antiretroviral treatment access study (MARTAS): a randomized controlled trial of the efficacy of a linkage-to-care intervention among HIV-positive patients in Ukraine. AIDS Behav. 2020;24:3142–54. https://doi. org/10.1007/s10461-020-02873-7.

19. Neduzhko O, Postnov O, Bingham T. Feasibility and acceptability of the modified antiretroviral treatment access study (MARTAS) intervention based on a pilot study in Ukraine. J Int Assoc Provid AIDS Care. 2019;18:2325958218823257. https://doi.org/10.1177/2325958218823257.

20. People-centered Approach to HIV Care. AHF Ukraine Odessa Test&Treat Clinic Model. Experience in Collaboration with Odessa Oblast Government, Ukraine. As presented at the meeting of national program managers of priority countries in WHO Europe Region. The Hague, the Netherlands. 16 May 2019.

21. *Test&Treat Clinic*: Наказ №6 03.01.2019 Про затвердження посадової інструкції медичної сестри. Order №6 03.01.2019 On approval of the job description of a nurse.

22. *Test&Treat Clinic*: Наказ №7 03.01.2019 Про затвердження посадової інструкції старшої медичної. сестри. Order №7 03.01.2019 On approval of the job description of a senior nurse.

23. *Test&Treat Clinic*: Наказ №8 від 29.01.2019 Про затвердження стандартів та протоколів сестринського огляду і системи оцінки якості їх виконання. Order №8 of January 29, 2019 On approval of standards and protocols for nursing examination and quality assessment system for their implementation.

24. *Test&Treat Clinic*: Наказ 28 від 25.06.19 Про затвердження клінічного маршруту пацієнта "Профілактика інфікування ВІЛ". Order 28 of 25.06.19 "On approval of the clinical route of the patient" Prevention of HIV infection.

25. *Test&Treat Clinic*: Наказ 29 від 02.07.2019 Про затвердження клінічного маршруту пацієнта з позитивним результатом обстеження на ВІЛ-інфекцію. Order 29 of 07/02/2019 On approval of the clinical route of a patient with a positive HIV test result.

26. AHF Ukraine: Test&Treat Clinic: Treatment: https://ahfclinic.org.ua/test-and-treat/en/treatment/. Accessed 22 Sept 2020.

27. AHF Ukraine: Test&Treat Clinic: Staff: https://ahfclinic.org.ua/test-and-treat/en/staff/. Accessed 20 Sept 2020.

28. AHF Europe: Test&Treat meeting internal documents: basic data and Cohort analysis. Presented on 16 Sept 2020.

29. Health 2020. A European policy framework and strategy for the 21st century. https://www.euro. who.int/__data/assets/pdf_file/0011/199532/Health2020-Long.pdf. Accessed 22 Sept 2020.

Chapter 7
Access to HIV Services for Key Populations: Leaving No One Behind

Ian Hodgson

Efforts towards universal health coverage should include a dedicated focus on reaching key populations and marginalised groups. People living with HIV and key populations need to be acknowledged as people whose care and well-being should be valued equally [1]

7.1   Introduction to the Chapter

Key affected and vulnerable populations (key populations, KAP) are people at increased risk of HIV, irrespective of the epidemic type or local context [2]. This is sometimes connected with high-risk behaviours, but there are also legal, political, or cultural factors that increase risk and inhibit access to services and support for HIV prevention, treatment, and care.

As a result, throughout the world, HIV prevalence is significantly higher among key populations [3]. A carefully targeted HIV response to reduce vulnerability and maximise support and care is required, based on the essential right to health. Health and community systems need to address the barriers that limit access to screening, treatment, and care, for those people especially vulnerable in the context of HIV, HIV comorbidities, gender expression, and the protection of sexual and reproductive health (SRH).

This chapter will discuss:

1. Who are the people defined as a 'key population', and why are they at more risk?
2. What are the barriers that inhibit access to services?
3. What works? Examples of interventions to improve access.
4. What can nurses do? The implications for nursing practice and recommendations for maximising access to treatment and care.

I. Hodgson (✉)
Freelance Global Health, Bingley, UK

European HIV Nursing Network, London, UK

© The Author(s), under exclusive license to Springer Nature   105
Switzerland AG 2021
M. Croston, I. Hodgson (eds.), *Providing HIV Care: Lessons from the Field for Nurses and Healthcare Practitioners*,
https://doi.org/10.1007/978-3-030-71295-2_7

7.2   Who Are the Key or Vulnerable Populations at Risk of HIV?

What should be emphasised is that there is no such thing as a 'high risk person'. It is context or behaviours, not people, that increase the risk of acquiring HIV infection. People may move in and out of HIV risk situations as their lives change. In the context of HIV, it is the risk behaviours and networks of specific populations and *their* networks that determine the dynamics of HIV epidemics, and it is key populations that are often most disproportionately affected by HIV [3].

It was estimated that in 2018 more than half of new HIV infections globally were among key populations and their sexual partners [4]. People disproportionately affected by HIV include:

1. Men who have sex with men (MSM).
2. People who inject drugs.
3. Sex workers.
4. Transgender people.

There are also groups considered vulnerable to HIV in certain situations. These include the following:

1. Young people and adolescents (especially girls in sub-Saharan Africa).
2. Migrant and mobile workers.
3. Women and girls.
4. People with disabilities.
5. Prisoners or others in a closed setting.

7.2.1   Why Are Key or Vulnerable Populations More at More Risk?

Key populations are 'key' for a reason [5]. Their increased risk of contracting HIV through physical, social, and structural factors combine to highlight that HIV, though technically a risk to all people, poses more of a threat to some than to others. According to UNAIDS in 2020, although they are a small proportion of the general population, key populations and their sexual partners accounted for more than 60% of new adult HIV infections globally in 2019 [6].

There are **biological** reasons for increased risk. HIV, compared with many other pathogens affecting human populations, is relatively difficult to catch. It is not airborne, it is not carried in the water supply, it cannot linger for long on surfaces, and is not carried by insects. However, in an infected, untreated person, HIV is present in large quantities in certain bodily fluids. Sexual activity is a key transmission vector, especially if with multiple partners. Also, unprotected penetrative anal sex is a higher risk than vaginal sex [7]. The sharing of needles by drug injecting users also poses increased risk of transmission from an infected to non-infected person [8]. However, important findings emerged in 2018 [9] consolidating previous studies confirming that, once successfully treated and with an undetectable viral load, the risk of a person living with HIV transmitting the virus is negligible. This is a significant development for HIV prevention. These and similar results are the driving force behind the U = U campaign (undetectable = untransmittable) [10].

Personal or interpersonal factors also play an important part. A person may not have the necessary information about how to protect themselves. For example, older MSM compared with younger MSM, the latter tending to have better access to more information [11]. There can also be restrictions on personal agency—the choice and freedom to act—to protect oneself. This can be the case in abusive relationships, strict religious communities, or where financial income depends on submitting to the sexual wishes and desires of another person. In the case of girls and young women, violence and unfavourable power relations can be attributed to a higher incidence of HIV infection [12] especially when associated with transactional sex.

There are also **sociocultural and structural factors** that exacerbate HIV risk or support and treatment for a person already living with HIV. For example, if a person is in a marginalised group, he or she may face barriers when seeking HIV prevention materials, especially if the group is viewed negatively by health providers, the general public, or policy and lawmakers. This can be seen in the case of sex workers [13] and MSM [14].

The same challenges would apply when trying to obtain an HIV test, or information on how to self-protect. In countries with a weak health system battling other health challenges, HIV mitigation—and support for sexual and reproductive health generally—may not be a high priority [15]. Or a person may belong to a group that is not clearly understood, or not seen to be at high risk of HIV, and therefore not prioritised by HIV prevention campaigns or services. This can be the case for people with disabilities [16]. There are also factors that diminish a person's ability to access the health system, such as those in mobile populations—migrants, refugees, and asylum seekers (especially if unregistered) can face significant difficulties [17].

Vulnerabilities can be increased when systems are under stress, such as during the COVID-19 pandemic in 2020. Here, many HIV community-based organisations reported that health and social services for many people were jeopardised. One report by APCOM, an LGBT advocacy and support organisation based in Southeast Asia, described the pandemic's impact on transgender people in Malaysia. Here, the economic downturn, requirement for social distancing, and difficulties accessing health and medical services because of a movement control order, all exacerbated this community's already fragile living conditions [18]. As stated by UNAIDS in July 2020 [19]:

> The COVID-19 pandemic has seriously impacted the AIDS response and could disrupt it more. A 6-month complete disruption in HIV treatment could cause more than 500 000 additional deaths in sub-Saharan Africa over the next year (2020–2021), bringing the region back to 2008 AIDS mortality levels. Even a 20% disruption could cause an additional 110,000 deaths.

And for Grace Violeta Ross, President of the Bolivian Network of People living with HIV:

> Those of us who survived HIV and fought for life and access to treatment and care cannot afford losing the gains that took so much effort to win. In some Latin American countries, we are seeing how HIV resources, medicines, medical staff and equipment are being moved to the fight against COVID-19 [19]

To summarise, key and vulnerable populations are at particular risk of HIV because they may:

1. Be at increased biological risk.
2. Lack information on how to protect themselves and other people.
3. Belong to a group involved in activities that are illegal in a particular country.
4. Belong to a group that is stigmatised and unpopular in a particular country or community.
5. Belong to a group that is disempowered in some way in a particular country, unable to make their own sexual health decisions and at risk of being controlled.
6. Belong to a group that has low socio-economic status, restricting their access to health and prevention services.
7. Belong to a group that is not seen by the community as being at risk of HIV, and therefore are unwilling or unable to take precautions to protect their sexual health.

Table 7.1 shows possible reasons for increased HIV risk for key and vulnerable populations.

> **Reflection Box 1:**
> Have you provided care for any of these groups? If so:
> • What were the main challenges?
> • What is the experience of people living with HIV who may be members of these groups?
> • How can nursing address their issues?

7.2.2 HIV Key and Vulnerable Populations: Focus on Europe

In the WHO European region there are 53 countries, 27 of which are members of the European Union (EU), and 18 that form part of central Asia. Health systems vary, as do the risks for key affected and vulnerable populations and the nature of the HIV response. Across Europe as a whole in 2018, according to the ECDC [24] new HIV infections resulted from sex between men [40%], heterosexual sex [33%], injecting drug use [4%], and vertical transmission [1%]. There are important regional and national differences to consider that shape HIV responses. Data below were released in 2019 and relate to 2018. Unless stated, data are from the ECDC [24].

In the 23 countries providing data in **western Europe** (including the UK, France, and Norway), new diagnoses were estimated to be 5.5 per 100,000 population. These were predominantly in sex between men (52%), more marked in the Netherlands, Ireland, and Spain. Heterosexual transmission accounted for 43%, with prominent countries being the UK, Belgium, France, and Italy, where heterosexual transmissions almost equals that of sex between men. HIV from injecting drug use is relatively low, holding at the European average of 4%, likely due to comprehensive harm reduction programmes available in many countries in this

Table 7.1 Key and vulnerable populations: specific risk factors [examples]

Key or vulnerable population	Possible reasons for increased HIV risk
MSM: 28× more at risk of HIV than the general population [8]	• Marginalised and stigmatised in many communities, and illegal in some countries • Biological and behavioural risk factors [unprotected anal sex; multiple sexual partners]
Sex workers: 13× more at risk of HIV than the general population [8]	• Illegal in some countries. Where sex work is legal the legislation rarely protects sex workers • Marginalised, and stigmatised, including by the police • Frequent unprotected sex is high risk—condom use can be erratic [sex workers often offered more money not to use a condom] • Other untreated STIs that can increase HIV risk • Can be multi-factorial risk—such as injecting drug use, being under 18, part of a migrant community, or the victim of human trafficking
People who inject drugs: 22× more at risk of HIV than the general population [8]	• Illegal in most countries, and heavily criminalised • Sharing needles and other drugs equipment is high risk • Can be associated with poverty, and other risk factors such as sex work, and gender-based violence) • Experience stigma, and when incarcerated exposed to other drug-related risks while detained • Can be associated with mental health issues that affects general health-seeking behaviour
Transgender women: 13× more at risk of living with HIV than the general population [8]	• Not recognised in most countries, with significant social and legal exclusion • Can have limited agency [freedom to act], low self-esteem, and disempowerment that limits capacity to negotiate safe condom use • Marginalised, and stigmatised (and/or simply not understood) by the general population • Risk is higher for transgender women [man>woman] than transgender men [woman > man] • Economic factors result in sex work for income, which adds increased risk • Self-administered hormone injections with shared/unsterilized equipment • Higher risks of poor physical health, disability, depression and perceived stress compared with the general population
Young people [10–24]: HIV is one of the top ten leading causes of death among adolescents [20]	• Affects girls/young women more than boys/young men • Can be infected early in life (vertical transmission) • Physical and emotional changes in adolescence, plus increasing freedom and independence is a time of exploration and experimentation (early sexual debut) • Intergenerational sex (especially sub-Saharan Africa) • Lack of information about sexual health, especially in restrictive religious and cultural settings • Unwillingness/incapacity to engage the health system • Multi-factorial—linked with other key population groups (young sex workers, young transgender people, young people who inject drugs, young MSM)

(continued)

Table 7.1 (continued)

Key or vulnerable population	Possible reasons for increased HIV risk
Women and girls: girls and young women [10–24] ×2 likely to be HIV+ than young boys and men [21]	• Biological factors • Increased vulnerability due to gender inequality and socio-economic status (poverty—which can force girls into marriage) • Child marriage • Sex-trafficking • Gender-based and intimate-partner violence and sexual coercion • Gender inequality means difficulty negotiating condom use • Lack of information/denied information about sexual health • Cultural attitudes towards sexuality and girls/women—denied access to services and information unless married • Transactional sex ['sugar daddies']
Migrants/displaced people [17, 22]	• The context of migration can lead to increased risk-taking • Fragmented access to health systems as they move through interim countries, or inability to pay for services • Increased HIV risk in final host country • Risk of stigma and discrimination in host country as a *migrant* or as a member of a particular group (e.g., MSM) • Increased risk of sexual violence and exploitation in migrant camps and urban settings
People with disabilities [risk of HIV the same or slightly higher than the general population] [23]	• Can face increased risk because of poverty • Especially for women, impact of gender inequality, vulnerability to sexual violence (can be directly related to dependence and need for additional physical support because of disability), intimate partner violence, and difficulties negotiating safe condom use • Exclusion from sex education • Problems communicating and/or cognitive impairment (dependant on disability) • General stigma and discrimination due to disability affecting willingness to attend services

sub-region [4]. What is of concern—where data about CD4 cell count on diagnosis are available—is that 49% of new infections in 2018 were classified as 'late presentation', with CD4 counts <350/mm. This alone strengthens the case for improved access to HIV testing and counselling.

In the **centre** of Europe (countries such as Poland, Bulgaria, and Albania), HIV prevalence is relatively low, and has been since the beginning of the epidemic. In 2018 it stood at 3.3 per 100,000 population. Across this sub-region, new infections are reported mostly in sex between men (28%) and heterosexual sex (28%). At the national level, in several countries MSM is the dominant group affected, such as Bulgaria, Hungary, Montenegro, and Serbia. In others, the heterosexual route is more common, such as Albania, Romania, and Turkey. Injecting drug users account for only 1% of new infections across the sub-region. However, data are not available for the route of transmission of 41% of new infections, so the true picture may be different, especially in Turkey and Poland. The trend in this sub-region suggests an increase in new diagnoses in MSM.

As with the west, many newly diagnosed people in the centre are late presenters (53%), particularly in nine countries, including Bulgaria and Croatia, and especially amongst injecting drug users. For gender, the highest male-female ratios were seen in Slovenia (35:1) and Hungary (25:1), two countries where most HIV diagnoses were reported between men who have sex with men. The lowest ratios were noted in Romania and Albania (both 3:1), meaning that in the latter, 25% of people newly diagnosed in 2018 were women.

Eastern Europe and central Asia, constituting 12 countries, has the highest prevalence of HIV in the European Region, in 2018 at 44.9 per 100,000 population. At the country level, the Russian Federation has the highest prevalence, at 59 per 100,000 population, followed by Ukraine (37.2). The lowest is Lithuania (5.7). Across the sub-region, heterosexual transmission is the dominant route (70%), and injecting drug use (23%). However, there are significant national variations—in Lithuania, 40% of new infections were among injecting drug users, with 35% in the same group in Latvia. No data are available for the Russian Federation on this statistic. New diagnoses in MSM were only 4%, though this was higher in Estonia and Georgia (10% or above). Late presenters accounted for 56% of new diagnoses in this sub-region. Trends suggest new diagnoses in injecting drug users are generally falling, and in MSM remain stable. Heterosexual transmission continues to climb on trend, however. Regarding gender, trends indicate that in some countries, HIV diagnoses among women are increasing at a faster rate, especially in Azerbaijan, Kazakhstan, and Kyrgyzstan.

7.3 Barriers Affecting Key Populations Accessing Services

Barriers to services for prevention and treatment support are noted in Table 7.2. One of the overarching factors that affects key populations in the community and health sector is stigma, which is often (though not always) associated with discrimination and prejudice. A second key component is political. Legislation and policy can have significant impact on the lives of some key populations and their freedom—or not—to access services. Finally, there is the capacity and skills of health workers themselves. How ready are they to support people who may be marginalised by the general population, or fall outside the usual route to gain access to services? These issues are addressed in the table below, and apply both to those at risk and people who live with HIV.

Reflection Box 2:
What about the country you work in?
- What kind of care is available for people living with HIV?
- How ready are nurses to provide that care?
- What is the experience of people living with HIV in the health and care system?

Table 7.2 Key populations: barriers to services [examples]

Group	Specific barriers to prevention and treatment services
MSM	• Health services not MSM-friendly • Difficulty getting prevention commodities [condoms, lubricants]
Sex workers	• Difficulties accessing general sexual health services, and hard for HIV prevention programmes to reach • Health services not welcoming to sex workers • Poor access to condoms or limited knowledge about HIV prevention in general
People who inject drugs	• Lack of access to harm reduction services, and difficulties entering general health system for treatment of drug-related illness and other health problems • Harm reduction services may not have capacity to deal with overlapping, multi-factorial problems
Transgender people	• Lack of access to tailored HIV services that address multiple risk and social factors
Young people [10–24]	• Health system can be unwelcoming, with no adolescent-friendly areas or trained personnel • Schools provide limited comprehensive sexuality education • The need to change behaviour and increase knowledge *before* sexual debut; afterwards can be too late • Limited support for transition to adulthood
Women and girls: girls and young women [10–24]	• Difficulties accessing services unless married • Schools failing to provide sufficient comprehensive sexuality education
Migrants/displaced people	• Difficulties for health systems to track the general health needs (including sexual health) of mobile populations • Language barriers • Inability to pay for health services and acquire HIV prevention commodities
People with disabilities	• HIV services and prevention programmes not prepared or able to support disabled people • People with disabilities not perceived as an HIV risk group

7.3.1 Attitudes Towards HIV and Key Populations: Stigma

7.3.1.1 Us and Them

We naturally generate our social world along a continuum, between people similar to us and those who are different. In many instances, this is a helpful method of creating a rapid mental picture of our networks. At other times, or when we cluster people into groups to construct a collective continuum, there is potential for harm. This is the basis of stereotyping, another common tool we use for arranging our social world, but one that leads to prejudice [25]. The roots of stigma—why a particular view is held—can be complex, and often based on inherited ideas from society, our peers, cultural beliefs, or religion.

Stigmatising people with certain illnesses is a constant and damaging social phenomenon, and can be manipulated to construct negative views towards certain groups, especially if they are already unpopular or marginalised:

> Reinforcing the fear of disease was a prejudice against strangers and all their strange ways.
> George Stewart in *Earth Abides* (1949, p. 277)

The standard definition of stigma was provided by Goffman in 1963 [26] as "an attribute that is significantly discrediting" which, in the view of others, serves to reduce the person who possesses it. They become unacceptable, tainted, and discounted. Stigma can be categorised into discriminatory, and internalised [27].

Discriminatory responses against groups and individuals can range from simple avoidance, to violence, and murder. In 2020, the global outbreak of COVID-19, caused by the SARS-CoV-2 virus, led to worldwide morbidity and mortality affecting millions, and highlighted the readiness to stigmatise those who are perceived a risk, or those from the country where the virus is assumed to have originated. There are many similarities with HIV, illustrating how a pathogen (virus) is readily conflated with a person and their social identity [28]. It also reminds us that throughout history people have been 'blamed' for their ailments, "[all] societies need to have one illness which becomes identified with evil, and attaches blame to its victims" [29], p. 42.

Culture plays a significant role in shaping responses to illness and, by extension, how we view people who are affected. Kleinman's explanatory model [30] provides useful insights into how 'disease' is defined by experts (practitioners) and is a relatively fixed concept, whereas 'illness' is defined by culture ('lay' people) and is more malleable. This can be based on subjective experience and prevailing belief systems, such as 'magical contagion' and over-cautiousness because a person is seen as a threat (rather than the pathogen he or she may or may not be carrying). If a person is deemed part of an unpopular group, contagion risk not only refers to a disease, but also the *personal qualities of an individual*. I can 'catch' what I believe to be their unacceptable behaviour. An added layer of stigma that applies in the context of key populations is the **social group** he or she belongs to. This can lead to double stigma in health care and is addressed in Sect. 7.3.3.

Reflection/Activity Box 3:
How might your beliefs be stigmatising?
- Do you think you have stigmatised people or groups without realising it?
- How could your personal views and opinions impact on the nursing care you provide?

Internalised stigma, or self-stigma, is the second major classification of stigma. It can be defined as the extent to which people endorse negative beliefs and feelings associated with their stigmatised attribute and apply them to self [31]. Self-stigma and illness have been studied in other health contexts, such as TB [32, 33], mental illness [34, 35], and obesity [36]. Self-stigma can be especially harmful because it influences affective, cognitive, and mental health outcomes, as well as healthcare behaviours. It affects a person's view of themselves and how they interact with the community and the health sector [37].

7.3.1.2   The Impact

Stigma changes how people engage with health systems. According to the ECDC [38], two out of three countries in Europe and Central Asia acknowledge that stigma and discrimination within key affected populations is a barrier to the uptake of HIV prevention and testing services. Stigma and discrimination among health professionals, particularly with respect to sex workers, men who have sex with men, and people who inject drugs, reportedly persists across the region and plays a role in preventing these key populations from accessing HIV prevention, testing, and treatment. Fear of stigma is associated with late diagnosis of HIV [39] from anxiety experienced by key populations caused by anticipated or experienced stigma. Late presentation for testing and subsequent treatment is associated with poorer health outcomes [40]. The experience of key populations can be especially acute, and this is discussed further in Sect. 7.3.3.

One of the positive outcomes of the COVID-19 outbreak during 2020 has been to illustrate the benefits of routine testing, perhaps decreasing stigma associated with HIV testing for key populations [41]. Whether or not this has long-term positive impacts remains to be seen.

7.3.2   Structure: Political, Legal, and Sociocultural Challenges

7.3.2.1   Some background to Structural Barriers

Whilst stigma and discrimination have serious implications for access to services, there are also *structural* factors that create difficulties. This can be associated with legislation (criminalisation of certain activities), social inequalities, gender inequality, and denial of essential human rights.

> In many countries, the criminalisation of sex between men, sex work, or drug use, and the lack of legal recognition of gender identities other than male or female, are a severe barrier to services. These are often made worse by illegal police practices such as harassment, arbitrary arrest, extortion, and violence. [42]

In the years leading up to 2020, we have seen across Europe an emergent conservative political movement supporting legislation that restricts (or bans) same sex relationships, drug use, and sex work, significantly affecting the HIV response. A marked rightward shift in the political and social landscape has, in many countries, seen a backsliding towards less tolerance and a strengthening of the notion of a 'core' (i.e., normal) society that conforms to powerful national or cultural identities.

Fundamental human rights have been increasingly under attack, posing significant threat to key populations. According to the OSI's Jonathon Cohen, speaking during the International AIDS Conference in 2018, Amsterdam, "Right wing politicians are looking for ways to close down NGOs" [43]. This approach is illustrated by Hungary's 'War in Drugs', where needle exchange programmes were closed down as part of a systematic political attack on harm reduction in general [44].

The far-right movement in Europe—often aligned with fundamentalist religious movements—also promotes mechanisms to ban abortion, restrict sexual and reproductive health services, and attempts to 'lock in' traditional family structures. A movement called 'Restoring the Natural Order: An Agenda for Europe' is a robust campaign aiming to ban same-sex marriage, divorce, gay adoption, the sale of pharmaceutical contraceptives, and in-vitro fertilisation (IVF). It will introduce "anti--sodomy legislation" and bans on "gay propaganda" alongside international bans on abortion, stem cell use, and euthanasia. It also seeks the abolition of equality legislation. 'Agenda Europe' is active in a number of European countries and subscribes to the view that there is a 'natural law' to protect life, protect the family, and protect religious freedom [45]. Another example of repression of minority groups in Europe can be seen in Chechnya in 2019, reported by Human Rights Watch [46].

This trend can also be seen in the Russian Federation. Here, the government promotes a socially conservative, hands-off, and often church-influenced approach to sexual and reproductive health and drug policy. This fuels the epidemic with state policies and inaction leading to more cases than ever of Russians contracting or dying from HIV/AIDS [47]. There is also aggressive criminalisation and extreme marginalisation of people who inject drugs. Many are denied access to information about HIV, and highly unlikely to access testing, prevention, or treatment services [only 10% in one study] [48].

Women living with HIV in the Russian Federation, especially young women, face multiple challenges and barriers to accessing HIV services, such as stigma, discrimination, gender stereotyping, violence, and barriers to sexual and reproductive health [49]. Certain laws regulate the availability of information to people under the age of 18 and access to comprehensive sexuality education materials. Sexuality education is not a distinct part of school curricula in the Russian Federation. Healthy lifestyle skills and hygiene are promoted, but the focus is very much on prevention. There is significant opposition to sexuality education from parents, church, traditionalists and some federal and local parliament members [50].

Reflection/Activity Box 4:
What about your own country?
- Are there policies and legislation in place that may impact directly on key populations?
- What can nurses do to address this and make sure the care and support provided for affected people is equitable and inclusive?

7.3.2.2 The Impact

Structural factors therefore directly impact on the well-being of key populations and their access to health services. For example, in many countries where **sex work** is criminalised, sex workers are exposed to to harassment by law enforcement [51]. Anti-prostitution legislation encourages violence towards sex workers which can include verbal, physical and sexual abuse; mandatory HIV testing; public 'naming and shaming' in media; forced evictions; and extortion [52]. Increased risk of violence can put sex workers at greater risk of HIV and other sexually transmitted infections (STI), but they also often face barriers accessing sexual and reproductive health services [3].

Drug users (including injecting drug users) are especially vulnerable, and this is one of the most heavily criminalised communities, a known factor affecting HIV prevention [53]. People who use drugs face unnecessary incarceration for victimless non-violent offenses, police brutality, and widespread violations to their right to health, including failure to provide adequate drug dependence treatment [54]. This can lead to marginalisation and social exclusion, pushing people away from jobs, education, and other health and social services. Crucially, the access of drug users to HIV prevention services—such as needle exchange and testing—can be affected by lack of policy initiatives, or even interest, in addressing the needs of this group. Women who use drugs can be especially affected when attempting to access sexual and reproductive health services, facing a 'double stigma', especially from policies largely being designed for and by men [55].

Men who have sex with men face stigma and discrimination in countries where same-sex relationships are criminalised [56], forcing them to hide their identities and avoid places they expect to be stigmatised, which can include health services. In Vietnam, for example, MSM experience stigma, are affected by poverty, and a lack MSM-friendly services [11]. Where there is specific legislation prohibiting sex between men—in some countries punishable by death—HIV responses are hampered by daily experiences of homophobia, discrimination, violence, and criminalisation. These can have severe and damaging effects on the physical and mental health of MSM and limit their access to and use of vital services [57].

Transgender people are amongst the most brutalized of all marginalised communities, with some countries outlawing transgender men and women altogether. They are at risk of being excluded and marginalised, not completing their education, and resorting to sex work for income. The risk of HIV faced by transgender people is high compared with other populations [58], and HIV response programmes often miss this group due to misclassification of transgender people as MSM or female sex workers [59], or structural stigma.

Banished from her home, Serina was forced to fend for herself and found a job as a bartender in a different town. Here she was able to present as a woman, and this was how the community knew her. Still, Serina's situation presented several challenges. Men in the bar often made advances towards her, but she knew this could put her in danger. "I knew I couldn't get so close to anyone because if they found out [my sex], they would hurt me instead," she said. [Source: Frontline AIDS, 'Serina's journey as a transgender youth in Uganda', https://frontlineaids.org/serinas-journey-as-a-transgender-youth-in-uganda/]

As a vulnerable group, **women and girls** face particular risks. The absolute number of women living with HIV is increasing in Europe, and half of women with HIV are diagnosed late [24]. There are limited data in Europe on the confounding effects of menopause and HIV, though evidence suggests women living with HIV might experience symptoms of menopause earlier [60]. Some girls and women will experience gender-based violence and sexual abuse [61]. Global estimates published by WHO indicate that about 1 in 3 (35%) of women worldwide have experienced either physical and/or sexual intimate partner violence or non-partner sexual violence in their lifetime. Violence negatively affects women's physical, mental, sexual, and reproductive health, and may increase the risk of acquiring HIV. Violence against women can be exacerbated in situations of conflict, post conflict and displacement, all of which may exacerbate existing violence, and lead to new forms of violence against women [62]. This has been evident during the COVID-19 pandemic in 2020 [63].

Blatant denial of rights can be enforced by the police, especially against **sex workers, drug users, asylum seekers, or due to sexual orientation**. Indeed, in many countries, law enforcement is complicit in stigmatising key affected populations and enacting discrimination that denies fair access to justice. According to Vanwesenbeeck [64]:

> Criminalisation (including oppressive anti-trafficking and migration policies) produces (sexual) abuse and exploitation of sex workers, because the whore-stigma legitimizes all sorts of presumptuous behaviour and supports a culture of impunity for violence and aggression.

This includes denying access for sex workers to justice if they are exploited by clients. Some of the issues around the denial of rights are more nuanced. For example, in the case of young people seeking access to sexual and reproductive health, this can in some countries be difficult if they are under 18 years, due to parental consent being required,[1] especially for girls.[2] In the case of MSM, rights are denied where government policies condone harassment and actions that restrict freedoms and support, for example in Jamaica where this has clear implications for the protection of human rights to ensure access to the HIV care cascade [65].

In addition, drug data are often male-focused. There is lack of information, for example, about interactions between the contraceptive pill and antiretroviral treatment (ART), the menopause and ART, and data on U=U in women. This shows a clear need for more women to be enrolled into HIV treatment trials so more information is available [66]. Indeed, this tendency towards the 'generic masculine' or

---

[1] This is the case in the majority of countries worldwide, according to UNAIDS: https://www.unaids.org/en/resources/presscentre/featurestories/2019/april/20190415_gow_parental-consent.

[2] IPPF (2014). Qualitative research on legal barriers to young people's access to sexual and reproductive health services. Available at: https://www.ippf.org/sites/default/files/ippf_coram_final_inception-report_eng_web.pdf.

'default male' is embedded in many cultures and dominates much academic research [67].

Finally, unequal gender norms continue to limit the agency and voice of women, reduce their access to education and economic resources, and "stifle their civic participation", all contributing to amplified HIV risk where there is high HIV prevalence [6].

7.3.3   Health Care: Is It a Safe Haven for Key Populations?

For key and vulnerable populations, when they access health care—once they have surmounted the obstacles—the experience is not always positive. The quality of this interaction is crucial, for it can determine acceptance of an HIV diagnosis and affect retention, especially when health care workers lack HIV knowledge [68]. There are many studies confirming that health care can be an unwelcoming and negative experience for key populations [69]. In the case of sex workers, there can be attribution of blame, pressure to adhere to sexual norms, lack of awareness, blame for an illness [70], and translocated stigma towards their children [71]. From all this there is therefore the possibility that affected people can be stigmatised on at least two levels—association with a virus (HIV), and association with an unpopular group (e.g., MSM, sex worker, or drug user). Chambers *et al* [72] identify particular strategies used in health care settings to manage HIV that can lead to negative outcomes: risk management, fear management, and moral management, coalescing into intersectional stigma.

Both kinds of externalised stigma—perceived and anticipated—have a detrimental effect on HIV reduction strategies, retention in care, and treatment adherence [73]. Reducing stigma can provide a solid foundation on which to develop effective interventions [74]. Constant attention is required to address stigma in health care—otherwise, through social entropy, there is an inevitable drift away from ideal, rights-based care towards exclusive and discriminatory care based on stereotyping and distancing [75].

Health care workers often exhibit the same tendency to categorise—and therefore potentially discriminate—as society in general. This can be based on religion [76], race [77], how 'worthy' is a person's contribution to society [78], or simply a lack of knowledge [79].

Many studies confirm that perceived or anticipated stigma affect access to health care. A priority for health policy in all countries has to be that health care workers are prepared and educated about HIV care generally, and how to support key and vulnerable populations in particular. This can be effective, and in India, for example, following training events, significant post-intervention improvements were seen in both knowledge and attitudes in nursing staff, and a higher tendency to improve than other health care workers [80]. Experience can also count, and in Laos stigmatising attitudes, including discrimination at work, fear of HIV, and prejudice, were lower in healthcare workers with more experience in treating patients with HIV [81].

As well as issues around stigma towards people affected by HIV, there is evidence to suggest health workers are not always suitably prepared for supporting particular key and vulnerable groups, often associated with negative attitudes. This has the potential for a damaging 'double stigma'. Studies suggest this can be directed at sex workers [82], implicit preference for heterosexual men over gay men [83], drug users [84], and transgender people [85]. For women drug users, there can be difficulties accessing sexual and reproductive health services, including HIV prevention and treatment, due to the negative attitudes of health care workers [86]. The situation is made more difficult in health systems that are hierarchical, doctor-led, and slow to adapt to change. In some Eastern European countries, this is a legacy from the Soviet Union.

One vulnerable group that experiences problems accessing HIV prevention and broader sexual and reproductive health services are adolescents. This can be due to unprofessional attitudes of nurses, [87], a lack of targeted and empowering services [88], and limited insights into the unique needs of a young person transitioning into adulthood [89].

In the European context, HIV-related discrimination in health care settings is reported by a number of studies. In one, with data from 14 countries, participants reported higher levels of discrimination by health care providers in Austria (35%), Poland (30%), and Greece (28%) [90]. According to the Stigma Index, from data collected during 2017, though nearly half of respondents in Greece reported supportive responses from health care workers on disclosure of their HIV status, 69 (15%) experienced discriminatory or very discriminatory reactions, and 48 respondents (11%) reported that they had been denied health services, including dental care, because of their HIV status at least once in the previous 12 months [91].

7.3.3.1 The Impact

If nurses specifically, or health systems generally, are not welcoming of people affected by HIV, there are consequences. There can be a dilution in the quality of care [92], implicit acquiescence of unprofessional activities [93], young people affected by HIV being less willing to attend for services [88], problems with treatment adherence [94], and a risk that key populations experience unnecessary suffering from untreated conditions, exclusion from healthcare and extreme psychological distress [70]. There is also a retrograde impact on health care workers themselves, living with stigmatising conditions and concealing their own health status [74].

7.4 Improving Access to Services for Key Populations

7.4.1 General Ways to Improve Services

An overarching principle is that, for prevention and effective ongoing care and treatment of people affected by HIV to be effective, responses have to **focus on those who are most vulnerable and face the greatest burden of disease**, specifically targeting key populations [95]. Key populations experience unnecessary suffering from untreated conditions, exclusion from healthcare, and extreme psychological distress. They also face existing health disparities that require care and support. For example, LGBT youth in the US are at higher risk for substance use, STIs, cancers, cardiovascular diseases, obesity, bullying, isolation, rejection, anxiety, depression, and suicide as compared to the general population [96]. There is also lack of disaggregated data on key populations accessing services, and more specifically their progress on the HIV care cascade [97]. The risk of clumping all key populations together in data reporting can be a barrier to obtaining a clear picture of progress.

There is a need for safe confidential environments, cultural sensitivity training, and public health strategies to reduce stigma and improve and increase access to healthcare for key populations [70]. A *challenge* for HIV prevention, and care delivery is to ensure **suitability for each key population** and adopting a *combination prevention* approach offering a variety of services [98]. Additional complexities are around structural challenges (for example, inequalities or negative attitudes defined by culture), or where factors intersect, for example where a transgender person may be exposed to multiple risks [99].

Therefore, it's vital to ensure support is **targeted.** For example, in the case of people who use drugs, an intervention combining nursing support and harm reduction can be effective in improving outcomes [100]. For adolescents affected by HIV, especially those attending for treatment, providing a 'youth friendly corner', age-appropriate information, and staff trained in supporting young people improves the quality of nurse-patient interactions and willingness to engage [88].

Addressing stigma should be a primary aim. Accepting the reality of stigma in *everyone* is central to this process [25]. Stigma is generic, and how people deal with this and block its translation into discrimination will be an ongoing process of self reflection. Overcoming **self-stigma** in people affected by HIV is also vital [33, 101].

7.4.2   Focus: A Rights-Based Approach

All interventions must be rooted in a rights-based approach. Barriers are often underpinned by a denial of rights. Human rights violations are a reality for many key populations, restricting their access for HIV prevention, care, support, and treatment services. Central to this is the need for information and data, such as the Rights-Evidence-Action initiative (REAct), a system designed by Frontline AIDS, an NGO supporting community-based organisations globally to systematically document human rights violations. This information can then be used to advocate for change.[3]

---

[3] More information is available here: https://frontlineaids.org/resources/reacting-to-reality-taking-action-on-human-rights-violations-against-key-populations/ Accessed 12 Jan 2021.

In many countries there is a great need for change, advocacy, and initiatives that work closely with all stakeholders, including policy makers and law enforcement, to address rights. These have been successful in some places. For example, in Vietnam, significant progress has been made in gathering government support for community-based harm reduction services, tied to the increasing prominence of universal health coverage in that country which, after intensive lobbying, included HIV prevention.[4]

7.4.3 Focus: Communities

Responses to HIV should be universal, contextual, informed, equitable, inclusive, and accountable. For nurses, **an awareness of the specific barriers to key populations accessing services** is an important starting point for how to address need and ensure accessibility. Working at the frontline of health systems, nurses are one of the main gateways for any person wishing to access care and treatment.

What's also important is that services should be **tailored to meet the needs** of key and vulnerable populations. A one-size-fits-all approach is not appropriate for everyone; groups are rarely purely homogenous, especially key populations, just as is the case for all patients, such as heterosexual men [102]. Just because a person is at increased risk of HIV does not mean they have a lot in common with other people at increased risk, apart from the risk itself. Lifestyles vary. Indeed, health care always faces the risk of applying universal interventions regardless of the recipient. This can be shown even in ensuring **men** access services, and more research is needed on male-centred approaches to increase engagement in HIV services, particularly later in the treatment cascade. Interventions targeting men who have sex with men are urgently needed in some countries [103].

One approach can be to **take the services to people in the community**, rather than waiting for them at the clinic door. The notion of using mobile clinics is not in itself new. Allied with innovations around rapid point of care testing over the past decade, community-based testing that provides facilities outside the clinical or health care setting is cost effective [104] and successful in reaching marginalised communities at increased risk of HIV [105]. They provide an important mechanism for expanding access—especially for LGBT people—to testing and support [106] and are an important route into health care and treatment [107]. They are also preferred by beneficiaries [69, 106]. What can be especially effective is to identify, with the community, 'hotspots' where target groups are likely to meet, for example near night clubs, or on beaches.

Some projects expand the services offered by mobile clinics, and include counselling on HIV and STI, distribution of LGBT-oriented education materials, male

---

[4] See: Aidsfonds: https://aidsfonds.org/story/how-to-ensure-communities-affected-by-hiv-in-vietnam-can-access-uhc . Accessed 12 Jan 2021.

and female condoms and lubricant, basic psychosocial counselling, and referral for HIV treatment, STI treatment, and professional psychosocial report. Key prevention messages can be provided for those receiving negative HIV test results, and guidance on being tested every three months, and—should a test be positive—rapid referral to health services, accompanied by staff member from the mobile clinic.[5] This person-centred approach is also a recommended intervention to link, or re-engage, existing HIV patients with care services [108].

Other initiatives that can reach out to communities include **community-based counsellors** that have a key role to play in reducing stigma, promoting resilience, support systems, and—ultimately—access to services [109]. Safe spaces for key populations are also beneficial, providing a safe haven from an intolerant world [110] and a place where people are able to express themselves without fear of being censured [111]. They can be empowering, providing knowledge, information, social networks, and encouragements to improve health seeking behaviour. This is linked to the benefit of community-based support groups—here, there is evidence that they are able to increase the capacity of groups to collectively cope with HIV stigma [112], building resilience for strengthening self-care and greater motivation to seek support and care, *in spite* of the barriers they may face.

7.4.4   Focus: Nurses and Health Care

Since the beginning of the epidemic, nurses have played a key role in providing care for people affected by HIV. They are pivotal in promoting a caring, engaging, and empathetic milieu, where—in theory at least—any person requiring health support can expect to be welcomed. The role of health care workers in the context of HIV should be no different to that of other health issues; approach the person as an individual, and planning interventions to meet identified needs. Even in the early days of HIV, nurses caring for what was then an unknown and fearful disease applied their existing knowledge and skills to care for those affected—the essence was no different, with patients' needs falling clearly into the nursing domain [113].

Historically, however, stigma of HIV and of key populations have proved barriers in ensuring treatment and care are available. Confidentiality, always a priority, is probably even more acute in the context of HIV: "confidentiality is important for people living with HIV because of the impact breaches have" [114], p. 16. Studies confirm that some HIV service users are afraid of confidentiality breaches [115].

What is known is that **nurse-led services** have proven effective in many countries. They improve the experience of patients just after diagnosis, maximise treatment management and adherence, have general comparable clinical outcomes as physician-led care, can improve mental health, and potentially improve overall

---

[5] An example of such a project is here: https://frontlineaids.org/we-have-an-impact-in/eastern-and-southern-africa/mozambique/ . Accessed 12 Jan 2021.

satisfaction [68, 116–118]. There is certainly scope for providing a greater proportion of routine care in nurse-led clinics, especially in the community, where there can be improved health outcomes [119]. Integrative or combination approaches to centralising services may also lead to stigma reduction and remove logistical barriers to meet the needs of key populations [120]. However, engaging with patients who are 'hard to reach' is a challenge for all those working in health care, and there is not always agreement on what this means [121]. Barriers to patients engaging with services have already been discussed, but, given that nurses are at the frontline, what can be done to maximise access?

Firstly, nurses should be **culturally competent,** for example around the lived experience of the LGBT community [122, 123]. To illustrate, nurses inadequately trained to support MSM discourage them from seeking HIV prevention and treatment [124]. There are many examples of interventions aimed at health care workers to ensure they are able to deliver high quality and equitable services for key populations. In the case of LGBT people, education can improve the quality of support provided by health care workers. In Mozambique, for example, a national project working specifically with LGBT communities provided targeted training for health care workers who are already experienced in providing HIV care in what is a generalised epidemic, but with limited experience of LGBT people.[6] This project also included the provision of safe spaces for LGBT people, which is highly valued by the community.

This is linked to the importance of shaping services to fit with clients' needs— this applies to all HIV nursing [125], not just when supporting marginalised groups. For example, in the case of young people, there can be a mismatch between adolescents' and health providers' views on youth-friendly services, service preferences, barriers and enablers of service use [87]. Here, service providers viewed physical and financial factors as the key barriers, whereas for adolescents it is the health care providers' attitudes that is the biggest hindrance. Indeed, services can also be tailored for people who experience problems with treatment, and beginning their second or third treatment regime, and this can have significant impact on adherence [126]. Shaping services to client needs can be as basic as flexible hours, follow-up visits, convenient and private access to care, and integrating testing and screening. For patients with logistical or financial problems due to their **immigration status**, additional mechanisms will need adding, and for undocumented migrants in particular, restricted access to ART is a real threat in some countries [127].

Second, there is a **moral imperative** to connect with key populations that naturally emerges from cultural competence and feeds directly into the notion of a **therapeutic relationship** with a person—the foundation of nursing interventions [128]. Nursing care is in a prime position to act *against* prevailing views, belief frameworks, and political expediency, in order to seek a meaningful relationship with patients who have specific and often complex needs. In the case of key populations, these needs

---

[6] Information about the programme is here: https://frontlineaids.org/our-work-includes/deep-engagement-mozambique/. Accessed June 2020.

are likely to be a web of physical, psychological, and socio-economic factors, often accompanied by ostracization from support systems, and memories of past negative experiences of health care. For them, violation of their rights is likely to be a common occurrence. In the context of advanced disease, "where clinical treatments have achieved all they can, what is left is human compassion and empathy" [113].

Underpinning all this, health care workers must be **educated** about HIV, the nature of risk, and ensure they are aware of the notion of universal risk, which assumes all people are potentially HIV infected. This prevents making assumptions about a particular individual's risk or non-risk. For example, in Zimbabwe, training and sensitisation events around sex workers for health care providers, especially targeting discriminatory practices, has been linked with improved access to HIV and sexual health services [129]. Studies suggest there are significant benefits resulting from sensitisation training [130], and have a positive impact on knowledge and some impact on attitudes, though these can be more intransigent [131]. Interventions to improve providers' skills in HIV services for MSM may not be met by the healthcare sector alone and may need policy and structural approaches— including community sensitisation—to promote effective care [70, 124]. Indeed, HIV nurse specialists may be best placed overall to provide care for all people affected by HIV [110].

An important part of the process of learning should be around self-awareness— addressing the unconscious, but still damaging, tendency for all people (including health care workers) to stigmatise, categorise, and avoid individuals and groups they may perceive as unacceptable or 'different' in some way, often tied with some form of judgement. It should never be assumed that a person working in healthcare, or for that matter any profession deemed to be altruistic, is necessarily free of a stigmatising tendency [25]. This is covered further in Chap. 14 of this text.

This can include training around patient engagement, and effective communication with people who may already feel marginalised and excluded from mainstream services. Offering the 'safe haven' of health care—consistent with moral and ethical imperatives—is something that needs to be worked on and maintained. This includes ensuring health care workers are satisfactorily prepared to provide whatever support is required for a person, regardless of their status and background. This seems a moot point, but sadly, as other parts of this discussion suggest, it is not. One study, Rouleau [128], highlights the various components required to ensure best practice in the promotion of ART adherence. One of these, building a therapeutic relationship with a people affected by HIV, is the foundation of HIV nursing care, and indeed **patient engagement** is crucial throughout the patient's journey. This can include shared decision-making, which takes into account the *patient's life and promote empowerment*, and effective communication, which takes into account the *patient's need for information to act and retain agency*. Shared decision making, an approach recommended by many nursing and medical guidelines, can be defined as:

> A process in which clinicians and patients work together to clarify treatment, management or self- management support goals, sharing information about options and preferred outcomes with the aim of reaching mutual agreement on the best course of action. [132]

Shared decision making is challenging for nurses because of organisational and health system factors [133], but has the advantage of allowing for the *patient's* needs, perspectives, and views to be taken into consideration. This is predicated on **effective communication**, where multiple methods of communication can enhance clinical outcomes [134], but where each on its own is likely to have less impact.

7.4.5   Case Study

All the initiatives above should, of course, be for all patients. For HIV key populations, who may already be experiencing complex lifestyles and facing a number of existing barriers, they are crucial. The following case study illustrates just some of these complexities in the context of human trafficking, shared by an HIV nurse based in Finland.[7]

7.4.5.1   Background: Human Trafficking

A human trafficker takes advantage of a vulnerable person, mainly financially. Trafficking in human beings often involves foreigners such as asylum seekers. A victim can be a woman, man, or even a child. He or she can be paperless, homeless or a drug user. A victim can be someone's spouse or relative. He or she can be sexually exploited in the sex trade. A victim may be pressured into criminal activity, forced marriages or begging. A victim of human trafficking is often dependent and subordinate to the abuser. A person may not have opportunity to understand how the situation could be overcome, and housing, food, and health care may only be possible through an exploiter.

7.4.5.2   The Experience of 'Mary'

Mary [not her real name] came to the Helsinki HIV Clinic in the summer of 2010. She was an asylum seeker from Nigeria. After coming to Finland, she lived in the immigration centre in the Eastern part of Finland, where she was diagnosed with HIV. Mary first moved from Nigeria to Spain in 2005, and according to her she was promised a better life there. She worked there as a sex-worker and says that she has always used a condom though, from time to time, this may not have been used properly. She has no family ties to Nigeria and says she hasn't used intravenous drugs.

After moving to Finland, Mary lived in an apartment with three men, paying her rent by cleaning. The social worker at the immigration centre made a home visit and

---

[7] Thanks to Helena Mäkinen, Triangle Hospital, Clinic for Infectious Diseases, Hospital District of Helsinki and Uusimaa (HUS), and board member of the Finnish Association of Nurses in AIDS Care, for compiling this case study.

found that the three slept on mattresses on the floor. When asked if Mary could store her HIV medication in the apartment, she said no, they are kept in her handbag.

7.4.5.3 Initial Support

At the clinic, I discussed HIV infection with her and the importance of taking medication regularly to reduce the viral load and increase her CD4 count. I also told her about the obligation to always tell sexual partners about HIV infection. I informed Mary about the activities and contact information of peer support at non--governmental organisations like Protukipiste unit, Hiv Finland and Hivpoint. Mary also asked about the possibility of pregnancy. She seemed to understand when I told her of the difficulties, and I gave her our contact numbers for if she has problems outside of office hours when starting medications or in case of post exposure situations.

At a later meeting, Mary says she's having trouble with her boyfriend, who is HIV-negative and has questions about when Mary became infected with HIV. Our psychiatric nurse was also offered help, but Mary didn't want this. She says there is a lot to think about.

7.4.5.4 Pregnancy

Mary did not appear for a planned meeting 3 weeks afterwards for her medication, laboratory test, and x-ray scan. I called Mary, but she could not speak properly, and it was hard to hear her clearly. Mary says she has a problem. She is pregnant. I asked if she has been taking her HIV medication, which should finish on the same day. She said they had finished this week. I asked her to come as soon as possible. The next day Mary comes to the clinic and is very unhappy about living with HIV. "Why her?" she asks. Mary says she is pregnant, and her roommate is the father. A condom had failed but Mary has decided to have the baby, which the father is happy with. There is currently no electricity in the home because the main tenant has not paid the electricity bill. Yesterday, Mary ate food at the store and was caught and fined. She later met with a doctor and is angry after the doctor expressed concerns are expressed about the health of Mary and the baby, especially if she does not take her medications regularly. Mary doesn't want to come here every day to take medication under supervision. She has moved to the Shelter Mona (Multicultural Women's Association), a non-governmental organisation. There she has her own room where she cooks the food. We arranged supervised medication at the shelter.

The following day, Mary has gestational nausea. We discuss how she can make it easier. Later, a nurse from the Shelter Mona calls saying that Mary has refused to take her HIV medication. After a long discussion with me, she took her medicine. Soon afterwards, Mary was moved to the third immigration centre, supporting victims of human trafficking and located 250 km from Helsinki.

7.4.5.5 6 Months Later: Relocation

A nurse from immigration centre called many times. Mary is not taking her HIV medication and her viral load has not decreased. The caesarean section is planned for just over a month. Mary is travelling to meet me in Helsinki next week. I also discussed about the situation with the doctors. We decided to continue to support Mary with HIV medication. We meet with Mary several times a week, and she is currently in Shelter Mona once again.

7.4.5.6 Delivery

Mary has the caesarean section and gives birth to a healthy child. But there are problems with treatment adherence. She lives in a shelter with the child, and I meet with Mary. Mary denies taking her HIV medication during pregnancy. I thought after reading the materials for Human trafficking training and I wondered if this was her only way and means decide on her own body and actions. Later she was adherent to medication.

Mary told me about her experience with voodoo. Perhaps a part of the refusal to take medication was caused by this. Often, she would say to me, "Drugs are poison. Things are spiritual, not physical."

7.4.5.7 Case Study: Questions for Reflection

1. As a person who has been trafficked, what were the barriers facing Mary accessing the health system? What were within her control, and what were outside her control?
2. What preparation would an HIV nurse need to care for someone in Mary's situation?
3. In your country, what options could be made available to support Mary?

7.5 Recommendations

This chapter has focussed on issues facing key and vulnerable populations accessing HIV care, prevention, and support services. Recommendations can be at three levels: for nursing, in the community, and for policy and planning.

7.5.1 Nursing

- Nurses are at the forefront to promote a service accessible to key populations, and nurse-led services are proven to be beneficial, especially in resource-poor areas. **Training** is vital to ensure they are suitably prepared, not just in the mechanics of HIV (including care for affected people, and in prevention), but in the best ways to work with key populations, some of whom will be members of groups that society already marginalises. Consideration of the **moral imperative** of nursing can be emphasised—a key factor in the early days of the HIV epidemic, and a continuing priority to ensure care is available and equitable.

- **Professional communication skills** are required to enable patients to share key aspects of identity and behaviour must be combined with enforcement of professional standards that require anti-discriminatory practice [70].
- The **environment** of care is important. How flexible is the service? Is it tailored to needs? Does it allow for a lifestyle that may be unpredictable? Is there suitable privacy? Are resources available? Drawing on current research on best practices for interventions studies [finding out what works best] should be a priority for retaining people in treatment and care, for example in the case of young people [135].
- **Networking** and information sharing are both vital, especially in the changing context of HIV.

7.5.2 Community

- **Point of care testing** is a proven methodology for improving access—taking the service to people in the community, rather than expecting them to attend a clinical setting. Explore and test multi-faceted interventions going *beyond health facilities* to address broader social barriers to adherence and retention.
- **Working with community leaders** to increase sensitisation and knowledge about HIV and the increased risk that faces key populations. Depending on the country, this can include liaising with law enforcement and policy makers to highlight ways that key populations can be protected and to promote more willingness for self-care, and enthusiasm to attend health services.
- **Working with community-based organisations** to provide integrated care and support services, and to learn what care interventions are best suited for particular people and groups.
- **Working with families** can be beneficial in reducing stigma and creating another support mechanism—especially in the case of young LGBT.

7.5.3 Policy and Planning

- Policy must enshrine non-discrimination for key populations with respect to access to public services [70].
- Explore a lifecycle approach:
  - Developing a more holistic and person-centred approach to care, integrating health and social systems, peer support services, and up-to-date technology for testing.

- Taking into account the impact of poverty, homelessness, gender-based discrimination, social exclusion, and isolation.

• Policymakers, those designing health professional training, and medical professionals, need to collaborate with organisations supporting key populations, who often have stronger groups/networks than health care workers.
• Consider the value of global initiatives, such as the drive for Universal Health Coverage (UHC), where all people and communities can use health services they need, that they are of sufficient quality to be effective, and not exposing the user to financial hardship. UHC has a key step relating to this chapter, 'Promote the right to health, including non-discrimination and gender equality', and has three objectives:

- Equity in access to health services.
- The quality of health services should be good enough to improve the health of those receiving services.
- People should be protected against financial risk, ensuring that the cost of using services does not put people at risk of financial harm.

7.6 Concluding Comments

This chapter has discussed issues facing key and vulnerable populations who face difficulties accessing HIV services. There can be a number of barriers, depending on location, the reason they are at increased risk in the first place, and the nature of services available to them. There are also powerful social and cultural reasons why it may be harder for this group to receive the care they require, such as the social and political environment, culture, and the influence of religion on shaping attitudes.

A number of solutions are offered that can improve access, though these are predicated on an educated and empathetic health care workforce committed to engaging with people in ways that may go against prevailing attitudes in the health system and the broader public domain. All approaches should be founded on the bedrock of human rights, which stands as a benchmark and gold standard against which all interventions can be measured. There is also a degree of self-learning required, as health care workers address their own ingrained attitudes. Willingness to begin this journey will be hard but will bear fruit—the quality of care and support for those at increased risk of HIV can only be strengthened. This includes prevention and will go some way towards meeting the ultimate goal of eradicating AIDS by 2030.

Learning Points

1. Whilst a risk for any person, certain key and vulnerable populations are at increased risk of HIV requiring effective prevention, support, and care services.

2. Key and vulnerable populations face particular challenges accessing HIV prevention and care services due to stigma, structural challenges, and an unprepared workforce.
3. Services require a rights-based, community-engaged approach that is ideally nurse-led to ensure all people requiring care and support have their needs addressed.
4. Health policies should reflect the principles of universal health coverage underpinned by principles of equity of access, quality-led, and holism to protect and improve the quality of life of all people affected by HIV, especially key and vulnerable populations.

References

1. UNAIDS. HIV and universal health coverage—a guide for civil society. Geneva: UNAIDS; 2019. https://www.unaids.org/en/resources/documents/2019/hiv-uhc-guide-civil-society. Accessed 12 Jan 2021.
2. Dingake OBK. The state of human rights in relation to key populations, HIV and sexual and reproductive health. Reprod Health Matter. 2018;26(52):46–50.
3. World Health Organisation. Consolidated guidelines on HIV prevention, diagnosis, treatment, and care for key populations. Geneva: World Health Organisation; 2016. https://www.who.int/hiv/pub/guidelines/keypopulations/en/. Accessed 12 Jan 2021.
4. UNAIDS. AIDS data 2019. Geneva: UNAIDS; 2019. https://www.unaids.org/sites/default/files/media_asset/2019-UNAIDS-data_en.pdf. Accessed 11 Jan 2021.
5. Osborne K. Human rights for key populations: words count and actions matter. Devex. 2016. https://www.devex.com/news/human-rights-for-key-populations-words-count-and-actions-matter-87515. Accessed 12 Jan 2021.
6. UNAIDS. Seizing the moment: tackling entrenched inequalities to end epidemics. Geneva: UNAIDS; 2020.
7. Centers for Disease Control and Prevention. HIV transmission. Atlanta: CDC; 2018. https://www.cdc.gov/hiv/basics/transmission.html. Accessed 11 Jan 2021.
8. UNAIDS. Miles to go: closing gaps, breaking barriers, righting injustices. Geneva: UNAIDS; 2018. https://www.unaids.org/sites/default/files/media_asset/miles-to-go_en.pdf. Accessed 11 Jan 2021.
9. Rodger AJ, Cambiano V, Bruun T, Vernazza P, Collins S, Degen O, et al. Risk of HIV transmission through condomless sex in serodifferent gay couples with the HIV-positive partner taking suppressive antiretroviral therapy (PARTNER): final results of a multicentre, prospective, observational study. Lancet. 2019;393(10189):2428–38.
10. The Lancet H. U=U taking off in 2017. Lancet HIV. 2017;4(11):e475.
11. Philbin MM, Hirsch JS, Wilson PA, Ly AT, Giang LM, Parker RG. Structural barriers to HIV prevention among men who have sex with men (MSM) in Vietnam: diversity, stigma, and healthcare access. PLoS One. 2018;13(4):e0195000.
12. Ziraba A, Orindi B, Muuo S, Floyd S, Birdthistle IJ, Mumah J, et al. Understanding HIV risks among adolescent girls and young women in informal settlements of Nairobi, Kenya: lessons for DREAMS. PLoS One. 2018;13(5):e0197479.
13. Decker MR, Crago AL, Chu SK, Sherman SG, Seshu MS, Buthelezi K, et al. Human rights violations against sex workers: burden and effect on HIV. Lancet. 2015;385(9963):186–99.
14. Frontline AIDS. A report of the SHARP Programme. Hove, UK: Frontline AIDS; 2016. https://frontlineaids.org/resources/a-report-of-the-sharp-programme/. Accessed 11 Jan 2021.

15. Germain A, Sen G, Garcia-Moreno C, Shankar M. Advancing sexual and reproductive health and rights in low- and middle-income countries: implications for the post-2015 global development agenda. Glob Public Health. 2015;10(2):137–48.
16. UNAIDS. The gap report: people with disabilities. Geneva: UNAIDS; 2014. https://www.unaids.org/sites/default/files/media_asset/11_Peoplewithdisabilities.pdf. Accessed 11 Jan 2021.
17. Ross J, Cunningham CO, Hanna DB. HIV outcomes among migrants from low-income and middle-income countries living in high-income countries: a review of recent evidence. Curr Opin Infect Dis. 2018;31(1):25–32.
18. Slamah K. Mama Tini talk of services for transgender women in Malaysia. Bangkok. 2020. https://www.apcom.org/mama-tini-talk-of-services-for-transgender-women-in-malaysia/. Accessed 10 July 2020.
19. UNAIDS. UNAIDS report on the global AIDS epidemic shows that 2020 targets will not be met because of deeply unequal success; COVID-19 risks blowing HIV progress way off course [Press Release]. Geneva: UNAIDS; 2020. https://www.unaids.org/en/resources/press-centre/pressreleaseandstatementarchive/2020/july/20200706_global-aids-report. Accessed 6 July 2020.
20. World Health Organisation. Global health estimates 2015: deaths by cause, age, sex, by country and by region, 2000–2015. Geneva: World Health Organisation; 2015. https://www.who.int/healthinfo/global_burden_disease/estimates_regional_2000_2015/en/. Accessed 12 Jan 2021.
21. UNAIDS. When women lead change happens. Geneva: UNAIDS; 2017.
22. Finnerty F, Azad Y, Orkin C. Hostile health-care environment could increase migrants' risk of HIV and prevent access to vital services. Lancet HIV. 2019;6(2):e76.
23. De Beaudrap P, Beninguisse G, Pasquier E, Tchoumkeu A, Touko A, Essomba F, et al. Prevalence of HIV infection among people with disabilities: a population-based observational study in Yaounde, Cameroon (HandiVIH). Lancet HIV. 2017;4(4):e161–e8.
24. European Centre for Disease Prevention and Control/WHO Regional Office for Europe (ECDC). HIV/AIDS surveillance in Europe 2019–2018 data. Stockholm: ECDC; 2019. https://www.ecdc.europa.eu/en/publications-data/hivaids-surveillance-europe-2019-2018-data. Accessed 12 Jan 2021.
25. Hodgson I. Stigma and HIV—Time for a New Paradigm? Stigma Res Action. 2011;2:42–5.
26. Goffman E. Stigma: notes on the management of spoiled identity. Englewood Cliffs, NJ: Prentice-Hall; 1963.
27. Earnshaw VA, Chaudoir SR. From conceptualizing to measuring HIV stigma: a review of HIV stigma mechanism measures. AIDS Behav. 2009;13(6):1160–77.
28. Logie CH, Lessons learned from HIV. can inform our approach to COVID-19 stigma. J Int AIDS Soc. 2020;23(5):e25504.
29. Sontag S. AIDS and its metaphors. Harmondsworth: Penguin; 1991.
30. Kleinman A. Patients and healers in the context of culture: an exploration of the borderland between anthropology, medicine, and psychiatry. Berkeley: University of California Press; 1980. xvi-427 p.
31. Link BG, Struening EL, Rahav M, Phelan JC, Nuttbrock L. On stigma and its consequences: evidence from a longitudinal study of men with dual diagnoses of mental illness and substance abuse. J Health Soc Behav. 1997;38(2):177–90.
32. Courtwright A, Turner AN. Tuberculosis and stigmatization: pathways and interventions. Public Health Rep. 2010;125(Suppl 4):34–42.
33. France NF, McDonald SH, Conroy RR, Byrne E, Mallouris C, Hodgson I, et al. An unspoken world of unspoken things: a study identifying and exploring core beliefs underlying self-stigma among people living with HIV and AIDS in Ireland. Swiss Med Wkly. 2015;145:w14113.
34. Maharjan S, Panthee B. Prevalence of self-stigma and its association with self-esteem among psychiatric patients in a Nepalese teaching hospital: a cross-sectional study. BMC Psychiatry. 2019;19(1):347.

35. Livingston JD, Boyd JE. Correlates and consequences of internalized stigma for people living with mental illness: a systematic review and meta-analysis. Soc Sci Med. 2010;71(12):2150–61.

36. Tomiyama AJ, Carr D, Granberg EM, Major B, Robinson E, Sutin AR, et al. How and why weight stigma drives the obesity 'epidemic' and harms health. BMC Med. 2018;16(1):123.

37. Pantelic M, Steinert JI, Park J, Mellors S, Murau F. Management of a spoiled identity: systematic review of interventions to address self-stigma among people living with and affected by HIV. BMJ Glob Health. 2019;4(2):e001285.

38. European Centre for Disease Prevention and Control/WHO Regional Office for Europe (ECDC). HIV/AIDS surveillance in Europe 2017–2016 data. Stockholm: ECDC; 2017. https://www.ecdc.europa.eu/en/publications-data/hivaids-surveillance-europe-2017-2016-data. Accessed 12 Jan 2021.

39. Gesesew HA, Tesfay Gebremedhin A, Demissie TD, Kerie MW, Sudhakar M, Mwanri L. Significant association between perceived HIV related stigma and late presentation for HIV/AIDS care in low and middle-income countries: a systematic review and meta-analysis. PLoS One. 2017;12(3):e0173928.

40. Sobrino-Vegas P, Moreno S, Rubio R, Viciana P, Bernardino JI, Blanco JR, et al. Impact of late presentation of HIV infection on short-, mid- and long-term mortality and causes of death in a multicenter national cohort: 2004–2013. J Inf Secur. 2016;72(5):587–96.

41. Relf MV. What's old is new! similarities between SARS-CoV-2 and HIV. J Assoc Nurses AIDS Care. 2020;31(3):263–5.

42. Global Fund. Technical brief on HIV and key populations Programming at scale with sex workers, men who have sex with men, transgender people, people who inject drugs, and people in prison and other closed settings. Geneva: The Global Fund; 2019. https://www.theglobalfund.org/media/4794/core_keypopulations_technicalbrief_en.pdf. Accessed 12 Jan 2021.

43. Cohen J. Civil society under threat: how can HIV advocates resist the impact? Conservative populism and social exclusion of civil society. Amsterdam: International AIDS Conference; 2018. http://programme.aids2018.org/Programme/Session/44. Accessed 12 Jan 2021.

44. Gyarmathy VA, Csak R, Balint K, Bene E, Varga AE, Varga M, et al. A needle in the haystack-the dire straits of needle exchange in Hungary. BMC Public Health. 2016;16:157.

45. Datta N. 'Agenda Europe': an extremist Christian network in the heart of Europe. Berlin: Gunda Werner Institute; 2019. https://www.gwi-boell.de/en/2019/04/29/agenda-europe-extremist-christian-network-heart-europe. Accessed 12 January 2021.

46. Human Rights Watch. Russia: new anti-gay crackdown in Chechnya. New York, 2019. https://www.hrw.org/news/2019/05/08/russia-new-anti-gay-crackdown-chechnya? Accessed 12 Jan 2021.

47. Cohen J, Friedman M. Russia's HIV/AIDS epidemic is getting worse, not better. Washington, DC: Pulitzer Centre; 2018. https://pulitzercenter.org/reporting/russias-hivaids-epidemic-getting-worse-not-better. Accessed 12 Jan 2021.

48. Heimer R, Usacheva N, Barbour R, Niccolai LM, Uuskula A, Levina OS. Engagement in HIV care and its correlates among people who inject drugs in St Petersburg, Russian Federation and Kohtla-Jarve, Estonia. Addiction. 2017;112(8):1421–31.

49. UNAIDS. Russian experts and civil society leaders join UNAIDS' Hands Up #HIVprevention campaign (Update). Geneva: UNAIDS; 2016. https://www.unaids.org/en/resources/presscentre/featurestories/2016/october/20161013_stpetersburg. Accessed 12 Jan 2021.

50. IPPF and BZgA. Sexuality education in the WHO European Region: the Russian Federation. Germany: The Federal Centre for Health Education (BZgA); 2018.

51. Human Rights Watch. Why sex work should be decriminalized. New York. 2019. https://www.hrw.org/news/2019/08/07/why-sex-work-should-be-decriminalized. Accessed 19 June 2020.

52. STOPAIDS. Factsheet: sex work, HIV and human rights. London: STOPAIDS; 2015. https://stopaids.org.uk/wp/wp-content/uploads/2017/06/STOPAIDS-factsheet-sex-work.pdf. Accessed 19 June 2020.

53. DeBeck K, Cheng T, Montaner JS, Beyrer C, Elliott R, Sherman S, et al. HIV and the criminalisation of drug use among people who inject drugs: a systematic review. Lancet HIV. 2017;4(8):e357–e74.
54. UNAIDS. Prevention gap report. Geneva: UNAIDS; 2016. https://www.unaids.org/sites/default/files/media_asset/2016-prevention-gap-report_en.pdf. Accessed 12 Jan 2021.
55. Frontline AIDS. Invisible and ignored: how can women who use drugs demand their sexual and reproductive health and rights? Hove, UK. 2019. https://frontlineaids.org/wp-content/uploads/2019/05/GCL-handout_formatted_updated.pdf. Accessed 12 Jan 2021.
56. Ferguson L, Nicholson A, Henry I, Saha A, Sellers T, Gruskin S. Assessing changes in HIV-related legal and policy environments: lessons learned from a multi-country evaluation. PLoS One. 2018;13(2):e0192765.
57. UNFPA. Implementing comprehensive HIV and STI programmes with men who have sex with men. Geneva: UNFPA; 2015. https://www.unfpa.org/sites/default/files/pub-pdf/MSMIT_for_Web.pdf. Accessed 12 Jan 2021.
58. Baral SD, Poteat T, Stromdahl S, Wirtz AL, Guadamuz TE, Beyrer C. Worldwide burden of HIV in transgender women: a systematic review and meta-analysis. Lancet Infect Dis. 2013;13(3):214–22.
59. Poteat T, Wirtz AL, Radix A, Borquez A, Silva-Santisteban A, Deutsch MB, et al. HIV risk and preventive interventions in transgender women sex workers. Lancet. 2015;385(9964):274–86.
60. Kang M, Fantry L. Menopause in HIV-infected women. J Clin Outcomes Manag. 2016;23:1.
61. European AIDS Treatment Group. Meaningful engagement of women in HIV treatment research [METRODORA]. Brussels: EATG; 2018.
62. World Health Organisation. Fact sheet: violence against women. Geneva: World Health Organisation; 2017. https://www.who.int/news-room/fact-sheets/detail/violence-against-women. Accessed 12 Jan 2021.
63. IPPF. COVID-19 and the rise of gender-based violence. London, IPPF; 2020. https://www.ippf.org/blogs/covid-19-and-rise-gender-based-violence. Accessed 12 Jan 2021.
64. Vanwesenbeeck I. Sex work criminalization is barking up the wrong tree. Arch Sex Behav. 2017;46(6):1631–40.
65. Logie CH, Lacombe-Duncan A, Kenny KS, Levermore K, Jones N, Marshall A, et al. Associations between Police Harassment and HIV vulnerabilities among men who have sex with men and transgender women in Jamaica. Health Hum Rights. 2017;19(2):147–54.
66. Curno MJ, Rossi S, Hodges-Mameletzis I, Johnston R, Price MA, Heidari SA. Systematic review of the inclusion (or exclusion) of women in HIV research: from clinical studies of anti-retrovirals and vaccines to cure strategies. J Acquir Immune Defic Syndr. 2016;71(2):181–8.
67. Criado-Perez C. Invisible women: exposing data bias in a world designed for men. London: Vintage; 2019.
68. Imazu Y, Matsuyama N, Takebayashi S, Mori M, Watabe S. Experiences of patients with HIV/AIDS receiving mid- and long-term care in Japan: a qualitative study. Int J Nurs Sci. 2017;4(2):99–104.
69. Bekker LG. HIV control in young key populations in Africa. Lancet Child Adolesc Health. 2019;3(7):442–4.
70. Hunt J, Bristowe K, Chidyamatare S, Harding R. 'They will be afraid to touch you': LGBTI people and sex workers' experiences of accessing healthcare in Zimbabwe-an in-depth qualitative study. BMJ Glob Health. 2017;2(2):e000168.
71. Willis BM, Hodgson I, Lovich R. The health and social well-being of female sex workers' children in Bangladesh: a qualitative study from Dhaka, Chittagong, and Sylhet. Vulnerable Children and Youth Studies: An International Interdisciplinary Journal for Research, Policy and Care. 2013.
72. Chambers LA, Rueda S, Baker DN, Wilson MG, Deutsch R, Raeifar E, et al. Stigma, HIV and health: a qualitative synthesis. BMC Public Health. 2015;15:848.
73. Nyblade L, Addo NA, Atuahene K, Alsoufi N, Gyamera E, Jacinthe S, et al. Results from a difference-in-differences evaluation of health facility HIV and key population stigma-reduction interventions in Ghana. J Int AIDS Soc. 2020;23(4):e25483.

74. Nyblade L, Stockton MA, Giger K, Bond V, Ekstrand ML, Lean RM, et al. Stigma in health facilities: why it matters and how we can change it. BMC Med. 2019;17(1):25.

75. Hodgson I. Attitudes towards people with HIV/AIDS: entropy and health care ethics. J Adv Nurs. 1997;26(2):283–8.

76. Reyes-Estrada M, Varas-Diaz N, Parker R, Padilla M, Rodriguez-Madera S. Religion and HIV-related stigma among nurses who work with people living with HIV/AIDS in Puerto Rico. J Int Assoc Provid AIDS Care. 2018;17:2325958218773365.

77. Stringer KL, Turan B, McCormick L, Durojaiye M, Nyblade L, Kempf MC, et al. HIV-related stigma among healthcare providers in the deep South. AIDS Behav. 2016;20(1):115–25.

78. Reidpath D, Chan KY, Gifford S, Allotey P. 'He has the French pox': stigma, social value and social exclusion. Sociol Health Illn. 2005;27(4):468–89.

79. Gagnon M, Cator S. Mapping HIV nursing core competencies in entry-level education: a pilot project. J Nurs Educ. 2015;54(7):409–15.

80. Machowska A, Bamboria BL, Bercan C, Sharma M. Impact of 'HIV-related stigma-reduction workshops' on knowledge and attitude of healthcare providers and students in Central India: a pre-test and post-test intervention study. BMJ Open. 2020;10(4):e033612.

81. Vorasane S, Jimba M, Kikuchi K, Yasuoka J, Nanishi K, Durham J, et al. An investigation of stigmatizing attitudes towards people living with HIV/AIDS by doctors and nurses in Vientiane, Lao PDR. BMC Health Serv Res. 2017;17(1):125.

82. Mtetwa S, Busza J, Chidiya S, Mungofa S, Cowan F. "You are wasting our drugs": health service barriers to HIV treatment for sex workers in Zimbabwe. BMC Public Health. 2013;13:698.

83. Sabin JA, Riskind RG, Nosek BA. Health care providers' implicit and explicit attitudes toward lesbian women and gay men. Am J Public Health. 2015;105(9):1831–41.

84. Lan CW, Lin C, Thanh DC, Li L. Drug-related stigma and access to care among people who inject drugs in Vietnam. Drug Alcohol Rev. 2018;37(3):333–9.

85. Stroumsa D. The state of transgender health care: policy, law, and medical frameworks. Am J Public Health. 2014;104(3):e31–8.

86. Sharma V, Sarna A, Tun W, Saraswati LR, Thior I, Madan I, et al. Women and substance use: a qualitative study on sexual and reproductive health of women who use drugs in Delhi, India. BMJ Open. 2017;7(11):e018530.

87. Onukwugha FI, Hayter M, Magadi MA. Views of service providers and adolescents on use of sexual and reproductive health services by adolescents: a systematic review. Afr J Reprod Health. 2019;23(2):134–47.

88. Hodgson I, Ross J, Haamujompa C, Gitau-Mburu D. Living as an adolescent with HIV in Zambia—lived experiences, sexual health and reproductive needs. AIDS Care. 2012;24(10):1204–10.

89. Ojwang VO, Penner J, Blat C, Agot K, Bukusi EA, Cohen CR. Loss to follow-up among youth accessing outpatient HIV care and treatment services in Kisumu, Kenya. AIDS Care. 2016;28(4):500–7.

90. Nostlinger C, Rojas Castro D, Platteau T, Dias S, Le Gall J. HIV-related discrimination in European health care settings. AIDS Patient Care STDs. 2014;28(3):155–61.

91. The Greek Association of PLHIV—Positive Voice. Stigma Index: Greece. Athens: The Greek Association of PLHIV—Positive Voice; 2017. https://www.stigmaindex.org/wp-content/uploads/2019/11/Greece_PLHIV-Stigma-Index-Report_2017_English.pdf. Accessed 12 Jan 2021.

92. Rahmati-Najarkolaei F, Niknami S, Aminshokravi F, Bazargan M, Ahmadi F, Hadjizadeh E, et al. Experiences of stigma in healthcare settings among adults living with HIV in the Islamic Republic of Iran. J Int AIDS Soc. 2010;13:27.

93. Nyblade L, Srinivasan K, Mazur A, Raj T, Patil DS, Devadass D, et al. HIV stigma reduction for health facility staff: development of a blended- learning intervention. Front Public Health. 2018;6:165.

94. Katz IT, Ryu AE, Onuegbu AG, Psaros C, Weiser SD, Bangsberg DR, et al. Impact of HIV-related stigma on treatment adherence: systematic review and meta-synthesis. J Int AIDS Soc. 2013;16(3 Suppl 2):18640.
95. Sharma A, Teltschik A, Davies L. HIV and key populations. Hive, UK: Frontline AIDS/GNP+/Stop AIDS Now! 2015. https://gnpplus.net/wp-content/uploads/2015/05/Community-Guide_I_HIV-and-key-populations-1.pdf. Accessed 12 Jan 2021.
96. Hafeez H, Zeshan M, Tahir MA, Jahan N, Naveed S. Health care disparities among lesbian, gay, bisexual, and transgender youth: a literature review. Cureus. 2017;9(4):e1184.
97. Risher K, Mayer KH, Beyrer C. HIV treatment cascade in MSM, people who inject drugs, and sex workers. Curr Opin HIV AIDS. 2015;10(6):420–9.
98. UNAIDS. Combination HIV prevention: tailoring and coordinating biomedical, behavioural, and structural strategies to reduce new HIV infections. Geneva: UNAIDS; 2010. https://files.unaids.org/en/media/unaids/contentassets/documents/unaidspublication/2011/20111110_JC2007_Combination_Prevention_paper_en.pdf. Accessed 12 Jan 2021.
99. Lacombe-Duncan A. An intersectional perspective on access to HIV-related healthcare for transgender women. Transgend Health. 2016;1(1):137–41.
100. Sereda Y, Kiriazova T, Makarenko O, Carroll JJ, Rybak N, Chybisov A, et al. Stigma and quality of co-located care for HIV-positive people in addiction treatment in Ukraine: a cross-sectional study. J Int AIDS Soc. 2020;23(5):e25492.
101. Yip JY. Self-stigmatisation among Chinese individuals with HIV in Hong Kong: understanding the sociological basis of spiritually and culturally sensitive care. HIV Nursing. 2019;19:31–5.
102. Makusha T, van Rooyen H, Cornell M. Reframing the approach to heterosexual men in the HIV epidemic in sub-Saharan Africa. J Int AIDS Soc. 2020;23(Suppl 2):e25510.
103. Sharma M, Barnabas RV, Celum C. Community-based strategies to strengthen men's engagement in the HIV care cascade in sub-Saharan Africa. PLoS Med. 2017;14(4):e1002262.
104. Heffernan A, Barber E, Thomas R, Fraser C, Pickles M, Cori A. Impact and cost-effectiveness of point-of-care CD4 testing on the HIV epidemic in South Africa. PLoS One. 2016;11(7):e0158303.
105. PEPFAR/ICAP. Expanding effective HIV prevention, care, and treatment for men who have sex with men in South Africa. Columbia: Columbia University; 2016.
106. Mullens AB, Duyker J, Brownlow C, Lemoire J, Daken K, Gow J. Point-of-care testing (POCT) for HIV/STI targeting MSM in regional Australia at community 'beat' locations. BMC Health Serv Res. 2019;19(1):93.
107. Arora DR, Maheshwari M, Arora B. Rapid point-of-care testing for detection of HIV and clinical monitoring. ISRN AIDS. 2013;2013:287269.
108. Jelliman P. Innovations in HIV: the liverpool community clinic. HIV Nursing. 2017;17:16–9.
109. Mburu G, Oxenham D, Hodgson I, Nakiyemba A, Seeley J, Bermejo A. Community systems strengthening for HIV care: experiences from Uganda. J Social Work End-of-Life Palliat Care. 2013;9(4):343–68.
110. Hodgson I. Empathy, inclusion and enclaves: the culture of care of people with HIV/AIDS and nursing implications. J Adv Nurs. 2006;55(3):283–90.
111. Stengal B, Weems L. Questioning safe space: an introduction. Stud Philos Educ. 2010;29:505–7.
112. Mburu G, Ram M, Skovdal M, Bitira D, Hodgson I, Mwai GW, et al. Resisting and challenging stigma in Uganda: the role of support groups of people living with HIV. J Int AIDS Soc. 2013;16(3 Suppl 2):18636.
113. McGarrahan P. Transcending AIDS: nurses and HIV patients in New York City. Philadelphia, PA: University of Pennsylvania Press; 1994.
114. National AIDS Trust. HIV: a guide for care providers. London: National AIDS Trust; 2015.
115. Dapaah JM, Senah KA. HIV/AIDS clients, privacy and confidentiality; the case of two health centres in the Ashanti Region of Ghana. BMC Med Ethics. 2016;17(1):41.

116. Kielly J, Kelly DV, Asghari S, Burt K, Biggin J. Patient satisfaction with chronic HIV care provided through an innovative pharmacist/nurse-managed clinic and a multidisciplinary clinic. Can Pharm J (Ott). 2017;150(6):397–406.

117. Van Camp YP, Van Rompaey B, Elseviers MM. Nurse-led interventions to enhance adherence to chronic medication: systematic review and meta-analysis of randomised controlled trials. Eur J Clin Pharmacol. 2013;69(4):761–70.

118. Wood EM, Zani B, Esterhuizen TM, Young T. Nurse led home-based care for people with HIV/AIDS. BMC Health Serv Res. 2018;18(1):219.

119. Piercy H, Bell G, Hughes C, Naylor S, Bowman CA. How does specialist nursing contribute to HIV service delivery across England? Int J STD AIDS. 2017;28(8):808–13.

120. Oldenburg CE. Integrated HIV prevention and care for key populations. Lancet HIV. 2019;6(5):e270–e1.

121. Jelliman P. Rules of engagement for 'hard to reach' patients living with HIV: a guide for nurses. HIV Nurs. 2019;19(4):BP9–BP12.

122. Felsenstein DR. Enhancing lesbian, gay, bisexual, and transgender cultural competence in a midwestern primary care clinic setting. J Nurses Prof Dev. 2018;34(3):142–50.

123. Margolies L, Brown CG. Increasing cultural competence with LGBTQ patients. Nursing. 2019;49(6):34–40.

124. van der Elst EM, Gichuru E, Muraguri N, Musyoki H, Micheni M, Kombo B, et al. Strengthening healthcare providers' skills to improve HIV services for MSM in Kenya. AIDS. 2015;29(Suppl 3):S237–40.

125. Pascoe SJS, Scott NA, Fong RM, Murphy J, Huber AN, Moolla A, et al. "Patients are not the same, so we cannot treat them the same"—a qualitative content analysis of provider, patient and implementer perspectives on differentiated service delivery models for HIV treatment in South Africa. J Int AIDS Soc. 2020;23(6):e25544.

126. Burns R, Borges J, Blasco P, Vandenbulcke A, Mukui I, Magalasi D, et al. 'I saw it as a second chance': a qualitative exploration of experiences of treatment failure and regimen change among people living with HIV on second- and third-line antiretroviral therapy in Kenya, Malawi and Mozambique. Glob Public Health. 2019;14(8):1112–24.

127. Deblonde J, Sasse A, Del Amo J, Burns F, Delpech V, Cowan S, et al. Restricted access to antiretroviral treatment for undocumented migrants: a bottle neck to control the HIV epidemic in the EU/EEA. BMC Public Health. 2015;15:1228.

128. Rouleau G, Richard L, Cote J, Gagnon MP, Pelletier J. Nursing practice to support people living with HIV with antiretroviral therapy adherence: a qualitative study. J Assoc Nurses AIDS Care. 2019;30(4):e20–37.

129. Aidsfonds. A story of change: treating each other with care and respect. Amsterdam: Aidsfonds; 2015.

130. Duby Z, Fong-Jaen F, Nkosi B, Brown B, Scheibe A. 'We must treat them like all the other people': evaluating the integrated key populations sensitivity training programme for healthcare workers in South Africa. South Afr J HIV Med. 2019;20(1):909.

131. Boakye DS, Mavhandu-Mudzusi A. Nurses knowledge, attitudes and practices towards patients with HIV andAIDS in Kumasi, Ghana. Int J Africa Nurs Sci. 2019;2019:11.

132. Coulter A, Collins A. Making shared decision-making a reality: no decision about me, without me. London: King's Fund; 2011.

133. Croston M, McLuskey J, Evans C. How do nurses facilitate shared decision making in HIV care? An exploratory study of UK nurses knowledge, perspective and experience of facilitating shared decision making in clinical practice. Eur J Pers Cent Healthc. 2016;4:4.

134. Storey D, Seifert-Ahanda K, Andaluz A, Tsoi B, Matsuki JM, Cutler B. What is health communication and how does it affect the HIV/AIDS continuum of care? A brief primer and case study from New York City. J Acquir Immune Defic Syndr. 2014;66(Suppl 3):S241–9.

135. Casale M, Carlqvist A, Cluver L. Recent interventions to improve retention in HIV care and adherence to antiretroviral treatment among adolescents and youth: a systematic review. AIDS Patient Care STDs. 2019;33(6):237–52.

Chapter 8
HIV Care in Rural Areas

Fiona Wallis

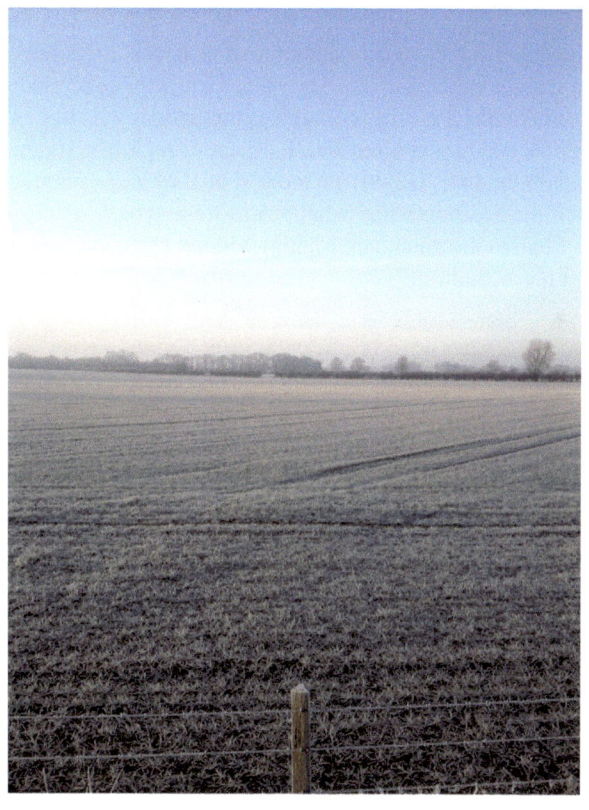

F. Wallis (✉)
York, UK

© The Author(s), under exclusive license to Springer Nature
Switzerland AG 2021
M. Croston, I. Hodgson (eds.), *Providing HIV Care: Lessons from the Field
for Nurses and Healthcare Practitioners*,
https://doi.org/10.1007/978-3-030-71295-2_8

8.1   The Context of Care in a Rural Setting

York and North Yorkshire is a large geographical area which is mainly rural, with small market towns. Over the last 30 years, there have been fantastic medical advances in HIV medicine, which allow patients to have a near-normal life expectancy. The patients who are sick with HIV are usually patients who present late for HIV testing, and therefore do not have timely access to antiretroviral medication or have disengaged from services. For many patients who do not test in a timely manner, this is due to lack of knowledge and/or stigma.

There are several patients for whom confidentiality and access to services are significant issues particularly in small remote communities, many patients live, work, and socialise within their community and have real worries over disclosure of their HIV status.

HIV is now considered a long-term condition, and the focus of care has shifted allowing patients to live well with the virus. In my experience, the nurse–patient relationship based on values of trust and mutual respect is fundamental to good care. In broadest terms, the nurse may have advanced knowledge of medication and their side effects, and the disease process; but it is the patient who has experience of living with the virus, and how it affects each aspect of their life. Essential to their care is shared decision-making (SDM) in order that they can continue with their life goals and reach their full potential whatever those maybe.

The Kings Fund in the document Making Shared Decision-Making a Reality. No decision about me without me (2011) [1] describe it as.

> *Shared decision-making is a process in which clinicians and patients work together to clarify treatment, management or self-management support goals, sharing information about options and preferred outcomes with the aim of reaching mutual agreement on the best course of action ... Shared decision-making explicitly recognises a patient's right to make decisions about their care, ensuring they are fully informed about the options they face. This involves providing them with reliable evidence-based information on the likely benefits and harms of interventions or actions, including any uncertainties and risks, eliciting their preferences and supporting implementation.*

Reflection Point
What does shared decision-making mean to you and how does it influence the care that you provide.

8.2   What Does It Mean to Provide Care in a Rural Setting?

In order to explore the appropriate care delivery system in a rural setting, it is important to consider what the term rurality means.

The Oxford Dictionary describes rural as 'in, relating to, or characteristic of the countryside rather than the town'.

A common definition and understanding of rural is not well described in England and Wales as compared to other developed countries such as Australia and Canada; this may be due to the shorter distances experienced between rural settings and urban conurbations in England and Wales [2].

> **Thinking Point**
> Take a couple of minutes to consider what a rural setting means to you? Can you identify any areas within your own country that you would consider rural? Consider how providing care in these areas could be challenging.

The Office of National Statistics defines rural as outside the settlements of more than 10,000 resident population [3].

Areas are further divided into six categories

- *Town and fringe*
- *Town and fringe in a sparse setting*
- *Village*
- *Village in a sparse setting*
- *Hamlets and isolated dwellings*
- *Hamlets and isolated dwellings in a sparse setting* [4]

The Nuffield Trust 2019 report into Rural Health Care identified that prior to 2007 there had been 30 definitions of rural across the United Kingdom. Generally, for the purposes of health, rural, and sparseness are identified by population size, population density, travel times to other hospitals, or a combination of other factors [5].

The 2017 Health and Wellbeing in Rural Areas Report by Public Health England and Local Government Association [6] identified eight main risks to health in rural areas

- *Changing Population. Patterns with outward migration of young people and inward migration of older people.*
- *Infrastructure. Remoteness of populations, and reduction in public transport incur increased transport costs and difficulties in accessing services.*
- *Digital Access. Exclusion due to lack of broadband and poor mobile network signal, this increases the socio-economic gap between 'the connected and not— the digitally excluded'.*
- *Air Quality. Deterioration due to increased vehicles on rural roads.*
- *Access to Health and related services. 'Due to distance and topography leading to "distance decay", where there is reducing use of service by rural residents due to distance'.*

- *Community support, isolation, and social exclusion. With an increasing older population and decreasing younger population, the social networks are breaking down which leads to social isolation which is a health issue.*
- *Housing and fuel poverty, house prices in 2017 were 26 prices higher in rural areas and there is limited social housing.*
- *Unemployment and under employment, unemployment, or seasonal work mean that many young people leave their families and rural areas to seek work elsewhere* [6].

8.3   HIV Care in a Rural Setting

All these background health risks impact on the delivery of services and care to people with HIV and access to testing. There is evidence from DEFRA in 2013 [7] that there is unmet health need in older rural residents who are reticent about discussing their health requirements; this can lead to delays in seeking advice until their needs are complex or not seeking advice even in an emergency situation. Some of the reasons given for this behaviour was 'a make do attitude' reluctance to make a fuss and fear of emerging and expressed ageing health issues [7].

Sowell et al. in his study of Resources, Stigma, and Patterns in Rural Women with HIV Infection in Georgia USA 1997 [8] recognised that rural communities are different but also recognised *'common features of limited access to healthcare, poverty and lack of transport, the study also recognised that there were common rural cultural attributes of self-sufficiency, concern about privacy and strong reliance on religious beliefs and sanctions'* [8].

My experience of working in rural settings recognises many of these behaviours especially self-sufficiency, such as the capacity to work, garden, provide community support, and/or fulfil a caring role. Many patients also find it important to adhere to the local cultural 'norms'. There are deeply held concerns about confidentiality and privacy.

The current health issues in a rural health setting also represent many of the HIV health issues in rural settings. The big challenge is to get HIV on the public health agenda both locally and nationally as the seroprevalence rates in rural areas are generally considered low. The HIV seroprevalence rate is based upon the number of infections per 1000 people. In areas of central London, the seroprevalence rate is >5 per 1000 people which is considered extremely high, in York and North Yorkshire the rate is 0–0.99 per 1000 people which is considered a low seroprevalence. See Box 1 a distribution Map published by Public Health England 2019. The enhanced HIV testing occurs in areas with a seroprevalence rate of 2 per 1000 people further discussion of this later in the chapter.

Diagnosed HIV prevalence (per 1,000 population aged 15 to 59 years): England,2018

Legend

    0-0.99
    1-1.99
    2-4.99 (high)
    5+ (extremely high)

London

18   HIV in the United Kingdom: 2019 Slide set (version 2.0, published 3 September 2019, updated 1 October 2019)

8.4 Stigma

In the previous section, rurality and low seroprevalence has been discussed; however people with HIV frequently face stigma and in rural areas this can feel omnipresent, as Tummala & Roberts 2009 [9] state *'In rural health care settings stigma takes on special importance because of the overlapping and interdependent relationships that exists in small communities'* [9].

The stigma index in the United Kingdom describes

- *'HIV-related stigma is commonly understood as a process of devaluation and may constitute:*
- *Self or internalised stigma: the acceptance of negative self-beliefs associated with being HIV positive*
- *Anticipated or perceived stigma: the awareness of negative beliefs and expectation of negative treatment amongst people living with HIV*
- *Discrimination: the negative and devaluing treatment of people due to their status. These may fall within the purview of the law'* [10].

The Positive Voices in 2017 surveyed 4442 people with HIV and found that internalised stigma and fear of discrimination were regularly reported by people with HIV.

- *16% of people surveyed worried about being treated differently due their HIV status.*
- *10% avoided seeking healthcare when needed due to their HIV status.*

- *5% of respondents felt they had been refused or had treatment delayed due to their HIV status.*
- *13% of those surveyed have not told anyone other than their healthcare professional about their HIV status* [11].

8.5   Practical Solutions to Address Stigma Within a Rural Setting

As a healthcare professional, there is a responsibility to challenge stigma through factual education and in a manner that does not further isolate the person living with HIV in a rural community. Isolation and lack of disclosure can complicate life and be risky to general health.

For example, some patients struggle to allow disclosure of their HIV status to their General Practitioner (GP), and this potentially can lead to problems with drug-to-drug interactions which can be harmful. Communication with the GP in small communities can cause difficulties, where friends or relatives can be employed by the GP practice.

Initially, it is important to understand the patient's reluctance to inform the GP and to also advise the patient that is good and normal practice to inform the GP as they have an overview of the patient's health. It allows for information on drug regimens to be shared and informs the GP of drug interaction websites should they need to prescribe other medication for unrelated conditions and thus prevents harmful drug-to-drug interactions. The HIV service can also communicate the need for flu vaccination and other relevant vaccinations at appropriate times and relevant information from national centres, such as caution with the use of HIV treatment during conception and the first trimester of pregnancy and annual cervical screening for women living with HIV.

For some patients, it is how the information gets to the GP that is the issue and who within the GP practice has access to the information; many rural practices are very aware of privacy issues due to other conditions such as mental health, incontinence, and reproductive health and the practice already has mechanisms in place to overcome these issues, for example, by addressing the letter to be opened by addressee only which alerts receptionists and secretaries to give the letter directly to the GP therefore reducing the access to personal information.

In my experience, it is essential that people living with HIV in rural areas have access to an empathetic GP service where the medical staff are aware of their HIV status. This is for the following reasons:

- Assists in breaking down stigma whether that be internalised, or anticipated stigma.
- Reduces reliance on an HIV clinic which could be a long distance.

- GPs in rural areas are mindful of rural healthcare issues and beliefs. Many surgeries adapt practices in recognition of these issues.
- Rural populations have an increasing ageing population so there is an increasing likelihood that people with HIV will have or may have future comorbidities which will require support and interventions from primary care. The GP can also be the conduit for further referrals such as to community memory clinics, weight loss programmes, smoking cessation, and mental health services.
- Rural landscapes and weather conditions at times does not allow a patient to access an HIV clinic or an HIV specialist to undertake a home visit so if there is an issue that needs rapid clinical attention the patient's GP is the best person locally to undertake the assessment. The GP is in an improved position to undertake the assessment if there is background knowledge of the patient's condition, current blood results and medication; and has clear contact details for the HIV team if advice or support is required.

A future strategy could be to use a secure email address for the GP. Ideally if broadband and network services allow (many rural areas have poor broadband and network coverage), web-based electronic records with patient access, could provide a way forward for patients in rural areas and allow real time information to be shared with all practitioners. The caveat being that there are secure safeguards for electronic access to the records; this could reduce the problems with written communication and privacy, real-time information would be available to all and it could prevent repetition of interventions and tests.

Case Study 1 John is a 55-year-old farmer who has recently been diagnosed HIV antibody positive; he has not disclosed this to any other person and has refused permission to inform his GP.

What issues do you think concern John?

As a healthcare practitioner consider what difficulties might this present in your practice?

How would you inform John of these difficulties and what ideas might you and the patient consider resolving the issues?

8.6 Living and Ageing Health and Well-Being in Rural Areas

Local Government and Public Health England in the document Health and Wellbeing in Rural Areas describe the changing population in rural areas of becoming an older population with lower levels of young people this is reflected in the HIV statistics in York and North Yorkshire as seen below.

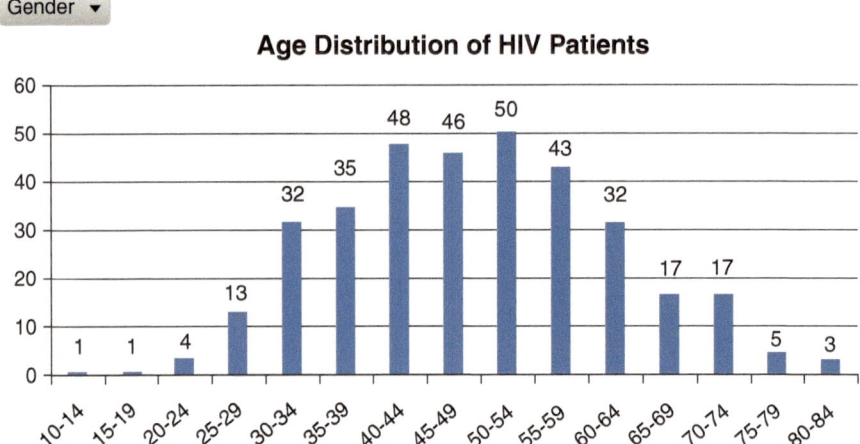

Age Distribution of HIV Patients

(Reprinted courtesy of Dr. I. Fairley York Teaching Hospital NHS Trust May 2020)

From the above Table 48% of the York and North Yorkshire population are 50 years or over years.

As with many patients who are ageing with comorbidities their partner and/or family often provide a carer role. Often the patient and or carer will have lived and worked in the community for many years and not disclosed any information about their HIV status; so, when the carer becomes unwell themselves and requires inpatient treatment, there can be a gap in the carer role. This can be problematic in small communities because of privacy and access to carers. In remote settings getting access to a carer is not always easy; this may be the lack of carers generally due to the changing demographic of rural areas and secondly the distances the carer may be required to travel. For example, patients with dementia may prefer to remain in their own home with familiar surroundings rather than have respite in unknown environment. This could involve up to four visits per day from the paid carers and not always the same personnel, which can be disorientating for the patient, and there may be concerns regarding the privacy of information, these are difficult decisions for patients and carers to make. It may be easier to discuss future care planning with the carer early on their carer role. In certain circumstances, the patient or carer may decide to disclose the HIV diagnosis to a trusted family member or friend who will provide the carer role during any hospitalisation of the carer. This may reduce the number of people coming to their home; it can also allow them to feel that there is more control over private information; and it can feed into the belief of self-sufficiency.

In cases such as this, it becomes important to have joint team working so that all health and social care staff are aware of the situation and the care plan as care and support nearer home becomes more significant for the patient. Prior to and during this time, it is important to assess and plan the support needs for the main carer.

Whilst many of the issues are similar for an ageing population in rural areas, there is the added concerns of confidentiality and stigma both to the patient and the main carer.

Case Study 2 Jane is an 87-year-old woman who lives on the outskirts of a small village; she lives independently with support from her daughter who is aware of her diagnosis and supports her with her medication and clinic appointments. The GP is aware of her diagnosis but no other members of the community or her family. The daughter needs to have a short inpatient treatment for her medical condition.

Consider

What are the key issues for Jane?

How would you plan Jane's care?

What support might Jane need?

How might you empower Jane's daughter?

8.7   Access to HIV Services

Infrastructure as discussed in the Health and Wellbeing document noted that sparsity in population with scarcity of public transport can significantly reduce access to healthcare services.

For people without private transport living in small villages with limited or no bus service attending clinic and hospital appointments becomes problematic. It is appreciated that for many people living in a similar geographical area they also would have problems with public transport. However due to the low seroprevalence of HIV, there are not several clinics for the same speciality at different times of day, the HIV clinic times also need to consider the timing and transportation of blood samples to regional laboratories. Outreach clinics need to understand the transport network and link the clinic timings where appropriate. These clinics can act as a one-stop clinic, for example, if a patient is co-infected with Hepatitis, it maybe that the Hepatitis team will attend clinic to see the patient or the HIV team will undertake the organisation of the relevant Hepatitis tests and vice versa.

Access to specialist HIV healthcare can be difficult for many patients in rural areas, and it is timely and costly for patients to visit HIV centres, and it is equally timely and costly for specialist staff to drive long distances for small clinics; however, it becomes increasingly costly if a patient falls out of care, develops advanced HIV disease, and requires hospitalisation. Models of care need to be developed that addresses these issues. Whist the internet and video consultations could provide a way forward for support and care this could for some patients reinforce their sense of isolation.

Thinking Point

How might you support patients to remain in care?

What models of care would be useful to implement to facilitate patient engagement?

The model of care developed in York and North Yorkshire was a 'hub and spoke' model. York is the hub, with satellite clinics; the Regional centres are at Leeds and Hull. A caseload management system was used in order that patients were cared for in a variety of settings hospital, clinic, community clinics, and at home. Each patient had an allocated Clinical Nurse Specialist and Consultant so that there was continuity of care, ease of accessibility both for the patient, and any other clinicians requesting specialist advice.

A key component in supporting good HIV care in rural areas is sustaining education and advice to primary care teams, and there are benefits for the patients. For example, the HIV Clinical Nurse Specialist provided a training seminar for Practice Nurses who work in geographically isolated locations following which there was a general discussion about vaccinations; a plan was agreed that with patient consent and in partnership with the Clinical Nurse Specialist that the Practice Nurses would check all the HIV patient's vaccination records and ensure that the relevant vaccinations were given in a timely manner to prevent any further infections and to reduce travel time and costs for patients. This programme allowed access to routine care closer to home and the patients felt supported by the primary care team. It enhanced the communication between the HIV clinic and primary care and in one instance allowed for therapeutic drug monitoring blood tests to be done in a remote location rather than the patient travelling long distances for this to be undertaken.

8.8   HIV Testing

Access is a problem for those that are diagnosed with HIV and have identified health issues but for those who have had an HIV risk and require testing without any other symptoms it may not be a priority to travel long distances for HIV testing. As previously discussed, privacy remains a big issue in rural areas and as HIV testing is not offered routinely in GP surgeries, it is incumbent on the patient to raise the issue of HIV testing, which is often difficult in small communities where GP staff are known to the patient. Home testing kits are available through some sexual health services and private providers if patients know how to access them and have enough privacy at home to receive them via the post. HIV testing using the indicator diseases can be problematic in low seroprevalent areas. The demographic of HIV patients in York and North Yorkshire are 48% of patients are 50 years or older, over 80% identify themselves as White British (May 2020), with a large self-identified heterosexual group see below.

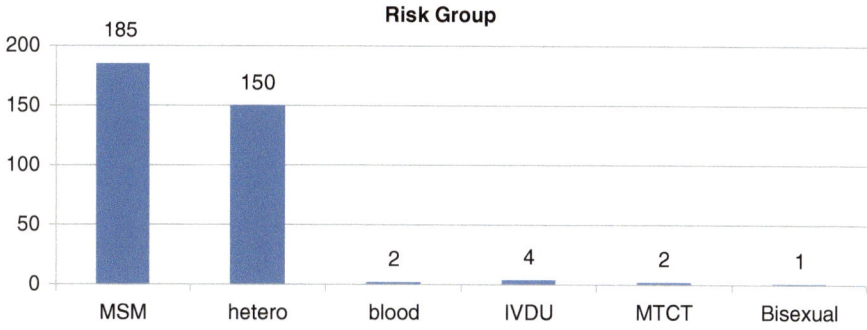

(Reprinted courtesy of Dr I Fairley York Teaching Hospital NHS Trust)

The community programmes for targeted HIV testing do not always incorporate this cohort of patients and many of the health prevention messages do not focus on the heterosexual older group of patients, consequently many patients perceive themselves at low risk. The lack of routine testing and relevant health prevention messages can lead patients to think that HIV may not be an issue for them. Youssef et al. in 2017 [12] found the main barriers to HIV testing in the 50-year-old and over was the patient perceived that they were at low risk, and the clinician's preconception that patients >50 years old were not at risk from HIV and their discomfort in discussing sexual activity with older patients; however, the offer of a test by a healthcare professional was the most cited reason for this older age group having an HIV test [12].

Reflection Point
Take a moment to pause and consider your thoughts on sexuality in older age.
    How comfortable are you discussing sexual risk with people over 50, 60, 70, 80.

In Cumbria another English rural area, Professor Matthew Philips, at the BHIVA Conference 2019 [13] discussed the initiation and support for HIV Point of Care Testing in local pharmacies. This intervention has had some good outcomes in that it can be a local accessible service conducted in private. It maintains anonymity as a patient could be seeing a pharmacist for many issues, so the patient is not identified as going for an HIV test. It has raised the awareness of HIV locally and approximately 35% of patients having an HIV test at the pharmacy have not previously had an HIV test [13].

Routine HIV testing within primary care and community facilities could provide some solutions for reduction in HIV transmission, prevention of late diagnosis, reduction of hospital costs, and finally could begin to break down some of the stigma associated with HIV.

8.9   Conclusion

In conclusion, HIV care in rural areas faces all the healthcare challenges experienced in rural areas but with the added challenge of stigma and the fear of loss of privacy. There are some suggested ways forward, in opening HIV testing in other settings, improving broadband and network access to allow for web-based records. One of the developments that needs to be continued is close liaison with primary care teams which allows access closer to home, challenges stigma, and can give patients confidence in local services.

Finally, HIV is nothing to be ashamed of; but stigma and prejudice disgrace us all.

Acknowledgments There are so many people to thank for their encouragement not only in writing this chapter but for their support in my role as a HIV nurse both in London and York. I am so appreciative and grateful to them.

I would like to thank Ruth Holt and Michelle Croston for supporting me and giving me the confidence to write this chapter.

My special thanks go to Dr. Ian Fairley and Professor Lacey for their support and guidance especially when I have been lone working in outreach settings. Virginia Russell and Jen Slaughter for allowing the nursing team to develop and explore new models of service delivery. Janet Jackson for her behind the scenes work and dedication. I especially would like to thank Peter Tovey, my colleague for his support, advice and joint ventures in the pursuit of excellence in HIV nursing care.

Finally, I would like to thank the HIV patients, on so many levels they are my teachers.

References

1. Kings Fund, Making Shared Decision Making a Reality. No decision about me without me; Coulter A, Collins A, 2011, p. 2. www.kingsfund.org.uk. Accessed Sept 2020.
2. Watts IA, Franks AJ, Sheldon TA. Health and healthcare of rural populations in the UK: is it better or worse? J Epidemiol Commun Health. 1994;48:16–21.
3. Government Statistical Service. 2011 Rural Urban Output Areas for England, 2011. https://www.ons.gov.uk/methodology/geography/geographicalproducts/ruralurbanclassifications/2011ruralurbanclassification. Accessed 20 May 2020.
4. Local Government Association & Public Health. England in Health & Wellbeing in Rural Areas Local Government Association. 2017. https://www.local.gov.uk/sites/default/files/documents/1.39_Health%20in%20rural%20areas_WEB.pdf. Accessed 20 May 2020.
5. Palmer B, Appleby J, Spencer J. Rural health care a rapid review of the impact of rurality on the costs of delivering health care. January 2019. Report prepared for the National Centre for Rural Health and Care. Nuffield Trust. https://www.nuffieldtrust.org.uk/files/2019-01/rural-health-care-report-web3.pdf. Accessed 19 May 2020.

6. Local Government Association & Public Health. England in Health & Wellbeing in Rural Areas Local Government Association. 2017. https://www.local.gov.uk/sites/default/files/documents/1.39_Health%20in%20rural%20areas_WEB.pdf. Accessed 20 May 2020.
7. Department of the Environment Food and Rural Affairs Connors C, Kendrick M, Bloch 2013 A Rural Ageing Research Summary Report of Findings TNS BRMB.
8. Sowell RL, Lowenstein A, Moneyham L, Demi A, Mizuno Y, Seals B. Resources stigma and patterns of disclosure in rural women with HIV infection. Public Health Nursing. 1997;14(5):302–12.
9. Tummala A, Roberts LW. Ethics conflicts in rural communities: stigma and illness. In: Nelson WA, editor. Handbook for rural health care ethics a practical guide for professionals. New England: University Press; 2009.
10. The People Living with HIV Stigma Survey UK Changes and Challenges; Actions and Answers. London 2015. http://www.stigmaindexuk.org/reports/2016/NationalReport.pdf. Accessed 25 May 2020.
11. Kall M, Kelly C, Auzenbergs M, Delpech V. Positive voices: the national survey of people living with HIV—findings from the 2017 survey. London: Public Health England; 2020. p. 14.
12. Youssef E, Cooper V, Delpech V, Davies K, Wright J. Barriers and facilitators in HIV testing in people age 50 and above a systematic review. Clin Med (Lond). 2017;17(6):508–20. https://doi.org/10.7861/clinmedicine.17-6-508.
13. Phillips M. HIV and Stigma in Rural Areas. Abstract 006. With increasing UK signatories to the Fast Track Cities Initiative, how can smaller urban and rural communities also achieve zero HIV-related stigma, infections and deaths by 2030? UK CA Community Session BHIVA Conference November 2019 www.bhiva.org. Accessed May 2020

Further Readings

Bell SA. Are HIV services in England accessible and acceptable to adults diagnosed with HIV at age 50 years and over? A mixed-methods study. PhD York University 2017. http://etheses.whiterose.ac.uk/17388/7/Sadie%20Bell%20-%20Final%20thesis.pdf. Accessed 25 May 2020.
BHIVA Conference. UK-CAB Community Workshop: HIV-related stigma; influencing and changing attitudes Dr Nina Pearson, Fiona Wallis, 2015. https://www.bhiva.org/Presentations150423. Accessed 24 May 2020.
BHIVA Conference. UK CAB Community Session: With increasing UK signatories to the Fast Track Cities Initiative, how can smaller urban and rural communities also achieve zero HIV-related stigma, infections and deaths by 2030? Andrew Evan, Anne Glew, Professor Matthew Philips, 2019. https://www.bhiva.org/Autumn2019Presentations Accessed 20 May 2020.
Dayan M. "Are parts of England 'left behind' by the NHS?" Nuffield Trust comment. 2018. https://www.nuffieldtrust.org.uk/news-item/are-parts-of-england-left-behind-by-the-nhs. Accessed 20 May 2020.
Gary Hart L, Larson EH, Lishner DM. Rural definitions for health policy and research. Am J Public Health. 2005;95(7):11491155. https://doi.org/10.2105/AJPH.2004.042432.
Gessert C, Waring S, Bailey-Davis L, Conway P, Roberts M, Van Wormer J. Rural definition of health: a systematic literature review. BMC Public Health. 2015;15:378. https://doi.org/10.1186/s12889-015-1658-9. Accessed 21 May 2020.
Mellor C, Fraser J, Hunter E. HIV care in North Cumbria: review of co-prescribed medications in primary care and associated potential drug drug interactions (PDDI). https://www.nhivna.org/file/5b4498b7d8719/Jane-Fraser.pdf Accessed 20 May 2020.
Towards Zero Stigma. A review of stigma in healthcare settings. https://www.nhivna.org/file/5b449958f3138/Mark-Roche.pdf. Accessed 20 May 2020.

Chapter 9
HIV and Ageing: Considerations for Older Adults Living with HIV

Jeffrey Kwong

9.1 Medication Considerations and Antiretroviral Therapy in Older Adults Living with HIV

9.1.1 Pharmacokinetics and Drug Metabolism

As part of the biological ageing process, body composition and metabolism change over time. In most individuals, the proportion of lean muscle to body fat changes with age. Older persons tend to have a higher proportion of body fat compared to lean muscle [1]. This can impact the absorption and distribution of medications. For example, medications that have a propensity to accumulate in adipose tissue, such as benzodiazepines, may be excreted more slowly. Therefore, the dose of benzodiazepines may need to be started at a lower dose in an older adult compared to a younger person. The principle of "*start low and go slow*", meaning starting treatment with the lowest possible dose and titrating the dose of medications slowly, is often used in geriatric prescribing [1]. Given that many drugs are processed by the kidneys and liver, monitoring renal function and hepatic function are a critical component of medication management [1]. When assessing renal function in older adults, it is important to remember that laboratory reference ranges need to be adjusted. Serum creatinine levels that may fall into a normal laboratory reference range may underestimate glomerular function as a person ages. Using a creatinine clearance or glomerular filtration formula, such as the Chronic Kidney Disease Epidemiology Collaboration (CKD-EPI) calculator or the Modification of Diet in

J. Kwong (✉)
Division of Advanced Nursing Practice, Rutgers University School of Nursing,
Newark, NJ, USA
e-mail: Jeffrey.Kwong@rutgers.edu

© The Author(s), under exclusive license to Springer Nature
Switzerland AG 2021
M. Croston, I. Hodgson (eds.), *Providing HIV Care: Lessons from the Field
for Nurses and Healthcare Practitioners*,
https://doi.org/10.1007/978-3-030-71295-2_9

151

Renal Disease (MDRD) equation, provides a more accurate estimate of renal function. These formulas use a combination of serum creatinine as well as age to better approximate renal function.

9.1.2 HIV Antiretroviral Therapy

Achieving virologic control of HIV and preserving immune function remain the primary goal in HIV treatment regardless of age. Evidence suggests that older adults are able to achieve similar virologic response to therapy as younger individuals [2]. However, in terms of CD4 cell response, older individuals tend to have a less robust CD4 cell response compared to younger individuals [2]. This supports the need to continue to screen and diagnose older adults who may be at risk of HIV infection in order to start them on treatment in a timely manner. In 2018, 24% of new HIV diagnosis in Europe occurred in persons over the age of 50 [3]. The fact that nearly a quarter of new infections occur in persons over 50 suggests that older adults may not perceive themselves at risk for HIV. Additionally, providers may not be screening older patients because they may assume that older adults do not engage in risk-taking behaviours [4]. It is important to continue to offer testing and assess for HIV risk, even in older adults.

The recommended HIV antiretroviral therapy regimens remain the same for persons ageing with HIV as those who are younger [5]. However, considerations with dosing, pharmacokinetics, metabolism, adverse effects, drug–drug interactions, co-occurring chronic diseases, and pill burden should be considered when initiating or switching HIV antiretroviral therapy in older adults. A few key principles of simplifying or switching HIV antiretroviral therapy in persons who may be on earlier generation treatment regimens is to check the patient's drug resistance history as well as their hepatitis B immune status [5]. If someone has any previous history of drug resistant mutations, this may limit their ability to simplify or switch HIV antiretroviral therapy [5]. Additionally, some of the HIV nucleoside reverse transcriptase inhibitors also treat chronic hepatitis B infection; therefore, it is important to know if someone has chronic hepatitis B before switching therapy to make sure they have adequate treatment of hepatitis B in their new regimen (Box 9.1).

Box 9.1 Things to Think About
- Although many individuals living with HIV may be able to take a single-tablet regimen, it is important to consider a patient's previous antiretroviral therapy history. Persons with a history of drug resistance to certain classes of antiretroviral therapy may not be able to simplify their treatment regimen.
- Many non-prescription medications and supplements can interact with HIV antiretrovirals.
- A thorough medication review is recommended for all patients.

9.1.3 *Polypharmacy*

In addition to HIV, other chronic conditions, such as diabetes or cardiovascular disease, are seen in the ageing population. Although some of these conditions can be managed with non-pharmacologic interventions, most individuals need to take other medications specific to each disease state. This in turn can lead to polypharmacy. Polypharmacy has been defined as taking multiple drugs for one or more condition [1]. The prevalence of polypharmacy among older persons living with HIV has been estimated to range from 37% to over 90% [6]. Although polypharmacy is an issue that affects persons without HIV, some studies indicate that persons living with HIV are more likely to take more than one medication for other co-occurring conditions at an earlier age compared to persons without HIV [7]. Polypharmacy not only increases the risk of drug–drug interactions, but it has also been associated with non-adherence to therapy, a greater risk for falls, cognitive impairment, and dementia [8].

One of the principles of managing medications in older patients is to minimize the use of drugs that may be unnecessary and stopping medications with high risk for adverse events [9]. Tools, such as the screening tool of older person's prescriptions (STOPP) tool, the Beer's Criteria, or the Good Palliative-Geriatric Practice (GPGP) can be used to identify high risk medications where the risks outweigh the benefits. Similarly, the screening tool to alert physicians to the right treatment tool (START tool) is an evidence-based tool to alert clinicians for medications that may be missing from a patient's medication regimen that may be of benefit [9]. Regardless of which screening tools are used, it is important for nurses and other providers to thoroughly review both prescribed and over-the-counter medications with patients regularly.

Reducing medication-related harm is considered one of the top three quality goals by the World Health Organization [10]. Several classes of HIV antiretrovirals, specifically non-nucleoside reverse transcriptase inhibitors (NNRTIs) and protease inhibitors (PIs), have the highest likelihood of drug–drug interactions [9]. These classes of drugs are metabolized primarily by the liver's cytochrome P450 enzyme system (CYP450). The CYP450 enzyme system processes not only HIV antiretrovirals, but other medications as well. Interactions with the CYP450 metabolic pathway can result in either higher levels of a drug (causing drug toxicity) or lower levels of drugs (resulting in sub-therapeutic levels). The integrase strand transfer inhibitor (INSTI) class can also interact with cation containing products, such as iron, magnesium, aluminium, or calcium, as well as medications such as metformin [5]. Therefore, a thorough medication review of patient's prescribed medications, supplements, herbs, and other non-prescription medications are an integral part of comprehensive care for geriatric patients.

9.2 HIV, Ageing, and Chronic Comorbidities

9.2.1 Pathophysiologic Effects of HIV on Ageing

Although there is still much to be learned about the cellular and pathophysiologic effects of HIV on ageing, various theories have been reported. One of the more commonly reported theories is that HIV induces chronic cellular inflammation which leads to a greater incidence of other comorbidities [11, 12]. Data suggests that even in persons who are on HIV antiretroviral therapy with an undetectable viral load, inflammation still occurs. The release of these cytokines and inflammatory markers lead to the development of diseases or conditions occurring at earlier ages in persons living with HIV compared to persons without HIV [13].

9.2.2 Cardiovascular Disease

Persons living with HIV have been shown to experience higher rates of cardiovascular disease (CVD), including atherosclerotic disease, dyslipidemia, hypertension, and myocardial infarction. Data suggest that the risk of developing CVD is 1.5–2 times greater for persons living with HIV compared to those without HIV infection [14]. Factors that have been associated with increased risk of CVD include use of certain HIV antiretroviral therapy, chronic inflammation, and tobacco use [14].

The European HIV clinical guidelines recommend regular assessment and management of CVD risk for persons living with HIV [5]. There are different risk calculators available to assist in predicting the probability of having a future cardiac event. Tools such as the Framingham Risk Calculator or the D:A:D risk score are tools used to predict the risk of a cardiac event and incorporate factors such as age, gender, blood pressure, cholesterol levels, and tobacco use. Regardless of which prediction tool is used, nurses can help reinforce and educate patients on the importance of lifestyle modification such as modifying or reducing tobacco use, maintaining a healthy weight, and incorporating a diet that is low in saturated fats and sodium.

For those with known CVD or those with significant risk factors, the use of statins, anti-hypertensives, anticoagulants, and/or antiarrhythmics may be used [5]. In these situations, awareness of drug–drug interactions is important. Certain brands of statins, antiarrhythmics, and anticoagulants are either contraindicated or need to be dose modified when co-administered with certain HIV therapies.

For patients with hypertension, current guidelines recommend a target systolic blood pressure for patients over the age of 65 as 130–139 mmHg with a diastolic less than 80 mmHg [5]. The target systolic blood pressure for those 18–65 years of age remains 120–129 mmHg. The threshold to initiate anti-hypertensive therapy older persons is slightly higher than younger adults. For patients 65–79 years of age, the threshold of start anti-hypertensive medication is $\geq$ 140/90 mmHg [15]. For those $\geq$80 years of age, given the risk of orthostatic hypotension and the overall risks and benefits of therapy, the threshold for starting anti-hypertensives is a blood pressure $\geq 160/90$ mmHg [15].

9.2.3   Diabetes

According to the International Diabetes Federation, nearly 28% of adults 65 years and older are living with diabetes [16]. However, in persons living with HIV, the prevalence of Type 2 diabetes is nearly four times greater [17]. Chronic inflammation, as well as co-infection with hepatitis C, and the use of HIV antiretroviral therapy have been associated as factors contributing to the higher rates of diabetes in persons living with HIV [17]. Current guidelines recommend that persons living with HIV be screened on a regular basis for diabetes with either fasting plasma glucose (FBG) or HgA1C at least annually [5]. However, it is important to note that abacavir, a nucleoside reverse transcriptase inhibitor, and some protease inhibitors can affect red blood cells resulting in underestimation of haemoglobin A1C(HgA1C). The use of a fasting blood glucose may be more appropriate in persons who have pre-diabetes or those at high-risk of diabetes [5]. Although A1C levels may underpredict mean glucose levels, treatment targets for those with confirmed diabetes remain the same. For individuals diagnosed with Type 2 diabetes mellitus, the goal is to keep or maintain HgA1C <7%; however, for older adults a target of <7.5% can be considered. Treatment for diabetes is the same for persons living with HIV as those without HIV and follow the recommendations established by the European Association for the Study of Diabetes [18].

9.2.4   Renal Disease

Chronic kidney disease (CKD), acute kidney injury, and HIV-associated nephropathy are forms of renal disease that disproportionately effect persons living with HIV [19]. HIV antiretroviral drugs, in particular indinavir, atazanavir, and tenofovir disoproxil fumarate [TDF], as well as conditions such as chronic hepatitis C and diabetes have been attributed to the higher prevalence of renal disease in persons living with HIV [19]. As noted earlier, regular assessment of renal function is important with regard to medication dose adjustments. Current guidelines recommend renal function monitoring every 3–12 months depending on an individual's medical history [5].

In persons with CKD who have an estimated glomerular filtration rate (eGFR) < 60 mL/min, TDF should be replaced with tenofovir alafenamide (TAF), which can be used in persons with an eGFR > 30 mL/min [5]. Other considerations include limiting nephrotoxic drugs, including non-prescription medications such as nonsteroidal anti-inflammatories, tobacco cessation, and screening and treatment of both dyslipidaemia and diabetes [5]. For those with CKD and evidence of proteinuria or who are in need of an anti-hypertensive, angiotensin-converting enzyme inhibitors or receptor blockers are considered the preferred drug choice [5]. As renal function declines, patients are typically co-managed in collaboration with a nephrologist.

9.2.5 Cancer

Persons living with HIV are known to have higher rates of lung, liver, anal, and pharyngeal cancers. Rates of breast and prostate cancer are comparable to persons without HIV [20]. Cancers traditionally considered AIDS-defining cancers (Kaposi's sarcoma, non-Hodgkin's lymphoma, and invasive cervical cancer), have declined in recent years due to effective HIV antiretroviral therapy [20]. Older individuals with HIV should receive recommended age-based cancer screenings according to national guidelines, keeping in mind overall life expectancy and the risks-benefits of screening [5]. Given the high prevalence of HPV-associated anal cancer in persons living with HIV, current guidelines recommend digital rectal exams with or without anal cytology every 1–3 years for men who have sex with men (MSM) and persons with HPV-associated dysplasia [5]. One of the common risk factors for all cancers is tobacco use. Therefore, an important component of providing care to all persons living with HIV regardless of age is to screen for tobacco use and assisting current users with cessation to modify their risk and mortality associated with cancer.

9.2.6 HIV-Associated Neurocognitive Disorder

It has been estimated that more than 50% of older adults with HIV will experience some degree of neurocognitive impairment [21]. HIV-associated neurocognitive disorder (HAND) refers to a spectrum of disorders that include asymptomatic neurocognitive impairment, mild neurocognitive disorder, and HIV-associated dementia. Persons living with HIV with HAND tend to experience poor medication adherence, worsening depression, and earlier mortality [21]. In persons with suspected cognitive impairment, it is recommended to assess for confounding aetiologies which may have similar presentations such as depression, psychiatric conditions, substance use, or potentially central nervous system-related opportunistic infections [5].

Screening tools for cognitive impairment are available, but there is a lack of consensus on what is the best tool to use in clinical practice because the majority of tools are imprecise at detecting milder forms of HAND. The International HIV

Dementia Scale (IHIVDS) is one screening tool that was adapted from the HIV Dementia Scale (HDS) to be used across different countries and cultures. The IVHDS assesses motor speed, psychomotor speed, and memory recall [22]. However, a recent analysis found that the IVHDS lacked specificity when tested in a 3000 person cohort of persons living with HIV in East Africa [23]. The Montreal Cognitive Assessment (MoCA) is a brief 10-min assessment that it has been used in persons living with HIV as well as those without HIV infection. The MoCA has been recommended by some as an initial screening test because it may have the best ability to detect more subtle signs of cognitive impairment compared to the other screening tools [24]. Regardless of which screening tool is used, individuals who screen positive should be referred for more extensive neurocognitive testing.

Unfortunately, treatment for HAND is limited. If an individual is not on HIV antiretroviral therapy, starting treatment is recommended [5]. There is some limited data on the benefits of exercise on preventing and delaying disease progression [25]. In situations where a patient has severe or worsening cognitive decline, lumbar puncture, and assessment of HIV viral load in the cerebral spinal fluid it is recommended [5]. If there is detectable HIV within the CSF, switching treatment is recommended.

9.2.7 Osteopenia, Osteoporosis, and Fractures

Osteopenia and osteoporosis result from the thinning of bone as individuals age. For persons living with HIV, the risk of developing either of these conditions is nearly double that of persons without HIV [26]. Multiple factors have been attributed to these higher rates in older persons living with HIV, including history of previous bone fracture, low body mass index, low body weight, hypogonadism, smoking, lower CD4 cell count, as well as the use of PIs and the nucleotide reverse transcriptase inhibitor, TDF [26].

In persons with osteoporosis, the major underlying concern is for the development of bone fracture which can impact morbidity and mortality in ageing individuals. Persons living with HIV have an estimated 60% greater risk of fracture as they age [26]. Assessment of fragility fracture with the Fracture Risk Assessment Tool (FRAX) is recommended for persons living with HIV 40–49 years of age [5]. Dual energy X-ray absorptiometry (DXA) is also recommended for men over 50, postmenopausal women, patients with a history of fragility fracture, patients receiving chronic glucocorticoid treatment, and patients at high risk for falls [5]. Treatment options for those with osteopenia and osteoporosis include minimizing or avoiding TDF and PIs, use of bisphosphonate therapy, optimizing calcium and vitamin D intake, limiting or reducing alcohol and tobacco, and incorporating weight-bearing exercise [5, 26].

9.3 Other Aspects of Caring for Older Persons Living with HIV

9.3.1 Mental Health

Among the ageing population, mental health conditions such as depression can develop as people experience isolation or changes in their overall health status. As a result, health-related quality of life may be negatively affected [27]. Prevalence of depression among persons living with HIV have been estimated to be 20–40% compared to 7% in the general population [5]. Annual screening for depression is recommended and can be easily done by asking two simple questions: (a) "Have you often felt depressed, sad, or without hope in the last few months?" and (b) "Have you lost interest in activities that you usually enjoy?" [5].

Other standardized depression screening tools exist for older adults, such as the Geriatric Depression Scale. Assessment of other psychosocial issues that may impact mental health, such as economic and financial issues, social engagement, and risk of violence should also be incorporated into an assessment [28]. Treatment of depression and anxiety is similar in persons living with HIV as those who are not living with HIV. Pharmacologic as well as non-pharmacologic options are helpful and effective interventions.

9.3.2 Substance Use

Substance use disorders, including alcohol abuse, are reportedly higher in older persons living with HIV compared to the general population [29]. The impact of substance use includes poor adherence, cognitive impairment, and risk of HIV transmission through sexual or injection drug use behaviours. Screening and assessment of substance use may help identify clients at risk [29]. Clients who screen positive for substance use abuse or misuse should be referred for treatment or assistance with a substance abuse specialist.

9.3.3 Mobility, Physical Function, and Frailty

Mobility and physical function are an integral part of quality of life for older adults. Decreased mobility and physical function has been associated with depression, multimorbidity, neurocognitive impairment, and low CD4 cell count in persons living with HIV [30].

Frailty is a phenomenon that occurs nearly twice as often in persons living with HIV compared to non-HIV populations [30]. Clinicians caring for older adults should assess for frailty as part of routine care. The European AIDS Clinical Society recommends measuring frailty with either the Frailty Phenotype or the Frailty Index [5]. The Frailty Phenotype assesses five specific features: (a) self-reported weight loss, (b) self-reported exhaustion, (c) low levels of physical activity measured by the Minnesota Leisure physical activity questionnaire, (d) measured 4 m walk speed time and (e) measured grip strength. The Frailty Index is calculated based on an extensive set of health deficits. For individuals identified as frail, a comprehensive geriatric assessment is recommended [31]. As part of this assessment, the patient's priorities are identified, and underlying or modifiable risk factors are addressed. The overall goal is to promote quality of life and maximize function (Box 9.2).

Box 9.2 Things to Think About
- Assessment of fall risk, mobility, and physical function are important indicators for quality of life.
- Exercise and physical activity have been shown to improve mood, cognition, and reduce risk for falls. Nurses can help educate patients on activities and exercises to maintain function, flexibility, and muscle strength.

9.3.4   Sexual Health

Sexual health remains an important issue for older adults but is often ignored during medical visits. Sexual health can be influenced by mood disorders, medication side effects, complications of other chronic illnesses, mobility, and physiologic changes such as vaginal dryness and erectile dysfunction [32]. Incorporating sexual health counselling as part of an overall assessment can normalize discussions about sex. For patients who report concerns about sexual function or libido, it is important to identify physiologic causes from non-physiologic causes, such as depression or anxiety [5]. Nurses can help support clients who may have issues that impact their sexual health by providing an unconditional, open environment to discuss these topics, and assist with referrals when indicated.

Although there are various ways of phrasing questions, it is important to begin a sexual history by reassuring the client that the responses to questions are confidential and that sexual health is an important aspect of one's overall health [33]. Normalizing the conversation is important. For instance, it may be helpful to begin by stating that "the next several questions are questions we ask all of our patients". During the history ask about partners (e.g. *"Can you tell me about your partners— do you have regular sexual partner or do you have more than one partner?"*). Inquire about the gender of their partners, if they know the HIV status of their partners, and whether or not any protective barriers, such as condoms or dental dams, are used. This can identify the need for counselling or education regarding risk for STIs as well as reinforce the importance of having an undetectable HIV viral load if they are having sex with others, especially those who may not have HIV. Scientific evidence supports that a person with an undetectable viral load is not able to sexually transmit HIV [34]. This concept is also referred to as "U = U" or undetectable equals untransmittable and is endorsed by the United Nations' UNAIDS programme [34]. Nurses can help reinforce information about U = U, which helps de-stigmatize living with HIV.

9.3.5 Recommendations for Nursing Practice

For nurses working with older adults living with HIV, it is important to incorporate and be aware of the various aspects of living with multiple chronic conditions as noted in the earlier sections of this chapter. A comprehensive geriatric assessment (CGA) is used by geriatric providers in order to obtain an overall picture of an individual's physical, mental health, and functional status [31]. Nurses play an integral role in completing parts of a comprehensive geriatric assessment. Box 9.3 provides an example of a CGA that incorporates unique considerations for persons living with HIV. It is important for nurses to not only take into consideration the physiological aspects of ageing, but to also recognize the importance of the social and psychological aspects of ageing with HIV. Many individuals who are now in their 6th, 7th, and 8th decades of life lived through the early years of the epidemic where they may have partners, friends, and entire communities. Issues such as survivor guilt and post-traumatic stress disorder can affect many older persons living with HIV. For individuals who are newly diagnosed later in life, many will experience the same range of emotions as younger individuals (shock, fear, anxiety) [35]. Nurses should provide emotional assistance and/or be prepared to refer clients to appropriate mental health services when needed.

Box 9.3 Nursing Approach to the Older Adult Living with HIV
- **General Health History**
    - Inquire about overall well-being (energy, mood, sleep, activity, nutrition).
    - Inquire about HIV treatment—assess for adherence issues to antiretrovirals, last HIV viral load, CD4+ cell count, liver function, kidney function.
    - Verify kidney function using a standardized renal function calculator (such as CKD-EPI or MDRD) which incorporates age as a factor when calculating results.
    - Inquire about adherence to any HIV-associated opportunistic infection prophylaxis (if needed).
    - Inquire about other chronic diseases (such as diabetes, hypertension, kidney disease, chronic hepatitis B).
    - Obtain a full list of medications (prescribed, over the counter, herbal supplements).

 - Review and assess for adherence to prescriptions.
 - Review medication list for any potential drug–drug interactions.
 - Review list for any drugs that can be eliminated and/or medications that may need to be started (STOPP/START protocol).

- **Assessment of Physical Function**

  - Inquire about mobility, ability to perform activities of daily living.
  - Inquire about any falls or injuries.
  - Inquire about any visual or hearing impairments.
  - Inquire about issues regarding urination, bladder control, or bowel control.

- **Assessment of Sexual Health**

  - Inquire and assess about sexual health—including any concerns about sexual function and STI risk.

- **Assessment of Mental Health, Cognition, Substance Use**

  - Inquire about issues with remembering things or cognition, including difficulty or trouble with managing a checkbook or paying bills.
  - Assess for depression, anxiety, isolation, social support.
  - Inquire about alcohol, tobacco, and other substance use.

- **Assessment of Preventive Health**

  - Inquire about vaccines and immunizations.
  - Inquire and assess if age-related health screenings (e.g. colon cancer screening, breast cancer screening, prostate cancer screening) are up to date.
  - Inquire about oral health, including any pain, mouth dryness, or difficulty chewing food which may impact nutrition.

- **Assessment of Social Needs**

  - Inquire about adequacy of financial resources, housing, transportation, and the ability to get and prepare food.

- **Assessment of Safety**

  - Inquire about any hazards in the home (e.g. leaving the stove on unattended, trip hazards such as rugs, availability of hand rails for stairs, challenges getting in and out of the tub or shower).
  - Inquire about any potential risk for abuse (such as financial exploitation, abandonment, physical, or psychological abuse).

- **Assessment of Goals of Care, Advanced Directives**

  - Inquire about expectations regarding goals of care, including end-of-life decisions or priorities.

Additionally, issues of isolation or loneliness may be greater among persons living with HIV due in part to the fact that many individuals may lack extended families or children to take care of them due to stigma or being cut off from families due to an HIV diagnosis [35]. Recognizing and incorporating those pieces of a patient's lived experience are important in developing a patient-centred plan of care.

As nurses, it is important to take a holistic approach to caring for older adults. Being able to assist patients in coordinating care is a vital role [36]. Many times, patients are referred to various specialists or services which can be confusing and overwhelming for some individuals. Additionally, as more and more providers become involved in the care of the older adult, there is an increased risk of miscommunication between providers, risk of potential drug interactions with prescriptions, or duplicate services or tests that are ordered. Being able to help patients navigate these complexities and ensuring that all providers are aware and in agreement with a patient's plan of care can help improve outcomes [36]. Furthermore, helping patients articulate their goals of care priorities is an important part of geriatric nursing. Often times, medical providers may be focused solely on specific clinical outcomes without taking into account a patient's quality of life or health priorities. Nurses can help patients and the patient's providers identify these issues when faced with treatment decisions or unanticipated medical complications. Although these skills are not unique to the care of older adults, it is an important aspect to keep in mind for persons living with HIV who may have had to deal with these similar issues previously, especially those who lived through the early days of the HIV crisis.

9.4   Chapter Summary and Conclusion

In conclusion, with improved therapies for HIV infection, the number of persons living with HIV ageing into older adulthood will continue to rise. Many of these individuals will receive care in a variety of health care settings, including primary care clinics, hospitals, and long-term care facilities. Nurses should be familiar with the health challenges experienced by older persons living with HIV. Given the complexities of ageing, HIV, and multimorbidity, nurses are ideally positioned to provide a holistic approach to help individuals age successfully into older adulthood.

Key Messages to Take Away
1. Ageing with HIV is complex due to the overlap of multiple chronic conditions.
2. Screening for and early detection of co-occurring conditions is a critical aspect of managing persons ageing with HIV.
3. Nurses should consider how physical health, mental health, and social support are all critical components of care when assessing and managing persons ageing with HIV.

Questions for Learning
1. Describe the considerations of ageing on the use of antiretroviral therapy.
2. Discuss the role of multiple chronic conditions in persons ageing with HIV.
3. List at least three interventions nurses can do to improve the overall quality of life for persons ageing with HIV.

Case Study
MZ is a 63-year-old male who was diagnosed with HIV in 1988. He was started on HIV therapy in 1991 when his CD4 cell count was 50 cells/μL and he was diagnosed with *pneumocystis* pneumonia. Since that time has changed medications several times, either due to drug resistance, side effects, or pill burden. He is currently on a multi-pill HIV regimen that he takes twice daily. His viral load has been undetectable for the past 10 years, and his CD4 cell count is currently 378 cells/μL. In addition to his HIV, he has Type 2 diabetes mellitus, hypertension, coronary artery disease, chronic kidney disease stage 3, and peripheral neuropathy due to HIV treatment that he was on in the early 1990s. At his most recent check-up, his viral load went from being undetectable to 50,000 copies/mL.

- What do you think could be contributing to this recent change in his viral load?
- What would you do to address this situation?
- Besides his HIV viral load elevation, what other issues are important to assess?

References

1. Katzung BG. Special aspects of geriatric pharmacology. In: Katzung BG (ed.) Basic & clinical pharmacology, 14e New York: McGraw-Hill; 2018. http://accessmedicine.mhmedical.com. proxy.libraries.rutgers.edu/content.aspx?bookid=2249&sectionid=175215168. Accessed 3 May 2020.
2. Jourjy J, Dahl K, Huesgen E. Antiretroviral treatment efficacy and safety in older HIV-infected adults. Pharmacotherapy. 2015;35(12):1140–51.
3. European Centre for Disease Prevention and Control/WHO Regional Office for Europe. *HIV/ AIDS surveillance in Europe 2019–2018 data.* https://www.ecdc.europa.eu/en/publications-data/hivaids-surveillance-europe-2019-2018-data. Accessed 3 May 2020.
4. Tavoschi L, Gomes Dias J, Pharris A. New HIV diagnosis among adults aged 50 years or older in 31 European countries, 2004-15:an analysis of surveillance data. The Lancet HIV. 2017;4(11):514–21.
5. European AIDS Clinical Society. *Guidelines version 10.0 November 2019.* https://www.eacsociety.org/files/2019_guidelines-10.0_final.pdf. Accessed 2 May 2020.
6. Livio F, Marzolini C. Prescribing issues in older adults living with HIV: thinking beyond drug-drug interactions with antiretroviral drugs. Ther Adv Drug Saf. 2019. doi: https://doi.org/10.1177/2042098619880122. Accessed 27 June 2020.
7. Ware D, Palella FJ, Chew KW, Friedman MR, D'Souza G, Ho K, et al. Prevalence and trends of polypharmacy among HIV-positive and -negative men in the multicenter AIDS Cohort Study from 2004 to 2016. PLoS One. 2018; https://doi.org/10.1371/journal.pone.0203890.
8. Freedman SF, Johnston C, Faragon JJ, Siegler EL, Del Carmen T. Older HIV-infected adults. Complex patients (III): polypharmacy. Eur Geriatr Med. 2019;10(2):199–211. https://doi.org/10.1007/s41999-018-0139-y.

9. Marzolini C, Livio F. Prescribing issues in elderly individuals living with HIV. Expert Rev Clin Pharmacol. 2019;12(7):643–59.
10. World Health Organization. *The third WHO global patient safety challenge: medication without harm.* https://www.who.int/patientsafety/medication-safety/en/. Accessed 3 May 2020.
11. Leng S, Margolick J. Aging, sex, inflammation, frailty, and CMV and HIV infections. Cell Immunol. 2020;348:104024. https://doi.org/10.1016/j.cellimm.2019.104024.
12. Marciel RA, Kluck HM, Durand M, Sprinz E. Comorbidity is more common and occurs earlier in persons living with HIV than in HIV-uninfected matched controls, aged 50 years and older: a cross-sectional study. Int J Infect Dis. 2018;70:30–5.
13. Babu H, Ambikan AT, Gabriel EE, Svensson Akusjarvi S, Palaniappan AN, Sundaraj V, et al. Systemic inflammation and the increased risk of inflamm-aging and ag-associated disease in people living with HIV on long term suppressive antiretroviral therapy. Front Immunol. 2019; https://doi.org/10.3389/fimmu.2019.01965.
14. Shah ASV, Stelzle D, Lee KK, Beck EJ, Alam S, Clifford S, et al. Global burden of atherosclerotic cardiovascular disease in people living with HIV. Circulation. 2018;138(11):1100–12.
15. European Society of Cardiology. *2018 ESC/ESH clinical practice guidelines for the management of arterial hypertension.* https://www.escardio.org/Guidelines/Clinical-Practice-Guidelines/Arterial-Hypertension-Management-of. Accessed 2 May 2020.
16. International Diabetes Federation. *Diabetes facts and figures.* https://idf.org/aboutdiabetes/what-is-diabetes/facts-figures.html. Accessed 2 May 2020.
17. Duncan AD, Goff LM, Peters BS. Type 2 diabetes prevalence and its risk factors in HIV: a cross-sectional study. PLoS One. 2018, 2018; https://doi.org/10.1371/journal.pone.0194199.
18. Davies MJ, D'Alessio DA, Fradkin J, Kernan WN, Mathieu C, Mingrone G, et al. Management of hyperglycaemia in type 2 diabetes, 2018. A consensus report by the American Diabetes Association (ADA) and the European Association for the Study of Diabetes (EASD). Diabetologia. 2018;61:2461–98.
19. Alfano G, Cappelli G, Fontana F, Di Lullo L, Di Iorio B, Bellasi A, et al. Kidney disease in HIV infection. J Clin Med. 2019; https://doi.org/10.3390/jcm8081254.
20. Reid E, Suneja G, Ambinder RF, Ard K, Baiocchi R, Barta S, et al. Cancer in people living with HIV, version 1.2018, NCC clinical practice guidelines in oncology. J Natl Compr Cancer Netw. 2018;16(8):986–1017.
21. Smail RC, Brew BJ. HIV-associated neurocognitive disorder. Handb Clin Neurol. 2018;152:75–97.
22. Sacktor NC, Wong M, Nakasujja N, Skolasky RL, Selnes OA, Musisi S, et al. The International HIV Dementia Scale: a new rapid screening test for HIV dementia. AIDS. 2005;19:1367–74.
23. Milanini B, Paul R, Bahemana E, Adamu Y, Kiweewa F, Langat R, et al. Limitations of the International HIV Dementia Scale in the current era. AIDS. 2018;32(17):2477–83. https://doi.org/10.1097/QAD.0000000000001968.
24. Rosca EC, Albarquoni L, Simu M. Montreal cognitive assessment (MoCA) for HIV-associated neurocognitive disorders. Neuropsychol Rev. 2019;29(3):313–27.
25. Quigley A, O'Brien K, Parker R, MacKay-Lyons M. Exercise and cognitive function in people living with HIV: a scoping review. Disabil Rehabil. 2019;41(12):1384–95.
26. Goh SSL, Lai PSM, Tan ATB, Ponnampalavanar S. Reduced bone mineral density in human immunodeficiency virus-infected individuals: a meta-analysis of its prevalence and risk factors. Osteoporos Int. 2018;29(3):595–613.
27. Rooney AS, Moore RC, Paolillo EW, Gouaux B, Umlauf A, Letendre SL, et al. Depression and aging with HIV: Associations with health-related quality of life and positive psychological factors. J Affect Disord. 2019;251:1–7.
28. Forstein M. Depression in the Aging HIV infected population. http://hiv-age.org/2016/01/26/depression-in-the-ageing-hiv-infected-population/. Accessed 3 May 2020.
29. Deren S, Cortes T, Vaughan Dickson V, Guilamo-Ramos V, Han BH, Karpiak S, et al. Substance use among older people living with HIV: Challenges for health care providers. Front Public Health. 2019; https://doi.org/10.3389/fpubh.2019.00094.

30. Bloch M. Frailty in people living with HIV. AIDS Res Ther. 2018;15:19. https://doi.org/10.1186/s12981-018-0210-2.
31. British Geriatric Society. *Comprehensive Geriatric Assessment Toolkit for Primary Care Practitioners*. https://www.bgs.org.uk/resources/resource-series/comprehensive-geriatric-assessment-toolkit-for-primary-care-practitioners. Accessed 27 June 2020.
32. White I. Sexual health and well-being in later life. Nurs Older People. 2020;32(3):32–40.
33. Wagner GT, Chaun M, Moyer D. *Sexual health: Tips for taking a geriatric sexual history*. https://www.uofazcenteronaging.com/care-sheet/providers/sexual-health-tips-taking-geriatric-sexual-history. Accessed 28 June 2020.
34. UNAIDS. Undetectable = Untransmittable: Public health and viral suppression. https://www.unaids.org/sites/default/files/media_asset/undetectable-untransmittable_en.pdf. Accessed 28 June 2020.
35. Brennan-Ing M. Diversity, stigma, and social integration among older adults with HIV. Eur Geriatr Med. 2019;10:239–46. https://doi.org/10.1007/s41999-018-0142-3.
36. Donelan K, Chang Y, Berrett-Abebe J, Spetz J, Auerbach DI, Norman L, et al. Care management for older adults:The roles of nurses, social workers, and physicians. Health Aff. 2019;38(6):941–9. https://doi.org/10.1377/hlthaff.2019.00030.
37. National AIDS Trust. *HIV in the UK statistics -2018*. https://www.nat.org.uk/we-inform/HIV-statistics/UK-statistics. Accessed 2 May 2020.
38. Centers for Disease Control and Prevention. *HIV and older Americans*. https://www.cdc.gov/hiv/group/age/olderamericans/index.html. Accessed 2 May 2020.

Chapter 10
Women Living with/or Affected by HIV: Frugality and the Politics of Deprivation

Christina Antoniadi

10.1 Introduction

Back in 1991, ACT UP at the International AIDS Conference introduced the slogan "Women Don't Get AIDS: They just die from it" [1]. It meant to highlight the delay in response to women's needs. As HIV first presented in men who have sex with men, it was originally thought to not affect women. Nevertheless, women in their roles as carers whether in official or unofficial capacities, responding to the epidemic, or just living their lives, were exposed to HIV and put their lives, health, and well-being at risk. Today, they represent 51% of the people living with HIV globally [2]. In recent years, Eastern Europe and Central Asia are one of the two regions that the overall prevalence of HIV has not declined [3] with adolescent girls and young women facing double the risk of HIV acquisition compared to their male counterparts [4]. Whether this is due to stigma, discrimination, lack of women-specific services, financial limitations, lack of social support, knowledge and certainly empowerment, or even intimate partner violence and cultural implications, women were traditionally, and remain to this day, equally exposed but with very limited access to support.

In the following pages, I intent to highlight differences between the sexes and gender-specific areas of deprivation. Identified good practice examples and recommendations or guidelines will be noted accordingly.

C. Antoniadi (✉)
Chelsea and Westminster Hospital, London, UK

M. Croston, I. Hodgson (eds.), *Providing HIV Care: Lessons from the Field for Nurses and Healthcare Practitioners*,
https://doi.org/10.1007/978-3-030-71295-2_10

10.2   The Biological Differences

HIV is affecting the CD4 cells and the body's ability to respond to threats by attacking the immune system of the individual. Biological differences including hormonal differences can interfere with prevention methods and/or treatments for HIV. Further evidence and data are required to fully understand the impact of hormones and other biological factors on HIV infection response and treatments developed, including sex, tissues examined, and age [5].

It is a documented fact that women living with HIV experience faster disease progression and premature ageing compared to their male counterparts [6] with increased numbers of myocardial infraction compared to non-infected women [7–9]. Moreover, women living with HIV present a 10–14 year increase in ageing markers including enhanced immune activation which can explain the early menopause as well as the higher incidence of inflammation-related diseases observed [10]. Accordingly, the female genital track has been identified as one of the reservoirs, one of the areas where HIV can survive in a latent form despite the use of antiretroviral therapy [5]. Meditz et al. highlighted an elevated risk of HIV acquisition in post-menopausal women by recognising increased levels of CCR5 expression in the CD4 cells of the cervix [11]. Increased risk of HIV acquisition appears to also be related to vaginal microbiota as well, with bacterial vaginosis, herpes, and HPV being the main implicated infections [12]. Finally, women living with HIV also suffer an elevated risk of miscarriage compared to non-infected women which in part can be attributed to differences in their immunoregulatory profile [13].

Despite the demonstrated equal treatment response for both sexes [14], the access to services and support in order for adherence to be achieved is not equal. In addition, several studies have suggested that women experience more adverse and side effects which seriously compromise their ability to take their treatment effectively [15]. Especially, the first- and second-generation antiretrovirals have demonstrated notable differences with women presenting more often skin rashes, mitochondrial toxicity, lactic acidosis, gastrointestinal intolerance, and lipodystrophy [16]. Similarly, women experienced more nausea with regimens containing efavirenz or rilpivirine while men experienced more diarrhoea and abnormal dreams [17] and cleared atazanavir much faster than men, leading them to experience treatment failure on an atazanavir containing regimens despite adhering to the treatment dosing [18].

10.3   Research Gaps

The above highlight the need for further research. Research that will not extrapolate results but rather produce them. It is a well-documented fact that clinical research is rather exclusive to women and these results can be extrapolated to women living with HIV. Mark Rapa in his paper "The participation of women living with HIV in

HIV clinical trials" [19] refers to the regulatory restrictions for women's involvement in clinical trials as well as the recent legal framework changes [20, 21] that will enable improved participation of women. In addition, he explains the barriers or perceived barriers that preclude women from taking part in clinical trials such as protectionism and the principle of beneficence [22], the principle of reproducibility [23], and economic costs [24]. Supporting the above, Westreich et al. [25] document a 38% women participation in HIV clinical research and only 4% pregnant women, while Curno et al. [26] document 23% women participants in 544 HIV studies, including prevention, treatment, and vaccine trials.

Alyson McGregor of Brown University has repeatedly written and spoken about the accuracy of science or the lack of it when medicine is not individualised and taking into consideration sex and gender differences [27]. One of her main proposals is to integrate sex and gender medicine into the official medical curricula and training. Mark Rapa's paper [19] suggests obligatory reporting for all research disaggregated by sex as per newer EU and US regulations, better inclusion of women in clinical trials in order to improve the science and provide better treatments for women, meaningful engagement of women from the first stages of trial design in order to better engage and improve recruitment and retention. To support the above findings and recommendations, and in line with current regulations, the FDA approved one particular medication as an option for PrEP in 2020 only in men and trans-gender women. The FDA refused to accept extrapolated results and indications for cisgender women, in essence forcing the company to run another clinical trial to evaluate efficacy and safety in cis gender women [28].

10.3.1 Best Practice Examples

GRACE Study (2006) [29]: multi-centre, open-label, phase IIIb clinical trial that examined the differences in effectiveness, safety, and tolerability of darunavir/ritonavir by sex and/or race over a 48-week period. The study managed to recruit 67% women by engaging with community very early in the design. According to The Well Project, the researchers combined methods such as enforcing specific recruitment strategies to the centres but also published information in community newsletters, while recruiting from community events [30].

MOXIE Study (2019) [31] is a phase II clinical trial that looked at the effects of the oestrogen receptor modulator (ERM) Tamoxifen in combination with a latency reversal agent (LRA) (Vorinostat) on the viral reservoirs of 31 post-menopausal women on ARV treatment. MOXIE was conducted by the AIDS Clinical Trials Group with an aim to examine if tamoxifen would enhance the effect of the LRA. Starting point for this clinical trial had been the recognition of increased viral activity in post-menopausal women. Even though MOXIE Study did not deliver the expected results, i.e. Tamoxifen did not enhance Vorinostat, it did highlight how easy it was to recruit women in an HIV Cure clinical trial from study sites across the USA.

ECHO Study (2015) [32]: is an open-label randomised trial which compared three contraception methods including a non-hormonal, to examine whether there is a link between those methods and higher risk of HIV acquisition. ECHO managed to recruit 7800 women in four countries; however, it did not prove increased risk for HIV acquisition with any of the methods used.

PRIME Study (2016) [33]: is a multi-centre, mixed-methods observational study which managed to recruit 1500 women living with HIV from 15 sites across England in order to document their experiences of menopause, gaps in the care delivery and clinical practice, and to propose possible public health interventions and/or improvements by informing the care of the individuals.

10.4   Social and Other Challenges

Socioeconomic factors influence the Quality of Life and the health outcomes for people living with HIV [34]. In the WHO European Region, new infections in women in 2018 reached almost 50,000 with 54% of them being diagnosed late [35]. A number of factors influence the increased vulnerability of women with lower socioeconomic status (financial hardship, non-employment, rented or unstable housing status, non-university education) being strongly associated with virologic failure and suboptimal adherence to treatment. Burch et al. [34] refer to the Swiss and Spanish cohorts that showed a correlation between educational level and undetectability, a finding not replicated in the Danish cohort, and the Italian cohort which associated unemployment with increased virologic failure risk. The "invisible no longer" [36] report highlights that 45% of the women in the UK who participated in the study were living below the poverty line while 17% never or rarely had money to cover basic needs. On the contrary, the PRIME Study [30] identified 89% of the participants to have enough money to cover basic needs at least some of the time. Moreover, non-adherence to treatment was also associated with lack of support networks, having children, not having a partner, having been born outside the UK and poor English language skills [34]. Eurosurveilance identified a positive correlation between older age and late diagnosis, obvious in the Dutch cohort, but also between older women and IVDU in Russia [35]. In addition, women are more vulnerable to gender based or intimate partner violence. According to WHO [37], women living with HIV are at least 1.5 times more likely to experience some form of violence. The findings from "Invisible no Longer" project [36] showcase that 58% of the participants had experienced some form of violence or abuse.

10.5   Sexual Health and Rights: The Pleasure Deficit

The British HIV Association in the publication "Standards of Care" [38] explicitly state "*People Living with HIV should be supported in establishing and maintaining healthy sexual lives for themselves and their partners*". The BHIVA standards further describe the processes for access to biomedical prevention and testing, partner notification support, and contraception and/or family planning services. In addition, the WHO published in 2017 [37] the "Consolidated Guidelines on Sexual and Reproductive Health and Rights of Women Living with HIV" where a holistic approach is adopted in order to present good practices and recommendations with worldwide effect. In essence, WHO strongly recommends that all women living with HIV should be given access to interventions that will empower them and maximise their self-efficacy around sexual health and rights as a means to improve their health outcomes. The guidelines also encourage the development of services that recognise intimate partner violence and offer support to women experiencing violence.

In the era of U=U (Undetectable = Untransmissible), it seems that women living with HIV have limited access to the benefits of the message. The evidence surrounding the data have been accumulating for the last 20 years starting with the prevention of vertical transmission in 1998 and moving forward with the Swiss Statement in 2008. Four major studies have been designed, delivered, and their results published [39] since then:

- HPTN 052 (2011) [40]: a study between 1763 heterosexual serodiscordant couples—transmission (in 17 individuals) only occurred in couples where the viral load was not undetectable or ART had not been initiated.
- PARTNER (2016) [41]: a study in approximately 900 European serodiscordant couples—no transmission was observed in the 58,000 sexual acts recorded provided the viral load was under 200 copies/mL.
- Opposites attract (2017) [42]: a study in 358 gay serodiscordant couples in Australia, Thailand, and Brazil—Again no transmission was observed when viral load was under 200 copies/mL.
- PARTNER 2 (2019) [43]: an extension to the partner study to include gay serodiscordant couples—no transmission was observed in the 77,000 sexual acts recorded provided the viral load was under 200 copies/mL.

Interestingly, Asa Melgren, in her presentation at the EACS Conference in 2017 [44] reporting on a Swedish cohort, highlighted that women's sexual satisfaction was unrelated to undetectable viral load. For Swedish women living with HIV, the prolonged exposure to ART and HIV were associated with decreased sexual satisfaction while it definitely correlated with physical and mental well-being. Compared to their male counterparts, women were more satisfied with their sexual lives (51.5%) regardless of age, raising a lot of questions about the expectations women actually have about their sexual satisfaction. The Sophia Forum in collaboration with Terence Higgins Trust in the UK, published the report [37] "Invisible no longer" based on women's experiences of HIV. The online survey of the project revealed that about one-third of the women were sexually active with 40% being dissatisfied by their sex lives. Wessman et al. [45] reviewing the sexual activity of Nordic women living with HIV highlights that 62% were sexually active while one-third of the sexually inactive women were in stable relationships. Marocco et al. [46] looked into an Italian cohort of women presenting Female Sexual Dysfunction and compared with an uninfected control group. FSD was present in 48% of the women living with HIV despite achieving virologic control and adherence to treatment compared to 18% of the negative controls.

Carlsson-Lalloo et al. [47] proved that women remain in fear of onwards transmission towards their children and sexual partners despite the effectiveness of the ART. They specifically describe a whole system of perceptions among women living with HIV, the society they live in and their healthcare providers that don't limit stigma but rather encourage it. Similarly, Wessman et al. [45] identified that 15% of the Nordic cohort of women believed the risk of vertical transmission to be higher than 2%. One reason for the above perceptions according to Jenny Higgins et al. [48] is the lack of sexual autonomy that signifies an increased risk for HIV, STIs, and unintended pregnancies in women. They highlight the focus of programmes on minimising the sexual harm and risk-taking behaviours instead of promoting positive parameters such as sexual pleasure that *"would acknowledge women as sexual agents rather than merely as sexual victims or as "targets" of contraceptive programmes and HIV prevention efforts"*.

10.5.1 Women of Reproductive Age

In addition to the above mentioned, women living with HIV should have access to contraception and family planning services [36, 38]. Pregnancy and the decision to become pregnant can be very stressful leading to increased levels of anxiety [49]. Furthermore, research has proven that support is required as an HIV diagnosis can often impact negatively on family planning for some women. Wessman et al. [45] report that in their cohort 8% had been sterilised after their diagnosis, 14% lost their interest to become mothers, and 44% presented an improved opinion about motherhood as the treatment options improved. Stigma and self-stigma can often be implicated for the change of heart many women experience towards fertility when living with HIV. Healthcare stigma and discrimination, friends and family critical attitudes in addition to other social determinants can also be attributing factors [49]. Better information and discussion about fertility desires has been shown to help change decisions influenced by an HIV diagnosis [47], which established in 42% of the women in the report "invisible no longer" [36], with 30% of the women asking the healthcare professionals to take the lead in the discussion [45]. Ivanova et al. [49] showed that stability in life including a full-time job, a partner, and an undetectable viral load were very significant factors that helped minimise stress for women who wanted to become pregnant. Wessman et al. [45] also picked up on another reason for increased stress and anxiety: possible difficulty in conceiving. A quarter of the Nordic cohort had tried to conceive without success, 28% of women in Spain were found to have tubal occlusion [50] while a 40% reduction in pregnancy incidence was reported from a study of 900 enrolled women living with HIV by Linas et al. [51].

Finally, monitoring for sexual health concerns and fertility should be part of a yearly review for women living with HIV [37, 45, 52] and become part of national and international guidelines and recommendations. An MDT of specialists should be involved throughout the antenatal period [40] in order to better support women.

10.5.2   Menopausal Women

Menopause is a transitioning and often challenging period for all women, including those living with HIV. Women often have to deal with physiological and psychological symptoms caused by the changes in hormone levels. Some of the menopause symptoms include (but are not limited to) lower sexual function [53], fewer orgasms, less sexual satisfaction, and diminished interest in sexual activity [46]. Those symptoms have also been confirmed by the "PRIME" study [33]. Tariq et al. managed to show that the increasing number of women transitioning through menopause and growing old with HIV has overlooked and unmet needs, including those related to sexual dysfunction: 69% of the women participating in the study reported at least one sexual problem lasting for more than 3 months and 68% reported vaginal dryness, urinary tract symptoms, and sexual problems. GPs would not be of much help to these women as they appear to have low confidence in managing menopause [54] with 79% being afraid additionally of possible drug–drug interactions [33].

On the other hand, Taylor et al. [52] managed to showcase that post-menopausal women living with HIV-experienced sex as more pleasurable after the age of 50, with increasing self-awareness and a sexual freedom that not only related to condomless sex as the risk of pregnancy was removed but also allowed them to move away from financial support and relationship status that were of great importance when the same women were younger. Condomless sex was also reported from a cohort of women in Italy [55] and was related to the updated evidence of Treatment as Prevention (TasP) but was also associated with lack of empowerment and difficulty negotiating condom use, a finding also evident in other studies [52].

10.5.3   The Role of Nurses in HIV Services

For the purposes of this chapter, the author invited four women living with HIV to contribute their views on HIV nursing care via an anonymised questionnaire. Two were under the age of 30, one a BAME member living in the UK, the other living in Romania. Two were over 30 years of age, living in the UK and Greece. Experience of HIV ranged from newly diagnosed, to living with HIV for nearly 30 years.

The responses showed women living with HIV express universal concerns towards their health and well-being that are not necessarily directly related to their HIV status. For example, the lack of personal time or the impact of the 2020 COVID-19 pandemic have become more important concerns for them. Their general experience of nurses is positive, rating their experience as very good or excellent. Kindness, availability, first point of contact, psychological support, and encouragement are among the qualities these women identify as important in HIV nurses. One of the women recalls having been helped to establish a personalised administration regimen to improve adherence, another describes nurses working in the 1990s as "fearless", especially before treatments were available. Another respondent, assisted in contacting other healthcare professionals, describes the nurses as their greatest "advocates". Finally, one respondent is in regular contact with nurses from her clinic, who are able to issue prescriptions for refills enabling the patient to skip queues; an act that improves the experience of the HIV clinic for service users.

When asked what improvements they would like to see in HIV care, they responded that nurses need to be more knowledgeable and educate patients better, offer smiles, patience and empathy, and to be in close proximity to communities in need. Nurse-led clinics are an available option for participants from the UK, where they have already established better communication with specialist nurses. Participants from Greece and Romania, where HIV care is still very medicalised and doctor-led, find limited application of nurse-led clinics, and would like more knowledgeable staff to run clinics. But they do recognise their benefit, especially for the newly diagnosed patients. Finally, all the women find the linkage between community services and HIV clinics important, with the "SHE" pan-European programme one of the best practices mentioned.[1]

10.6 Conclusion

Women living with HIV despite belonging to a very vulnerable group have managed throughout the years to make their voices heard. Through community organisations like the Sophia Forum they are conducting their own research and are clarifying their unmet needs and gaps in their care that will guide and inform future clinical trials and possibly transform services. However, all research has indicated that programmes with further investment in building community knowledge and capacities are needed in order for these women to become agents of change and to take control of their own health, while enhancing their relationships, especially the sexual ones.

Key Learning Points
- Women living with HIV (WLHIV) are a particularly vulnerable, nevertheless resilient, group that requires targeted interventions and recognition of risk in order to be provided with effective prevention and treatment options.

---

[1] More information on the SHE programme can be found here: https://www.prnewswire.co.uk/news-releases/she-day-the-strong-hiv-positive-empowered-women-she-faculty-and-bristol-myers-squibb-celebrated-four-years-of-she-a-first-of-its-kind-programme-addressing-the-specific-challenges-faced-by-women-living-with-hiv-in-europe-265166141.html. Accessed Jan 2021.

- WLHIV are faced with higher rates of socioeconomic disparities that often influence their health outcomes negatively.
- WLHIV develop better control of the virus but have higher rates of poor adherence and treatment failure which in many instances can be attributed to socioeconomic factors and adverse reactions to medication.
- Clinical research needs to better engage WLHIV in all the stages, from design, recruitment, and retention to interpreting results.
- Clinical research as is conducted in recent years with limited female representation raises very serious questions about scientific accuracy.
- Sexual pleasure and fulfilment have not been investigated systemically for WLHIV (or without HIV to be fair).
- Some evidence is becoming available about the experience of menopause in WLHIV. Keeping in mind that WLHIV are faced with premature ageing this is of outmost importance in order to be supported appropriately throughout this transition.
- Female Sexual Dysfunction presents more often in WLHIV as is impaired fertility. Early identification during yearly check-ups can improve the health outcomes and quality of life for WLHIV.
- Pregnancy and natural birth are experiences appropriate for most WLHIV. The risk of vertical transmission in recent ART is less than 2%.
- Post-menopausal WLHIV experience sex as more pleasurable after the age of 50, with increasing self-awareness and sexual freedom.

Recommendations for Nursing Practice *Empathy*—It is vital for HIV nursing to create an environment of trust and acceptance. Often, our opinion as healthcare professionals will not be in line with the priorities of our patient/client. We need to realise that and put ourselves in our patient's/client's shoes in order to help them manage their health condition as best as possible.

Knowledge—it is our obligation and prerogative to increase our knowledge on the area we work in, probably HIV if you are reading this book. Scientific updates can be available through professional bodies (such as NHIVNA) and national or international conferences. A lot of the available training and updates has been made available online in an effort to continue delivering support for healthcare professionals during the COVID times.

Advocates—Being a patient's advocate or even better ensure our patients are being supported appropriately to advocate for themselves! Patient education is at the core of our nursing practice. Accompanied with empowerment and support programmes can lead WLHIV to have their voices heard and become agents of change, take the lead managing their health condition, and support themselves.

Holistic care—Caring for WLHIV often includes caring for entire families and communities. It is unthinkable to expect any kind of adherence or retention in care when the survival of the person and their family/loved ones is threatened. As women are often subjected to poverty, unemployment, unstable housing and violence, addressing those issues is vital to ensure good health outcomes and well-being into old age.

Research—As shown above research that doesn't include women is just bad science. Improving the representation of women in clinical research can happen by involving women in early stages as researchers, in boards and other decision-making positions, in the design. Recruitment and retention can be significantly improved if it is targeted and supported by community representatives. Patient information leaflets and consent forms need to be designed and checked by community people to ensure lay persons are able to understand the context.

Stigma and discrimination—Despite the fact healthcare professionals are trained to provide care that is free of judgement or discrimination, in reality this is not always the case. Healthcare professionals have an obligation to themselves and their patients/clients to be aware of their inherited biases and shortcomings and to practice in a conscious way that will be addressing them.

References

1. Taylor-Brown S. Women don't get AIDS: they just die from it. Affilia. 1992;7(4):96–8.
2. World Health Organisation. Global Health Observatory data, HIV epidemic. Size of the epidemic. Geneva; WHO 2020. https://apps.who.int/gho/data/node.main.620?lang=en. Accessed Oct 2020.
3. UNICEF. Children, HIV and AIDS. Regional Snapshot: Eastern Europe and Central Asia. 2018. https://data.unicef.org/wp-content/uploads/2018/11/EECA-regional-snapshot-2018.pdf. Accessed Jan 2021.
4. UNAIDS. Women and HIV—a spotlight on adolescent girls and young women. 2019. Geneva; UNAIDS. https://www.unaids.org/en/resources/documents/2019/women-and-hiv. Accessed Jan 2021.
5. Fiscus SA, Cu-Uvin S, Eshete AT, et al. Changes in HIV-1 subtypes B and C genital tract RNA in women and men after initiation of antiretroviral therapy. Clin Infect Dis. 2013;57:290–7.
6. Addo MM, Altfeld M. Sex-based differences in HIV type 1 pathogenesis. J Infect Dis. 2014;209(Suppl 3):S86–92.
7. Triant VA, Lee H, Hadigan C, Grinspoon SK. Increased acute myocardial infarction rates and cardiovascular risk factors among patients with human immunodeficiency virus disease. J Clin Endocrinol Metab. 2007;92:2506–12.
8. Lang S, Mary-Krause M, Cotte L, et al. Increased risk of myocardial infarction in HIV-infected patients in France, relative to the general population. AIDS. 2010;24:1228.
9. Fitch KV, Srinivasa S, Abbara S, et al. Noncalcified coronary atherosclerotic plaque and immune activation in HIV-infected women. J Infect Dis. 2013;208:1737–46.
10. Martin GE, Gouillou M, Hearps AC, et al. Age-associated changes in monocyte and innate immune activation markers occur more rapidly in HIV infected women. PLoS One. 2013;8:e55279.
11. Meditz AL, Moreau KL, MaWhinney S, et al. CCR5 expression is elevated on endocervical CD4+ T cells in healthy postmenopausal women. J Acquir Immune Defic Syndr. 2012;59:221–8.
12. McKenna C, et al. Vaginal microbiota and susceptibility to HIV. AIDS. 2018;32(6):687–98.
13. Richardson K, Weinberg A. Dynamics of regulatory T-cells during pregnancy: effect of HIV infection and correlations with other immune parameters. PLoS One. 2011;6:e28172.
14. Moore AL, Kirk O, Johnson AM, et al. Virologic, immunologic, and clinical response to highly active antiretroviral therapy: the gender issue revisited. J Acquir Immune Defic Syndr. 2003;32:452–61.

15. Currier JS, Spino C, Grimes J, et al. Differences between women and men in adverse events and CD4+ responses to nucleoside analogue therapy for HIV infection. The Aids Clinical Trials Group 175 Team. J Acquir Immune Defic Syndr. 2000;24:316–24.
16. Ofotokun I, Pomeroy C. Sex differences in adverse reactions to antiretroviral drugs. Top HIV Med. 2003;11:55–9.
17. Hodder S, Arasteh K, De Wet J, et al. Effect of gender and race on the week 48 findings in treatment-naive, HIV-1-infected patients enrolled in the randomized, phase III trials ECHO and THRIVE. HIV Med. 2012;13:406–15.
18. Smith KY, Tierney C, Mollan K, et al. Outcomes by sex following treatment initiation with atazanavir plus ritonavir or efavirenz with abacavir/lamivudine or tenofovir/emtricitabine. Clin Infect Dis. 2014;58:555–63.
19. Rapa MJ. The participation of women living with HIV in HIV clinical trials. Brussels: European AIDS Treatment Group Metrodora Project; 2018.
20. European Commission. Council Regulation (EC) 536/2014 Article 36. https://ec.europa.eu/health/sites/health/files/files/eudralex/vol-1/reg_2014_536/reg_2014_536_en.pdf. Accessed Jan 2021.
21. FDA. Food and Drug Administration Amendments Act of 2007 Article 2(A) (I) (bb). https://www.fda.gov/media/70258/download. Accessed Jan 2021.
22. Bosnjak S. The declaration of Helsinki—the cornerstone of research ethics. Arch Oncol. 2001;9(3):179–84.
23. Brown BA, et al. Challenges of recruitment: focus Groups with research study recruiters. Women Health. 2000;31(2-3):153–66.
24. Schmotzer G. Barriers and facilitators to participation of minorities in clinical trials. Ethn Dis. 2012;22:226–30.
25. Westreich D, et al. Representation of women and pregnant women in HIV research: a limited systematic review. PLoS One. 2013;8(8):e73398.
26. Curno MJA. Systematic review of the inclusion (or exclusion) of women in HIV research: from clinical studies of antiretrovirals and vaccines to cure strategies. J Acquir Immune Defic Syndr. 2016;71(2):181–8.
27. McGregor AJ, et al. Advancing sex and gender competency in medicine: sex & gender women's health collaborative. Biol Sex Differ. 2013; 4: 11. doi: https://doi.org/10.1186/2042-6410-4-11
28. Editorial. For the HIV epidemic to end so must gender inequality. Lancet HIV. 2019;6(7):E411.
29. GRACE Study: clinicaltrials.gov: NCT00381303.
30. The Well Project: Lessons from GRACE: A US study focused on women living with HIV, 20-03-2019. https://www.thewellproject.org. Accessed Jan 2021.
31. MOXIE trial: Selective Estrogen Receptor Modulators to Enhance the Efficacy of Viral Reactivation with Histone Deacetylase Inhibitors. clinicaltrials.gov: NCT03382834.
32. ECHO Study: The Evidence for Contraceptive Options and HIV Outcomes Trial (ECHO). clinicaltrials.gov: NCT02550067.
33. Tariq S, et al. PRIME (Positive Transitions Through the Menopause) Study: a protocol for a mixed-methods study investigating the impact of the menopause on the health and well-being of women living with HIV in England. BMJ Open. 2019;9:e025497.
34. Burch LS, et al. Socioeconomic status and treatment outcomes for individuals with HIV on antiretroviral treatment in the UK: cross-sectional and longitudinal analyses. Lancet. 2016;1(1):e26–36.
35. Mardh O, et al. HIV among women in the WHO European Region—epidemiological trends and predictors of late diagnosis 2009-2018. EuroSurveilance. 2019;24(48):pii=1900696. https://doi.org/10.2807/1560-7917.es.2019.24.48.1900696.
36. Sophia Forum and Terrence Higgins Trust. Women and HIV: Invisible No Longer. 2018. https://www.tht.org.uk/sites/default/files/2018-04/women-and-HIV_summary_final.pdf. Accessed Jan 2021.

37. World Health Organisation. Consolidated Guidelines on Sexual and Reproductive Health and Rights of Women Living with HIV. 2017. https://apps.who.int/iris/bitstream/handle/10665/254634/WHO-RHR-17.03-eng.pdf;jsessionid=2D7FE794457E743E5AB2B7746A1D3BB2?sequence=1. Accessed Jan 2021.
38. BHIVA. Standards of Care for People Living with HIV. 2018. https://www.bhiva.org/standards-of-care-2018. Accessed Jan 2021.
39. Collins S. The evidence for U = U (Undetectable = Untransmittable): why negligible risk is zero risk. HIV i-base. October 2017. https://i-base.info/htb/32308. Accessed January 2021.
40. Cohen MS et al. Final results of the HPTN 052 randomized controlled trial: antiretroviral therapy prevents HIV transmission. IAS 2015, 19–22 July 2015, Vancouver. MOAC0101LB. https://doi.org/10.7448/IAS.18.5.20482.
41. Rodger AJ, et al. Sexual activity without condoms and risk of HIV transmission in serodifferent couples when the HIV-positive partner is using suppressive antiretroviral therapy. JAMA. 2016;316(2):1–11.
42. Grulich A et al. HIV treatment prevents HIV transmission in male serodiscordant couples in Australia, Thailand and Brazil. IAS 2017, Paris. Oral abstract TUAC0506LB. http://programme.ias2017.org/Abstract/Abstract/5469. http://jama.jamanetwork.com/article.aspx?doi=10.1001/jama.2016.5148. Accessed Jan 2021.
43. Rodger AJ, et al. Risk of HIV transmission through condomless sex in serodifferent gay couples with the HIV-positive partner taking suppressive antiretroviral therapy (PARTNER): final results of a multicentre, prospective, observational study. Lancet. 393(10189):2428–38.
44. Meligren A et al. Self-reported physical and psychological well-being, but not treatment outcome, are factors associated with sexual satisfaction in HIV Infected Individuals—a Swedish National Cohort Study. EACS 2017 Oral presentation, http://resourcelibrary.eacs.cyim.com/mediatheque/media.aspx?mediaId=34845&channel=28172. Accessed Jan 2021.
45. Wessman M, et al. Perception of sexuality and fertility in women living with HIV: a questionnaire study from two Nordic countries. J Int AIDS Soc. 2015;18:19962.
46. Marocco R et al. PE10/7—Differences in sexual health among HIV infected and uninfected women of child-bearing age. EACS 2019 oral presentation. http://resourcelibrary.eacs.cyim.com/mediatheque/media.aspx?mediaId=78696&channel=28172. Accessed Jan 2021.
47. Carlsson-Lalloo E, et al. Sexuality and childbearing as it is experienced by women living with HIV in Sweden: a lifeworld phenomenological study. Int J Qualit Stud Health Well-Being. 2018;13(1):1487760.
48. Higgins J, et al. The pleasure deficit: revisiting the "sexuality connection" in reproductive health. Int Fam Plan Perspect. 2007;33(3):133–9.
49. Ivanova EL, et al. Correlates of anxiety in women living with HIV of reproductive age. AIDS Behav. 2012;16:2181–91.
50. Coll O, et al. Fertility assessment in non-infertile HIV-infected women and their partners. Reproduct Med Online. 2007;14(4):488–94.
51. Linas BS, et al. Relative time to pregnancy among HIV-infected and uninfected women in the Women's Interagency HIV Study, 2002–2009. AIDS. 2011;25(5):707–11.
52. Taylor TN, et al. "The pleasure is better as I've got older": sexual health, sexuality, and sexual risk behaviours among older women living with HIV. Arch Sex Behav. 2017;46(4):1137–50.
53. Wilson, et al. HIV infection and women's sexual functioning. J Acquir Immun Deficien Syndr. 2010;54:360.
54. Toorabally N, et al. Association of HIV Status with sexual function in women aged 45-60 in England: results from two national surveys. AIDS Care. 2020;32(3):286–95.
55. Cicconi P, et al. Inconsistent condom use among HIV-positive women in the "Treatment as Prevention Era": data from the Italian DIDI study. J Int AIDS Soc. 2013;16:18591.

Chapter 11
Ageing with HIV: Lifestyle Interventions Towards Health

Catarina Esteves Santos

11.1 Introduction

HIV has been transformed from a fatal disease into a chronic condition where the majority of HIV-infected individuals can look forward to a full and active life. This is due to an increased understanding of the disease and its management, but above all, to the unprecedented improvement in antiretroviral drugs. Current comprehensive HIV management strategies can no longer be limited to suppressing HIV RNA levels but must help to guarantee an active, satisfying, and long life for the people living with HIV (PLHIV).

Effective antiretroviral treatment is a reality, which is why many PLHIV live longer. However, longer life is not synonymous with quality of life. Although there is now much more hope, HIV infection influences all areas of a person's life, affecting how much and how they live [1].

Diseases that are typically diagnosed in HIV-negative people between the ages of 60 and 70 are more likely to occur in PLHIV between the ages of 40 and 50. This reality brings the issue of ageing with HIV to the centre of care. In fact, 5.8 million people living with HIV worldwide are over 50 years old [2].

Several factors can make people more prone to illnesses and age-related conditions with greater intensity and younger ages. PLHIV are more predisposed to some risk factors, which play important roles in increasing rates of diseases and conditions related to ageing than HIV-negative people, leading them to have more diseases as they get older. These can include:

C. E. Santos (✉)
Hospital de Cascais Dr. José de Almeida, Cascais, Portugal

M. Croston, I. Hodgson (eds.), *Providing HIV Care: Lessons from the Field for Nurses and Healthcare Practitioners*,
https://doi.org/10.1007/978-3-030-71295-2_11

- The side effects of antiretroviral treatment, some of which may contribute to bone loss, kidney damage, redistribution of fat and elevated cholesterol and triglycerides [3].
- Viral hepatitis co-infection, which increases the risk of hepatocellular carcinoma, liver failure, kidney disease, and diabetes [4].
- Human papillomavirus (HPV), which can cause cervical and anal cancer, as well as head, neck, and throat cancer [5, 6].
- Tobacco use is present in many users, a major cause of heart disease, cerebrovascular accidents (strokes), lung cancer, and emphysema [7].
- Rates of mental illness and substance abuse that are often higher than in people who do not have HIV [8].
- HIV can directly infect important tissues in bone, brain, circulatory system and elsewhere, and can cause inflammation-related damage to the heart, nervous system, liver, and kidneys [9].

11.2   Comorbidities: The Persistent Challenge

As the person living with HIV gets older, other comorbidities can appear. Consequently, more medication is prescribed. In practice, this means having a distinct health and medication team for each pathology diagnosed, with many people polymedicated. Many comorbidities are not specific to HIV itself but are associated with ageing. These can include [1, 2]:

- Cardiovascular disease
- Chronic obstructive pulmonary disease
- Frailty
- Liver disease
- Non-AIDS cancers
- Neurocognitive dysfunction
- Non-AIDS infections
- Osteoporosis
- Renal disease
- Thromboembolic disease
- Type II diabetes

Chronic non-communicable diseases are one of the major public health challenges of the twenty-first century, generating negative economic and social impacts [10]. This group of diseases, which includes cardiovascular, cancer, diabetes, and chronic respiratory diseases, is the main global cause of death, responsible for 70% of cases in the world and 86% in Portugal, corresponding to 91,800 cases [11].

These diseases have modifiable risk factors, such as smoking, inappropriate eating habits, physical inactivity, and excessive alcohol consumption, which in turn can lead to the onset of the disease [2].

In the context of the Global Burden of Diseases study by the World Health Organisation, risk factors that most contribute to the total years of healthy life lost by the Portuguese population are inappropriate eating habits, arterial hypertension, high body mass index, and smoking. These are the main risk factors, often modifiable and, therefore, avoidable for oncological diseases, of the circulatory system, and for a wide group of diseases, led by diabetes, endocrine, haematological, and genitourinary diseases [11].

Chronic non-infectious diseases require guidance and intervention strategies in the areas of health determinants, risk and protective factors for non-infectious diseases, evaluation of the effectiveness of health interventions, and health literacy. For all these reasons, the ideal management of non-infectious disease for PLHIV may differ from that for an individual without HIV infection.

The focus of health care provided to PLHIV under treatment requires new research on epidemiology, pathophysiology, prevention, and treatment of complications from other chronic diseases and, the translation of such research into guidelines, development of uniform policies and procedures in health education, disease prevention and care.

11.3   Preventing Risk Factors and Reducing the Morbidity Associated with PLHIV is a Priority

In the ART era, several large cohort studies found that HIV infection is associated with an increased risk of acute myocardial infarction, ischemic stroke, and heart failure [12–14]. Although total mortality has decreased by a decade among PLHIV, mortality from cardiovascular disease (CVD) increased significantly in the same period [15].

The underlying mechanism that drives the excess risk of CVD is unclear. It may involve a combination of factors including the virus itself, the side effects of ART, and risk factors for coronary artery disease (e.g., smoking, drinking, habits inadequate diet) and non-traditional risk factors (e.g., hepatitis C, substance use, or abuse). In the first part of the ART era, observational studies reported that ART is an important risk factor for CVD in people infected with HIV [16].

The concern about the excess risk of CVD associated with ART was one of the findings leading to Antiretroviral Therapy (SMART) Treatment Strategies, a randomized controlled trial that examined ART-guided CD4+ cell count interruption (i.e., less ART) versus continuous ART (i.e., less HIV virus) and the risk of opportunistic infections, death and other adverse events, including CVD [17]. SMART clearly demonstrated that episodic ART did not reduce the risk of opportunistic infections, death or adverse events, including CVD, which were associated with ART. In addition, the results suggested that the unrepressed HIV virus plays a greater role in the risk of cardiovascular events than ART.

Arterial hypertension is the most important modifiable risk factor for diseases of the circulatory system (stroke and ischemic heart disease), which are the leading cause of death in Portugal and, with a proven direct relationship with excessive salt intake in food and physical inactivity [11].

In Portugal, the consumption of foods with excessive levels of salt is one of the main public health problems. The daily intake of salt by the Portuguese (10.7 g) is almost double that recommended by the WHO (less than 5 g). On the other hand, our fruit consumption is low (less than three pieces of fruit per day), being the preventable food risk that most contributes to the loss of years of healthy life [11].

The promotion of physical exercise throughout the life cycle, adequate eating habits are absolutely fundamental and irreplaceable as protective factors for health.

Smoking takes on pandemic contours, contributing to six of the eight main causes of death seen annually. Tobacco use is the cause or worsening factor of the most prevalent non-communicable diseases, in particular cancer, respiratory diseases, brain and cardiovascular diseases, and diabetes. Smokers have a two to three times higher risk of death, which translates into an average loss of 10 years of potential life expectancy [11]. The time devoted to smoking cessation interventions allows for considerable health gains.

The smoking rate in PLHIV is two to three times higher than in the general population. PLHIV who smoke face an increased risk of death from cardiovascular disease and cancer compared with non-smokers, as well as an increased risk of AIDS-related death [2, 4].

Depression is a common, but often undiagnosed, feature in PLHIV. To find a strategy for detecting depression in a non-specialized clinical setting, the overall performance of the Hospital Anxiety and Depression Scale (HADS) [18] is effective, as are the depression identification issues proposed by the European HIV Society (EACS) guidelines [19].

Lifestyle changes can help to decrease the risk of developing a comorbidity and reduce the impact of existing comorbidities. Agreement about the best course of action with realistic goals can be facilitated with other members of the care team.

The key to successful lifestyle changes, and indeed HIV infection, is empowerment of the central figure in the process—the PLHIV. Most PLHIV can do much to prevent the appearance of age-related illnesses.

The prevention of disease and the promotion of protective health behaviours within the health sector is part of the model that advocates a continuum of care and approach to individuals. It focuses on changing personal and social behaviours and practices in order to promote individual and collective health.

Although the rates of age-related illnesses are much higher in PLHIV, this does not mean that all PLHIV will experience other illnesses when they reach 50 years of age. In fact, the actual rates of some age-related illnesses remain well below 10% in PLHIV [20]. What remains unclear is who will be most at risk of what illnesses, how vigilant we need to be in screening for various illnesses and whether the treatment for any disease will need to be different in people with HIV.

The need to create a more differentiated approach allows the identification of areas that require attention or monitoring and provides individual care plans in the medium and long term, focused on: early detection of potential health complications, empowerment, health knowledge, disease prevention, combat illiteracy, and encourage the user's active participation in health gains.

11.4 The Role of the Nurse

A nursing consultation should focus on education and health promotion of protective factors against non-communicable diseases, based on the assessment of the therapeutic regime, through the tools:

- Monitor sleep
- Monitor meals
- Monitoring of tobacco, alcohol, and drug use
- Evaluate concomitant medication and over-the-counter medications, multivitamins, natural products
- Assess adherence to the drug regime: side effects, adherence, and drug interactions
- Validation of use of contraceptive methods
- Evaluation of anthropometric parameters (such as weight monitoring, abdominal circumference, body mass index, blood pressure)
- Assess adherence using the Treatment Adherence Measure (MAT) [21] and Treatment Adherence Measure, specific for HIV/AIDS infection (CEAT-HIV) [22, 23]
- Quality of life assessment in four domains: psychological, physical, social relations, and environment
- (WHOQOL-Bref) [1]
- Anxiety and depression assessment (HADS) [18]
- Health education in promoting a healthy and balanced diet and physical exercise
- Promote resilience in teaching effective coping and anxiety management strategies
- Monitor the capacity for performance [24] that assesses the person's level of independence in performing Instrumental Activities of Daily Living
- Monitor the ability to perform self-care [25], which assesses the level of independence of individuals in ten life activities

Monitoring is constant in each consultation, with quarterly (minimum) and half-yearly (maximum) evaluations, and others that are carried out annually. Teamwork is essential, as well as the electronic registration of everything that is addressed and carried out with the user, in order to continue quality care.

The centre of nursing care is the user, and currently must be focused on health promotion and disease prevention in the person seen as a whole, inserted in the family and community and interacting with health professionals, and health education has become increasingly important in nursing.

Every nurse must, as part of their duties, be a health educator. The Quality Standards of Nursing Care [26] defined by the Order of Nurses emphasizes the importance of playing the role of health education agent. In the permanent search for excellence in professional practice, nurses can help clients achieve the maximum health potential. In this sense, the nurse's role involves enabling autonomy, creating opportunities, reinforcing convictions and skills, respecting users' decisions and learning rhythms, in a process of growth and development.

Respect for autonomy is important in the context of health as it is central to person-centred care [27].

Autonomy is the ability of an individual lives according to personal values, beliefs, and preferences. In health, this involves the person who uses services making informed decisions about the care, support, or treatment that he or she receives [28].

The process of individualized risk assessment, communication, and informed decision-making is key.

Nurses are also responsible for teaching patients about the prevention and management of medical conditions, particularly true in chronic illness. By transmitting information, nurses help patients to control their health care and ensure commitment to health gains.

Patient education is a significant part of the nurse's job [27]. Education empowers patients to improve their health. When patients are involved in their care, they are more likely to be involved in interventions that can increase their chances of positive results, being linked to care and compliance with the therapeutic plan.

The benefits of patient education include [11]:

- Prevention of non-infectious medical conditions such as obesity, diabetes, or heart disease.
- Decrease in the possibility of complications, teaching patients about medications, lifestyle changes.
- Reduction in the number of patients readmitted to the hospital.
- Maintaining independence by learning self-sufficiency.

Without proper education, the patient can go home and resume harmful health habits or ignore the management of his medical condition. These actions can lead to worsening of the disease and eventually to hospitalization.

To educate patients, nurses can instruct them on the following:

- Self-care measures they need to take.
- Why they need to maintain self-care and retention in care.
- What to do if a problem occurs.
- Who to contact in case of doubt.

Many patients are unaware of health. Nurses should assess their patients to identify the best way to educate them about their health and determine how much they already know about their medical condition. They need to build a relationship with patients by asking questions to address concerns. Nurses may have to adjust their teaching strategies to meet the patient's preferences. Many patients want detailed information although some may request only a checklist.

A practical approach is essential to ensure that the patient understands the information provided. Nurses should also teach the patient's family, friends, or caregivers at home, if the user authorizes it.

11.5   Seeking Health

Health is a fundamental factor for human development, training, and adaptability to changes. Its promotion takes on a variety of outlines, dimensions, and responsibilities, including surveillance and individual investment, through the positive valuation of the factors that determine it. Health promotion and health education are both the responsibility of nursing.

Health professionals, educators, researchers, and policy makers are focusing on shared decision-making (SDM) at the national and international levels [29, 30]. SDM is described as the optimal outcome between the partnership between the healthcare provider and the patient characterized by a collaborative two-way exchange of information and discussion involving negotiation leading to a shared decision [31]. SDM happens when there is a relationship between two participants—in this case nurse and patient, participative, collaborative, open, respectful, and trustworthy.

The use of SDM in the daily practice of nurses working with HIV is evident and embedded, and while SDM is aimed at in the context of chronic disease management to facilitate long-term health outcomes, there are still challenges to be overcome [32].

Shared decision-making can only be adopted if it improves patient outcomes. It is necessary to change attitudes with recognition of the role of nursing in SDM, more training and improvements in the knowledge of SDM are necessary for the imperatives of policies to be carried out at the structural and organizational level [32].

11.6   Conclusion: Points for Learning

- HIV infection is a chronic disease and ART is effective and allows people living with HIV to live longer.
- The long-term side effects of HIV treatment and ageing with HIV, can lead to the appearance of age-related illnesses earlier.
- Care models with multidisciplinary teams must be adapted and focused on the early detection of signs and symptoms of diseases associated with ageing.
- The centre of care is the patient and currently must be focused on health promotion and disease prevention.
- Interventions should focus on promoting positive responses at the individual level, disease prevention, and health gains for the person as a whole, inserted in the family and the community.

References

1. Canavarro M, Pereira M. Avaliação da qualidade de vida na infecção por VIH/SIDA: Desenvolvimento e aplicação da versão em Português Europeu do WHOQOL-HIV-Bref. Laboratório de Psicologia. 2011;9(1):49–66. I.S.P.A.
2. Teeraananchi S, Keer SJ, Amin J, Ruxrungtham K, Law MG. Life expectancy of HIV-positive people after starting combination antiretroviral therapy: a meta-analysis. HIV Med. 2017;18:256–66.
3. Max B, Sherer R. Management of the adverse effects of antiretroviral therapy and medication adherence. Clin Infect Dis. 2000;30:S96–S116.
4. Soriano V, Barreiro P, Nuñez M. Management of chronic hepatitis B and C in HIV-coinfected patients. J Antimicrob Chemother. 2006;57(5):815–8.
5. Wigfall L, Bynum S, Brandt H, Sebastien N, Ory M. HPV-related cancer prevention and control programs at community-based HIV/AIDS service organizations: implications for future engagement. Front Oncol. 2018;8:422.
6. Konopnicki D, Wit S, Clumeck N. HPV and HIV coinfection—A complex Interaction resulting in epidemiological, clinical and therapeutic implications. Futur Virol. 2013;8(9):903–15.
7. Altekruse S, et al. Cancer burden attributable to cigarette smoking among HIV-infected people in North America. AIDS. 2018;32(4):513–21.
8. Klinkenberg W, Sacks S. Mental disorders and drug abuse in persons living with HIV/AIDS. AIDS Care. 2004;16(Suppl 1):S22–42.
9. Nasi M, et al. Ageing and inflammation in patients with HIV infection. Clin Exp Immunol. 2017;187(1):44–52.
10. World Health Organization. Global status report on noncommunicable diseases. Geneva, Switzerland: WHO; 2014. https://apps.who.int/iris/bitstream/handle/10665/148114/9789241564854_eng.pdf?sequence=1. Accessed Jan 2021.
11. World Health Organization. Noncommunicable diseases progress monitor. Geneva, Switzerland: WHO; 2018. https://www.who.int/nmh/publications/ncd-profiles-2018/en/. Accessed Jan 2021.
12. Freiberg M, et al. VIH infection and the risk of acute myocardial infarction. JAMA Intern Med. 2013;173:614–22.
13. Marcus J, et al. VIH infection and incidence of ischemic stroke. AIDS. 2014;28:1911–9.
14. Butt A, et al. Risk of heart failure with human immunodeficiency virus in the absence of prior diagnosis of coronary heart disease. Arch Intern Med. 2011;171:737–43.
15. Feinstein M, et al. Patterns of cardiovascular mortality for VIH-infected adults in the United States: 1999 to 2013. Am J Cardiol. 2016;117:214–20.
16. Friis-Moller N, et al. Combination antiretroviral therapy and the risk of myocardial infarction. New Engl J Med. 2003;349:1993–2003.
17. El-Sadr W, et al. Strategies for management of antiretroviral therapy. New Engl J Med. 2006;355:2283–96.
18. Pais-Ribeiro J, et al. Validation study of a Portuguese version of the Hospital Anxiety and Depression Scale. Psychol Health Med. 2007;12(2):225–35.
19. European AIDS Clinical Society. EACS HIV guidelines 9. 2017; 68.
20. National Institues of Health. HIV, AIDS, and older people. 2016. https://www.nia.nih.gov/health/hiv-aids-and-older-people. Accessed Jan 2021.
21. Delgado AB, Lima ML. Contributo para a Validação Concorrente de uma Medida de Adesão aos Tratamentos. Psicologia, Saúde e Doenças. Sociedade Portuguesa de Psicologia da Saúde. 2001;2:81–100.
22. Remor E. Valoración de la adhesión al tratamiento antirretroviral en pacientes VIH+. Psicothema. 2002;14(2):262–7.
23. Reis A, Lencastre L, Guerra MP, Remor E. Adaptação portuguesa do questionário para avaliação da adesão ao tratamento anti-retrovírico—VIH (CEATVIH). Psicologia, Saúde & Doenças. 2009;10(2):175–91.

24. Araújo F, et al. Validação da escala de Lawton e Brody numa amostra de idosos não institucionalizados. In: Leal I, et al., editors. Atas do 7° Congresso Nacional de Psicologia da Saúde. Lisboa: ISPA; 2008. p. 217–20.
25. Araújo F, et al. Validação do Índice de Barthel numa amostra de idosos não institucionalizados. Revista Portuguesa de Saúde Pública. 2007;25:59–66.
26. Padrões de Qualidade dos Cuidados de Enfermagem. Ordem dos Enfermeiros. 2001. https://www.ordemenfermeiros.pt/media/8903/divulgar-padroes-de-qualidade-dos-cuidados.pd. Accessed Jan 2021.
27. Kany I. Groundwork of the metaphysics of morals. Trans. M. Gregor. Cambridge: Cambridge University Press; 1998.
28. Slowther AM. The concept of autonomy and interpretation in healthcare. Clinical Ethics. 2007;2:173–5.
29. Institute of Medicine. To err is human: Building a safer health system. Washington, DC: National Academies Press; 2000.
30. Salzburg Global Seminar. Salzburg statement on shared decision making. 2011. https://www.salzburgglobal.org/fileadmin/user_upload/Documents/2010-2019/2010/477/Salzburg_Global_Shared_Decision_Making_Statement__2013_design_.pdf. Accessed Jan 2021.
31. Charles C, Gafni A, Whelan T. Shared decision-making in the medical encounter: what does it mean? (or it takes at least two to tango). Soc Sci Med. 1997;44(5):681–92.
32. Croston M, McLuskey J, Evans C. How do nurses facilitate shared decision making in HIV care? An exploratory study of UK nurses knowledge, perspective and experience of facilitating shared decision making in clinical practice. Eur J Pers Cent Healthc. 2016;4:4. https://nottingham-repository.worktribe.com/OutputFile/971484. Accessed Jan 2021.

Chapter 12
Bringing Compassion to HIV Care: Applying the Compassion-Focused Therapy Model to Healthcare Delivery

Stuart Gibson, Jane Vosper, Sarah Rutter, and Chris Irons

The role of compassion in healthcare has become increasingly important, especially since it is now considered one of the six "Core Values" in the United Kingdom's National Health Service [1]. This chapter will present a psychological theory and approach which places building compassion (for self and others) at the heart of its aims: Compassion Focused Therapy (CFT) [2, 3]. The role of building compassion for people living with HIV and health professionals working in this field will be explored.

12.1 Introduction

While there are many definitions of compassion, it is described in CFT as "an awareness and sensitivity to distress and a commitment to relieving or preventing it" [3]. CFT integrates theoretical approaches from cognitive behavioural therapy, evolutionary psychology, neuroscience, Jungian approaches, attachment theory and

S. Gibson
Barts Health NHS Trust, London, UK
e-mail: stuart.gibson5@nhs.net

J. Vosper
Royal Holloway, University of London, London, UK

S. Rutter (✉)
North Manchester General Hospital, Manchester, UK
e-mail: Sarah.Rutter@pat.nhs.uk

C. Irons
Balanced Minds, London, UK
e-mail: Chris@balanceminds.com

© The Author(s), under exclusive license to Springer Nature
Switzerland AG 2021
M. Croston, I. Hodgson (eds.), *Providing HIV Care: Lessons from the Field for Nurses and Healthcare Practitioners*,
https://doi.org/10.1007/978-3-030-71295-2_12

Eastern philosophy as well as therapeutic approaches from a range of different psychological therapies to help people build compassion for themselves and others. CFT also promotes a non-judgemental understanding of psychological difficulties with an aim of bolstering confidence and competence at alleviating or preventing distress. In this chapter, we discuss how CFT is applicable to the field of HIV care, with examples of how the theory and practice may help both patients and staff develop compassion and improve quality of life.

Our focus on CFT is to help developing a deeper understanding of why we sometimes struggle in facing psychological difficulties [2, 4]. The evolutionary theory behind CFT is described at the beginning of this chapter, with a focus on how our "tricky brains" have evolved. We present a model of emotions that can be very helpful to understand how our emotions work (Three Systems Model), and the three "Flows of Compassion" (compassion for self, compassion from others, and compassion for others). The second part of the chapter focuses on how CFT relates to the mental health of people living with HIV and how building compassion can help relieve shame and distress. The end of the chapter considers the need for compassion for health professionals, with a review of research on the risk of compassion fatigue and burnout.

12.2 Compassion Focussed Therapy

One of the key drivers for the development of CFT came from observations of people who displayed high levels of shame and self-criticism in psychological therapy [2, 5]. Although clients could see the benefits of trying to think of more evidenced-based thoughts (e.g., "I know that I'm not to blame for my abuse"), Gilbert noticed that these more rational thoughts did not necessarily make people feel better (e.g., "… but I still *feel* like I'm to blame and that I'm a bad person"). On further exploration, Gilbert noticed that many clients were engaging in these alternative thoughts with a hostile, angry, and critical inner voice tone. Clients recognised that this was not a voice tone they would use when trying to be supportive to friend or family member who was struggling. But while guiding clients to bring a more kind, caring inner voice tone to their supportive thoughts, Gilbert noticed that many of his clients found this new comforting and reassuring emotional tone strange, alien, uncomfortable, or even triggering of unpleasant feelings.

In HIV settings, health professionals frequently witness similar self-critical tones in their patients, especially when discussing their diagnoses. Despite trying to convey positive and hopeful messages of good health and longevity, health professionals can sometimes hear their patients blame themselves in harsh tones. This might especially be the case when trying to reassure patients about their diagnoses not reflecting anything bad or shameful about their character. Despite such positive and reassuring statements, many people living with HIV might still struggle to "hear" them and certainly struggle to reassure themselves with warmth and kindness.

Psychological theories and therapeutic approaches looking directly at understanding and reducing shame are extremely important in HIV care. Another observation made by Gilbert was that people who demonstrated high levels of shame and self-criticism often reported difficult early years and/or early trauma [3]. Highly threatening childhoods were often reported (physical, verbal, or sexual abuse) as well as insufficient safeness, care, and soothing from others during their development. These observations from therapy led Gilbert to adapt aspects of Attachment Theory to CFT, with a focus on emotional systems that promote bonding, soothing, and connection rather than relying on "rational thought" alone. Given that people living with HIV also tend to report a relatively higher incidence of trauma than the general population [6, 7], CFT appears relatively useful and appropriate in HIV care. It can help with those who self-shame and struggle in caring for themselves because of their trauma backgrounds.

CFT is a relatively new psychological therapy, using evolutionary theory, cognitive theory, and neuroscience to build an understanding of psychological difficulties [2, 5]. The therapy itself integrates a variety of approaches to help clients build compassion. For example, CFT encourages clients to become aware of their difficulties so they can try to understand them (engagement). It also focuses on building confidence and competence in addressing such difficulties to improve quality of life (action). At the beginning of therapy, "formulations" of problems are developed with clients which aim to de-shame and normalise their psychological difficulties. From this, strategies are then introduced to help clients act compassionately towards themselves. This can help them to start soothing themselves when needed, challenge themselves if appropriate, and work towards developing more connected and fulfilling lives [8].

CFT has been used to help with a number of different psychological difficulties, including depression [9], eating disorders [10], bipolar disorder and psychosis [11], and persistent pain [12]. A systematic review reported an emerging body of evidence for CFT, particularly for people who are highly self-critical [13]. There is increasing interest in using CFT in physical health settings [14] with some studies supporting its usefulness for people living with HIV [15, 16].

12.2.1 Evolutionary Stance – Normalising Difficulties

CFT uses evolutionary theory to understand and explain why people experience psychological difficulties [5]. Evolution does not result in "perfect" systems. What we have instead are systems that have adapted to varying environments at different points in time. According to CFT, our emotional responses have adapted to develop an effective "fight, flight, or freeze" response to challenging situations that are an imminent threat to our safety or wellbeing (e.g., when being chased by a predator). But this threat response system is less adaptive and often not very helpful when feeling challenged or threatened in other situations more common in the modern world (e.g., during social interactions) [2, 5].

Our brains and bodies often react using these older threat response systems. For example, when we freeze in the middle of giving a lecture or case presentation. The CFT approach suggests that the evolution of our brains has led to a "tricky brain" rather than a "perfect brain" [3]. It uses a biopsychosocial model to understand how we feel and behave, with the message that our difficulties are "not our fault", as we have brains and bodies that are the result of millions of years of evolution, reacting to a variety of different social environments that we did not choose. However, once we become aware of our distress, it is our responsibility to then move towards alleviating it [3]. Rather than presenting depression, anxiety, and other psychological difficulties as "abnormal", a therapist presents these as understandable reactions given the way our brains and bodies have evolved. This normalising formulation aims to challenge the shame and self-criticism associated with psychological difficulties. In the context of HIV, where shame, stigma, and self-criticism can be major issues and a very real threat, an approach that is de-shaming from the outset seems highly appropriate.

12.2.2   Tricky Brain

The "tricky brain" in CFT draws on a key component of evolutionary theory that evolution can only move forward; we cannot de-evolve older parts of our brain [17]. New adaptations are linked with existing structures if they can provide an added benefit to a species. Evolutionary theory suggests that we still have parts of our brains that were highly adaptive in early species, such as reptiles and amphibians (fight-flight-freeze, seeking and consuming food, and sex). However, other parts of our brain have evolved in species who nurture their young or live together in groups such as birds and mammals (attachment between infants and parents, care of other, safety in numbers and altruism). More recent evolution of our human brains has given us newer structures such as the frontal and temporal lobes, giving us language, logical and abstract thinking, problem-solving and future thinking. These newer functions of the brain have developed "on top of" the older areas. While we gain new abilities and functions (e.g., rationale thought), we do not get rid of older functions (e.g., fight/flight/freeze) [2].

To illustrate this idea in CFT terms, we can make a distinction between the "old brain" and "new brain". The old brain includes the limbic system, which is important in controlling immediate emotional reactions to events to help us survive (food, territory, and safety) and reproduce (sex). The new brain includes frontal areas, which are important in generating rational and logical thought, mentalisation, theory of mind, and self-monitoring [3]. In other species, the limbic system (old brain) is only triggered when there is an external stimulus (e.g., predator). However, with the addition of newer areas of the brain, our old brain (limbic emotional response) can also be triggered by internal thoughts and mental images of the past or a potential future. We have evolved this ability as it is helpful in many circumstances (e.g., planning to avoid future threats) [2].

However, it also means our emotions can be continually activated even when there are no real external threats. While other species will feel scared or angry if attacked or feel distressed if they are separated from their young or their social group, these feelings only happen *in the situation.* As far as we know, they do not happen before the situation and do not continue afterwards. However, for humans, we might become anxious and scared about possible health consequences of HIV in the future that might never happen. We might feel scared about the *potential* to be excluded and rejected should others become aware of your HIV diagnosis. We can definitely feel angry towards the person who you suspect may have placed you at risk for contracting HIV, even when they are no longer a part of your life. We can develop an "inner critic" that criticises us even when no-one else is around [4]. These functions are not the brain malfunctioning; rather, it is the result of our brains trying to keep us safe. From a CFT perspective, we keep in mind that both our old brain and new brain work tirelessly to keep us safe. However, these two brain systems rarely work together in a perfectly coordinated way.

It is not surprising that we experience anxiety, depression, and other difficult feelings such as shame given how our brain systems have evolved. Our new brain can trigger worries for the future and regrets about the past, which can then activate difficult feelings generated by our old brain. Once these difficult feelings get noticed our new brain tries to make sense of them, resulting in a "perpetuating loop" that keeps suffering active and present in our minds.

Case Example: Melissa

Melissa (a 37-year-old woman originally from Ghana) attends her regular HIV clinic appointment. She reports feeling very low and often struggling to leave her house. She has not told anyone about her diagnosis and feels very alone. She also hints at having experienced a difficult childhood. She then describes herself as lazy and stupid, criticising herself strongly that she is unable to work as hard as she should.

A health professional could advise her (in a well-meaning way) that she should join a social support group for people living with HIV, do some enjoyable activities and reassure her that she will eventually feel better. However, Melissa may then feel even worse when she is not able to "comply" with the advice she is given. As health professionals, sometimes we can feel frustrated when patients like Melissa don't engage in activities that we think would make them feel better. However, from a CFT perspective we can understand how there are strong evolutionary reasons for Melissa's feelings of shame that can inhibit, block or impede progress.

From a CFT perspective, we might note that these "old brain" emotions are very strong and might take considerable time and *compassion* to alleviate. Encouraging her with messages that she is *not* lazy or stupid and that it is understandable that she is struggling can be the start of the process. *"It's not your fault"* can be a very powerful message to give.

12.3 Three Systems Model of Emotional Regulation

CFT aims to understand basic emotions and their purpose from an evolutionary perspective. One of the first steps with clients in therapy is to map out which emotions appear to be most dominant and which are less active. A Three Systems Model can be used, which describes how different types of emotions evolved to help us manage our world. These three distinct systems are based on (1) detecting and responding to threat (e.g., fear, anger, disgust), (2) seeking out resources and reward (e.g., energetic excitement, joy), and (3) resting and care-based systems, non-wanting (e.g., content, soothed, safe) [2, 18] (Fig. 12.1).

These systems have evolved to help us survive a difficult world. The *Drive* system activates us to find food, territory, and sexual opportunities whereas the *threat* system signals danger and the *Soothing-Affiliative* system encourages us to rest, digest, and nurture bonds (e.g., between caregiver and infant and/or within groups) [3, 4, 19].

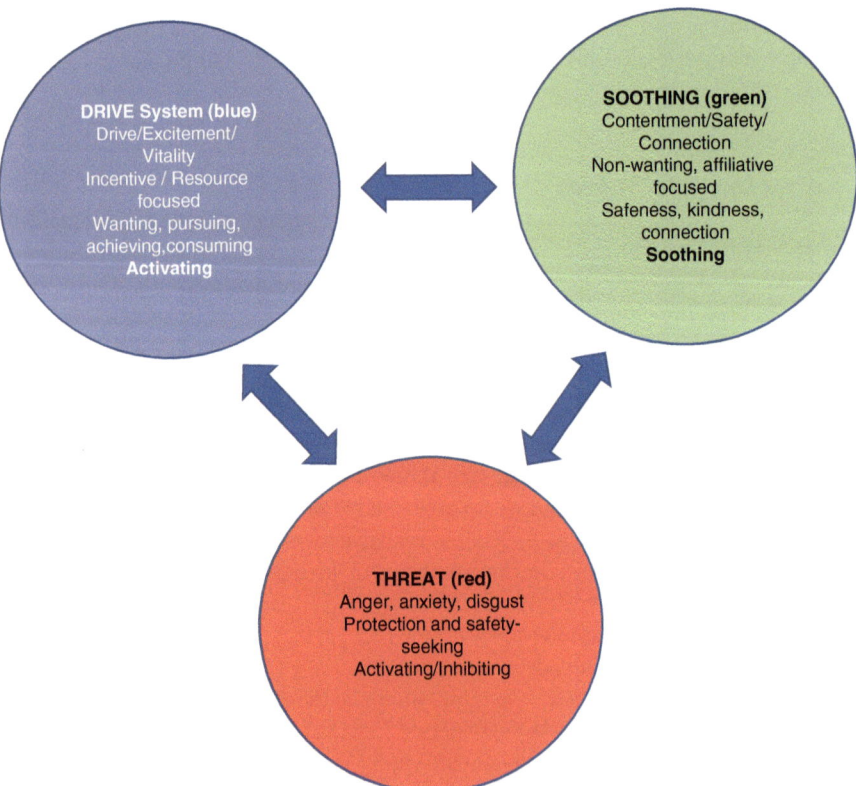

Fig. 12.1 Three systems model adapted from Gilbert (From *The Compassionate Mind* [4], reprinted with permission from Constable & Robinson Ltd.)

12.3.1   Threat System

The threat system was extremely important in survival for our ancestors and continues to help us navigate the world. We might not particularly like experiencing these emotions; however, we cannot get rid of them and they remain important for us (albeit different circumstances to our ancestors). If we are in physical danger, then feeling fear while running away is a very helpful response. If food is rotten, we need to feel disgust to stop us eating it. If we need to defend ourselves, then anger helps us fight. In some circumstances, the most helpful response is "freezing" to avoid being seen (e.g., zebras when hunted by lions) or for our body to "switch off" and play dead to discourage a predator. Illness has always been a threat for humans and other species. A fear response to receiving a diagnosis of an illness (either our own or another) is very understandable. The threat system is also activated when there is a social threat, as being excluded by a social group or abandoned by a caregiver would have been fatal for our ancestors [2]. This kind of threat can activate any of the threat system emotions and can result in a complex emotion of shame. Shame is a social emotion; while experiencing shame is extremely unpleasant, its underlying function is to keep us in groups or connected to others who keep us safe [3].

If people experience repeated adversity and threat in their environment (particularly during childhood), the threat system response can build up to become the "go-to" system [2]. It is then the system that is most easily activated, guiding actions and behaviour (and dominates over the other systems). This is the brain adapting to its environment, by promoting responses that are most helpful. It is not the brain being "abnormal" or malfunctioning. In the case of HIV, receiving the diagnosis may activate the old brain response of fear. However, the social context and fear of exclusion by others should they discover the diagnosis can also be activated. It is not surprising that the "old brain" threat system response may be very strong for people when they are diagnosed. If people have already experienced repeated trauma before their diagnoses, it is not surprising that the threat system response dominates.

12.3.2   Drive System

The drive system is our activating "get up and go" system. This is the set of emotions that can make us feel great when we get something we want (e.g., food, sex, territory ... or in today's world all sorts of material goods that we *want*) [2]. The satisfied feeling you experience when you acquire something (from a new phone to a new partner) is from the activation of the drive system. This system is also activated when you achieve something, like passing an exam, getting a new job, or winning a competition. In these situations, we experience positive feelings such as joy, a surge, and flow of energy—feelings most of us like to experience. The drive system is part of our "old brain", that has activated all species to seek out things we need to survive [3]. While most of us enjoy experiencing these drive emotions, it is not something we can necessarily rely on to feel good all of the time. We cannot win every competition and obtain material objects whenever we want. We cannot find new partners just to keep us happy for short periods of time before we *want* something new. When we feel an emotion in the threat system (e.g., anger or fear), the drive system can be used to "turn down" the threat system [2]. If you feel anxious about something, you might get some short-term relief from the worry by purchasing something or from working hard to achieve a goal. However, the buzz from the good feeling wears off. To continue turning down the threat system with drive system activity, you would have to keep acquiring or competing at a rate that is unsustainable.

Both the threat and drive systems activate the sympathetic branch of the autonomic nervous system (ANS). This keeps our minds and bodies physiologically activated. This is fine in short bursts. However, when over-used for prolonged periods of time, both our minds and bodies will become fatigued and worn out [3, 20]. The threat system can also activate the parasympathetic branch of the autonomic nervous system (ANS) that is responsible for shutting down and immobilising us in frightening situations (e.g., freeze response) [20].

12.3.3   Soothing System

The *activating* drive and threat systems are important for our safety and survival. However, a trade-off or balance between these energising states is required. The ability to slow down, rest, recuperate, and reserve energy is necessary, as being constantly activated by threat and drive is not sustainable. This natural tendency to "rest and digest" is controlled by the parasympathetic branch of our ANS. This soothing system is associated with feelings of calmness and contentment that occur while resting. However, humans and other mammalian species who live in groups and/or care for young have developed another cluster of emotions than are triggered by restful situations. These emotions involve attachment to others. Circumstances involving care, affection, and affiliation can also activate this soothing system when you feel safe and secure with another person and/or group.

Generally, we enjoy these feelings but they are very different feelings from the drive or threat system. These feelings have helped our species survive by keeping parents and infants together and/or keeping us in groups [2]. The need for care and connection with important others has led to systems in our brain that promote bonding (e.g., oxytocin), whether bonding with a parent/infant, between partners or among a group. We feel *connected, safe,* and often *soothed* when we are with a caring parental figure who is looking after us. We also feel *connected, safe, and soothed* when we are with a compatible and caring partner or mate.

Feeling *connected, safe, and soothed* also happens when we believe that we belong to a group and we are accepted and valued by its members [2]. In terms of infant/parent bonding, infants require a parent to keep them safe and nourish/support them until they are able to fend for themselves. Positive feelings associated with bonding helps to keep parents and infants together so the infant can survive. In a context where parents provide safety on a consistent and unconditional basis, these positive feeling are experienced again and again by infants [2]. In time, these positive experiences of being held and cared for become internalised within infants. As a result of such learning, they can then create such positive feelings for themselves, should they need to reassure and soothe themselves when feeling anxious, irritated, or even sad.

12.3.4 *Three Systems Interacting:* Balance

These systems constantly interact with one another. Sometimes one system can activate (up-regulate) another system, while at other times one system can deactivate (down-regulate) another system. Ideally, these systems are flexible; each being activated when corresponding external and internal events occur [8]. When threat is high, a sense of safeness can help to down-regulate it (e.g., when there is a group or caregiver conveying a sense of safety). However, for individuals who find it difficult to create a feeling of safeness and contentment within relationships, it may be easier to rely on the drive system to manage threat (e.g., working hard to achieve goals or compete). In time, these emotional systems can become unbalanced, with one or two systems dominating over each other leading to emotional difficulties [2, 18, 21].

12.3.5 *Soothing Threat and Shame*

As we described earlier, connections with a group and/or caregivers have helped us survive as a species, and we have very strong mechanisms to try to maintain these connections. For example, the possibility of being excluded from a social group will ignite strong feelings of fear and potentially shame, which is a complex and unpleasant emotion. We will often do anything to avoid exclusion as, from an evolutionary perspective, exclusion may well lead to not surviving. For people living with HIV, the perceived stigma of the diagnosis can lead to an extremely strong fear of being excluded, triggering strong feelings of shame. With our "tricky brain", just the thought of this rejection and exclusion will trigger very strong emotions to try to prevent the possibility of exclusion. However, as mentioned earlier, this can lead to unintended consequences [5, 8].

From the case example, if we map out Melissa's emotions it appears her threat system is very dominant over her other emotional systems (see Fig. 12.2). Her soothing system is down-regulated (feeling calm/safe/connected), as well as her drive system (action/excitement/wanting). To help these systems become more balanced and flexible, we would have to build strategies to help activate Melissa's soothing and drive systems. In this example, the health professional had a sense of this imbalance. However, when a threat system is highly dominant it can take time

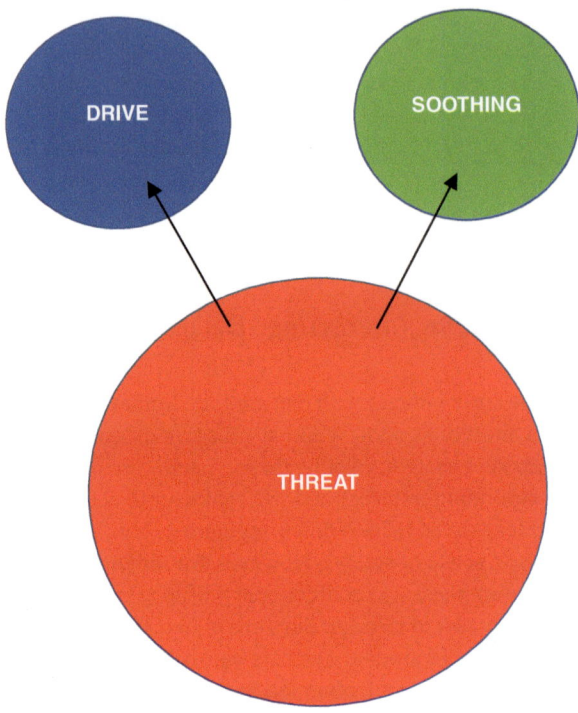

Fig. 12.2 Melissa's three systems

with understanding, commitment, and considerable compassion to help re-balance the systems. The next section introduces "competencies of compassion", which Melissa may build on over time and with support and guidance from others.

12.4   Building Compassion: Engagement and Action

CFT aims to help people build a range of "competencies of compassion" [3, 8]. People are encouraged to look at their difficulties with wisdom and without judgement (compassionate engagement) and to act in ways that can alleviate or even prevent suffering (compassionate action). The biopsychosocial and evolution informed theory of CFT is used to help build an understanding of difficulties that we all face as humans. CFT is also used to guide our actions in helpful ways to promote compassionate responses. For example, we can identify, explore, and map out the emotional systems that have become relatively more dominant and the ones are less active. Once this is done, we can identify and design various actions that can build upon those systems that can become more active [3, 8].

In CFT, engagement is referred to as the "first psychology of compassion" as it promotes awareness and understanding of distress. Engagement refers to a willingness to look at and greet distress rather than distract or turn away from it. In doing so, CFT suggests six core competencies—care for wellbeing, sensitivity to distress, sympathy, distress tolerance, empathy, and non-judgement (see inner circle in Fig. 12.3 below).

When someone feels a strong sense of shame, they may criticise and blame themselves for experiencing such shame instead of being non-judgemental about it (as in the example of Melissa). When people feel alone with a difficulty, it can be very difficult to build understanding, as there may not have been an opportunity to gain knowledge and wisdom from others in a similar situation. For people living with HIV, a sense of shame may inhibit some from talking to those who could help offer awareness and understanding. A first step in building compassion is to be able to look at one's distress *non-judgementally*. Health professionals working in HIV can help with this process by noticing when a patient is in distress and demonstrating an understanding and non-judgemental stance towards the distress.

Action is referred as the "second psychology of compassion" which involves building wisdom and learning a variety of skilful ways to alleviate suffering. It can also involve developing ways to prevent it from happening in the first place. CFT suggest six core competences which interventions may target—attention, reasoning, behaviour, sensory focus, emotion, and imagery. Different methods can be used to help build on these skills, from challenging an "inner critic" to building on soothing system where this may be less active (using imagery or breathing) [8].

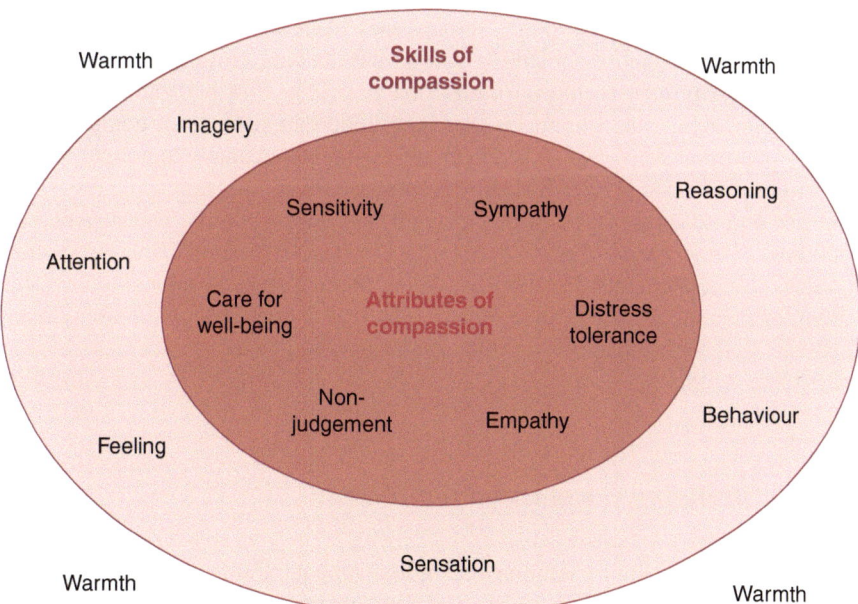

Fig. 12.3 Competencies of compassion. (From *The Compassionate Mind*, [4] reprinted with permission from Constable & Robinson Ltd.)

12.4.1   Flows of Compassion

When beginning to build on compassionate engagement and action, we can explore the "flows of compassion". This refers to compassion directed from self to others, from others to self, and from self to self (otherwise known as self-compassion) [22, 23]. Often, health professionals can meet people in clinic who are very compassionate to others—but clearly struggle when turning that compassion inwards. For example, Melissa may find it very natural to be supportive and encouraging to her sister, providing wise advice when needed in addition to displaying strength, stability, warmth, and kindness. However, she may find it difficult or nearly impossible to turn this compassion inward towards herself. Some may also struggle in accepting compassion from others, whereas others may become "blocked" in all flows of compassion. For example, sometimes people living with HIV can display very negative and rejecting views about other people living with the same condition. Part of the work in building compassion is to look at where compassion is flowing to and where it is blocked—and then to gradually and gently get compassion flowing in *all directions*.

12.4.2   Blocks to Compassion

There are numerous ways in which the flows of compassion can become blocked [19]. For example, when some people hear the word "compassion", they may regard it as something "fluffy" or "soft". Perhaps they have learned to avoid, dismiss, or even reject and trivialise something that is only natural. However, compassion is more that warm fuzzy feelings. Compassion is variable, flexible, and multifaceted. Without a doubt, warmth and kindness are important features of compassion in some circumstances. However, strength and courage are equally important in other situations. For example, firefighters will demonstrate compassion while preventing injuries and suffering by showing strength and courage while entering burning buildings. There probably is not very much kindness or warmth displayed in those compassionate moments. For Melissa, taking the first steps by attending a support group or meeting up with a peer mentor may take a huge amount of strength and courage. In this circumstance, a strong and encouraging inner voice represents compassionate action.

12.4.3   Building Compassion for Yourself

CFT can assist us in understanding and normalising painful feelings such as shame and other psychological difficulties. The competencies of compassion can also be developed in various ways. We present a few ideas and suggestions in the next sections of this chapter. However for readers who would like to build their own practice of compassion, there are a number of books and online resources available which describe numerous CFT techniques and strategies [8, 24–26].

We have introduced the CFT model to understand how our brains and bodies have evolved and why humans may be predisposed to experience psychological suffering. The next section of this chapter looks in more detail at the experiences of people living with HIV and how CFT can be used to understand the psychological difficulties they may experience.

12.5   Applying the Three Systems: HIV, Mental Health and Trauma

It well known that there are many associations between HIV and mental health, and it is frequently documented that anxiety and depression are more prevalent in the HIV population than they are in the general population [27]. This is likely to be linked to high levels of trauma experienced by people living with HIV, whether this be prior to or after their diagnosis [28, 29]. This condition tends to disproportionately affect people who belong to marginalised communities due to factors such as race, ethnicity, sexuality, and environmental displacement or social disadvantage, where there can be layers of powerlessness and multifaceted trauma. An HIV diagnosis brings an additional stigma to groups already having to cope with discrimination [30]. This stigma sits within a heavy history of HIV, where there can be an intense fear of death and/or an explicit and often expressed hatred of people who had acquired the condition. We described earlier that our brains and bodies have adapted to manage the threats in our environment: the people we see in clinic have often experienced multiple threats in their worlds. If the threat system in their brains becomes dominant, it is an understandable and potentially necessary reaction, albeit with some adverse consequences. Although with the incredible advancements of medication, the actuality of death is removed for those able to engage with treatment. Unfortunately, stigma and discrimination persist, both in society, and at times within the healthcare system itself [31]. This appears to be due to factors such as a lack of updated HIV-related knowledge and "moral" judgements around engagement with sex and substance use. It is easy to comprehend how shame can damage the self-esteem and emotional wellbeing of many people who are living with the condition [32, 33].

As explored in the previous sections, shame is rooted in our evolutionary need to be accepted by and belong to social groups. This is to increase our sense of safety in the world through the connection with others and, therefore, the protection of being in a group. Shame is associated with negative self-evaluations (self-criticism, self-blame, etc.), which can lead to experiences of "social threat", whereby people assume that others will share these negative perceptions. Because we have evolutionary-based needs for belonging to ensure physical safety, we can struggle with concerns and worries about being rejected by valued relationships and important social support systems. These fears of rejection can reduce psychological safety

	Self-protection action	Unintentional consequence
Experience of HIV-related (self) stigma and shame	Withdrawing from friends, family and intimate relationships	Loneliness and isolation low mood
	Constantly trying to please or appease others to make up for **perceived flaw** of having HIV)	Own needs not met Resentment and anger Controlling/abusive relationships
	Thinking over and over again (ruminating) about **perceived flaw** of having HIV	Reinforcement of skewed negative idea of self Loss of confidence Low mood and increased anxiety

Self-attacking increases sense of shame

Fig. 12.4 Adapted in part from CFT model [5]

and wellbeing [25]. Such concerns then trigger the threat system and associated overwhelming thoughts and emotions. This can lead to a range of behaviours designed to self-protect. Many people try to protect themselves from distress by avoiding certain situations, trying not to think about difficult things, or using alcohol or substances to block things out. However, attempts to self-protect can sometimes result in unwanted consequences that are detrimental to wellbeing. It is also often the case that people can then go on to criticise themselves further ("self-attacking") for the unintentional consequences of behaviours designed to self-protect. This can have a further negative impact on emotional wellbeing and may even contribute to triggering or deepening self-stigma [5]. Consider the following examples in Fig. 12.4:

The interplay between HIV, trauma, and emotional wellbeing is a complex one, occurring on intrapersonal, interpersonal, and wider social levels. Risks and impacts can be understood as sitting within the intersections of a whole range of social categorisations and are inextricably linked to the differing levels of power that individuals and groups hold within a society [34], with this in mind, we will utilise the Three Systems Model to understand some of the processes through which a history of trauma can make people more vulnerable to contracting HIV, how HIV can be (re)traumatising and how post-HIV diagnosis distress can impact health-related life quality, including health outcomes.

12.5.1 Existing Vulnerabilities: The Increased Risk of Contracting HIV

When people are not cared for sufficiently in childhood, this can lead to mental health issues later in life as well as problems in relationships. When "good enough" care is provided (children's needs are responded to in a caring and fairly consistently way), children learn to understand and label their emotions and develop coping strategies for managing distress. They learn to regulate their three emotional systems (drive, threat, and soothing) in a flexible and balanced way. However, when caregivers do not respond consistently to children's expressed needs, or are abusive and neglectful, this impacts emotional and cognitive development and is detrimental to self-esteem, as the child learns to believe they are not worth caring for [35–37]. Feelings of worthlessness and historical experiences of abuse are synonymous with feelings of shame [38, 39]. To manage an aversive childhood, the threat system becomes dominant, as the soothing system cannot be relied on for safety. Abusive and neglectful early care experiences often lead to the person entering into relationships with expectations that others will not notice or care for them, or may hurt them in some way, which results in the development of a range of self-protection strategies. These may include strategies such as appeasing or avoiding others (to avoid harm), high expression of needs (to ensure a response), or constantly seeking connection with others (to feel valued/loved) (Crittenden, 2006). Again, we may see this as the brain adapting to its environment, but with adverse consequences in the long term.

When thinking about this in terms of intimate relationships, people with early trauma histories and low self-worth may be less able to keep themselves safe [40]. For example, a person with low self-esteem and feelings of shame may lack the confidence to negotiate safer sex practices. Also, if they have not been cared for in the past, they might have little idea of how to care for themselves, which includes self-protection. They may also submit to the demands/requests of sexual partners in order to maintain positive regard, or avoid negative responses/rejection, which can result in sexual risk-taking behaviours. Additionally, a constant search for the connection and love that was lacking in their early life might result in people pursuing multiple partners. Sex may be driven by needs to self-soothe and/or seek pleasure as a way to reduce threat. In the short term, the emotional systems may feel more balanced, but threat may continue to dominate in the long term. If there are tendencies towards pleasing others, then it follows that people are vulnerable to such sexual risks [41, 42]. Perpetrators of abuse and control are particularly adept at identifying vulnerable people [43], and we can easily see how the above can apply within situations of coercive, abusive, and physically violent relationships. Although the strategies described are designed to protect the person psychologically in the moment, sexual risk taking clearly increases the likelihood of HIV acquisition [44].

It is also well known that people who have lived through adversity and neglect in early care relationships are more likely to use alcohol and substances later on in life as a way to avoid the trauma-related distress that they were never helped to manage in the first place. Again, substance use helps to avoid distress and reduce feelings of threat in the short term. It helps to stimulate feelings of drive or soothing which reduce threat. However, the using alcohol and substances excessively exacerbates mental health issues in the longer term [45]. It can become the main way people access soothing and drive emotions. This can lead to chaotic lifestyles and an ongoing lack of control over consciousness. When this happens, the ability to monitor behaviour and make safe choices diminishes. When sexual contact or drug use that might lead to the sharing of equipment is involved, then the risks of contracting HIV are higher [46]. We can think about issues such as these using the Three Systems Model. Consider the example below:

Case Example: Stefan
Stefan lacked care and secure attachment in his early life. As a young adult, he went to great lengths to find intimacy, love, and affection as an adult. The strong need to be noticed, feel loved, worthwhile, and connected for Stefan lead to the threat system being constantly triggered by the fear and/or shame of feeling unlovable. Stefan experienced distress related to his loneliness as he did not feel close to anyone. Attempts to soothe his distress involved a constant search for intimate relationships, perhaps leading to many sexual encounters. Stefan developed a passive, "people pleasing" stance to avoid jeopardising his social connections in any way. If questions arise around safe sex, Stefan's threat system gets triggered by worries about expressing opinions opposite to that of his sexual partners because he fears negative judgement and rejection. In this case, Stefan may submit to pressures from his sexual partners and suppress his own preferences to ease his overwhelming distress associated with his deep-seated fear of loss of the connection. This deep-rooted fear of rejection may be much more powerful than any fears associated unprotected sex. If this pattern is repeated, interactions between the three systems mean the risk of acquiring HIV accumulate over time, as well as the risk of onward transmission should Stefan become positive and not get tested and/or fail to start suppressive anti-retroviral medications.

Stefan's *THREAT* system is often activated by the *fear* of being alone and the *shame* of being unlovable. In combination with an under-developed *SOOTHING* system, Stefan's heightened *DRIVE* state motivates him to seek love and connection. However, his *THREAT* system activates again in response to negotiating safer sex, where *fear* of rejection leads to submission to the others' needs. When this happens, Stefan feels temporarily *soothed* by keeping the connection and deferring to the desires of his sexual partners for condomless sex (see Fig. 12.5).

12.5.2 Triggering the Threat System: HIV as (Re)traumatising

There is a general consensus in the literature that being diagnosed with HIV can be traumatising [29, 47]. Although vastly improved anti-retroviral treatment (ART) means that (as long as diagnosis is not too late) people can live a normal lifespan, not everyone has this updated knowledge. Due to the widely known history of HIV

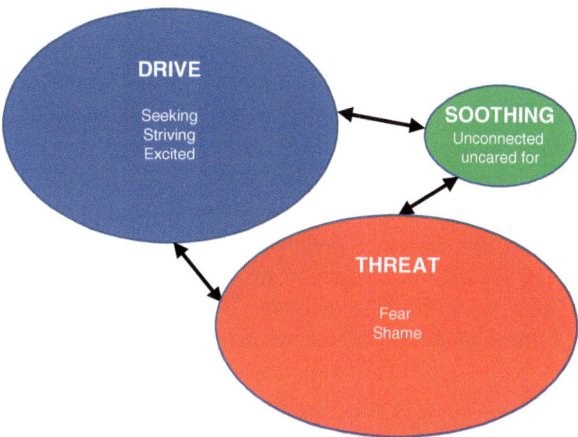

Fig. 12.5 Three systems model example of vulnerability to acquiring HIV

at the beginning of the epidemic before 1996, the diagnosis is strongly associated with the fear of death, which clearly creates the conditions for a trauma response [48]. Even those who are aware of the improved treatments, they still might feel traumatised by the fact they are carrying something in their body which could kill them. As we discussed earlier, illness is very likely to trigger old brain systems and emotions.

Then there is the powerful influence of shame. As we described earlier, shame is the outcome of very powerful old brain systems. HIV is a highly stigmatised condition and for many people who are affected by it, the anticipation of shame or the actual experience of it is an everyday reality. So is the possibility of internalising shame which then becomes even more corrosive [31]. Shame can be powerful [49]. In clinics, we see many people who express ideas such as being "a biohazard" or "riddled with the virus", identifying themselves as a shameful risk to others. This triggers the threat system with fears of losing valued social relationships. For those who are affected by feelings of shame, the impact is not simply after the diagnosis event. It continues and persists with an ongoing need to conceal the condition. Continuing to hide the HIV diagnosis within existing relationships and when forming new intimate partnerships can have the psychological effect of breeding a sense of shame. The act of concealing the condition reinforces the idea that HIV is something to be ashamed of. The threat system is then triggered constantly and becomes traumatising. The impact of such constant trauma on emotional wellbeing becomes cumulative [25, 49].

As suggested above, the effect of HIV-related stigma is perhaps even more marked for people who belong to already marginalised communities [30]. The diagnosis just adds to existing burdens of stigma often encountered by people from these groups, which creates (unfair and unfounded) shame attached to self-identity. An early illustration of this within the epidemic was the reference to HIV as "the gay plague", where further stigma was attached to an already socially maligned gay community. The transgender population, who already carry multiple layers of stigma and discrimination with increased exposure to trauma, can also feel the heavy impact of an HIV diagnosis. Trying to negotiate a world with rigid boxes around identity can create low self-worth and shame, and adding HIV as another potential cause for negative judgement can trigger an already sensitised threat system [25, 50]. For people belonging to BAME communities, the experience of racism may have already resulted in a range of traumatic experiences and feelings of socially based shame. HIV will exacerbate both anticipated and enacted shaming external judgements from others. This can then translate to internalised stigma [31, 51]. For those who are seeking asylum, they may be already subjected to messages that they are not welcome in society. An HIV diagnosis may feed into these prejudiced narratives that they are bringing problems and utilising resources. This might deepen a sense of shame that may already exist due to prior trauma [25, 52].

Another group of people who may be more intensely impacted by an HIV diagnosis are survivors of sexual abuse. It is well known that this traumatic experience is associated with the development of feelings of shame, often due to the strategies used by abuse perpetrators to silence their victims. These might include messages designed to induce negative self-evaluations and shame, such as implying that there is something inherently wrong with the person, that they are to blame for the abuse and that nobody will believe them if they speak out [43]. Existing negative thoughts about the self can then be compounded by receiving a diagnosis of HIV that is synonymous with ideas about being "dirty" and "infected". These hurtful ideas may be related to "moralistic" societal views of sex and substances. This can feed often held beliefs about being "damaged goods" for those who have lived through abuse [39, 53]. Additionally, the historical "brushing under the carpet" of child sexual abuse [43] might connect with the sense that HIV must be concealed. Such concealment might (unjustly) validate or confirm longstanding feelings of shame. Again, ongoing difficult thoughts and feelings in relation to shame may keep the threat system constantly activated [25]. The potentially traumatic impact of an HIV diagnosis on a person's interpersonal relationships is explored below.

Case Example: Carla

Carla has a history of trauma in early relationships. As a result, she has fragile self-esteem and low self-worth. Her recent HIV diagnosis becomes an immense threat to her identity and the way she views herself through the eyes of others. Before her diagnosis, Carla already had thoughts such as *"I am dirty"*, *"I am damaged goods"*, or *"nobody will want me"* because of her difficult history of being a survivor of sexual abuse. There is a strong drive then for Carla to self-protect from the possibility of other people forming these opinions should they find out about her HIV diagnosis (due to HIV-related stigma). Carla develops strategies that involve self-isolation to conceal her diagnosis. She avoids intimate and sexual encounters. Although such actions do provide relief from anticipatory distress in the short term, it means that the "certainty of rejection" is never challenged for Carla. Thus, her beliefs that she is damaged and unlovable are never changed as she is unable to experience an outcome different to her predictions and expectations of rejection. Carla's beliefs are experienced as "facts" rather than thoughts, which feeds a sense of shame and fuels the threat system. Additionally, the continued avoidance of relationships is likely to affect many areas of Carla's life, such as impacting her ability to pursue other goals and incentives for her life. Therefore, such avoidance and isolation have a detrimental impact on Carla's wellbeing in the long term.

In this example, Carla's **THREAT** system (already sensitised by early trauma) is constantly re-triggered by fears and shame related to the HIV diagnosis. Trauma in early life is likely to result in an under-developed **SOOTHING** system. Carla's beliefs are based on her lived experience. Relationships are not safe and people cannot be trusted. Unfortunately, the unintended consequence of the need to self-protect, results in withdrawal, which limits the **DRIVE** system and Carla's general ability to achieve and thrive in life (see Fig. 12.6).

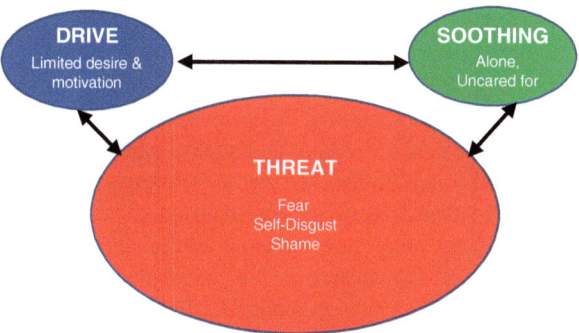

Fig. 12.6 Three systems model example of HIV diagnosis as socially traumatising

12.5.3   Trauma and the Problem of Self-Care: HIV Health and Wellbeing Outcomes

With the considerable advancement of HIV treatments over the last 25 years, it is incredible that we are now in a place where people can live a healthy life with an average life expectancy, if they are diagnosed early enough and are able to adhere to their treatment. However, what we know from the UNAIDS 90-90-90 initiative [54], is that some people, although diagnosed and engaged with care, are not able to adhere to their treatment. This then leads to poor health outcomes, and in extreme cases, mortality. Where there are issues with taking treatment, these are generally related to psychological, emotional, and social issues [55].

As outlined in the section above, an HIV diagnosis can trigger intense feelings of fear and shame. If experienced as (re)traumatising then, as is the nature of trauma, anything that reminds a person of their HIV status can lead to a response of over-whelming distress. Given the intense discomfort of this, a person may go to great lengths to avoid such reminders. Such avoidance may be deliberate or it may occur outside of awareness. These emotional triggers often include taking ART and attend-ing HIV healthcare appointments. Each tablet and consultation may bring attention back to the diagnosis producing unbearable emotional responses. Disengaging from care and treatment can be ways of reducing triggers to the threat system [29, 56]. As people do not always become immediately unwell with HIV, they can continue to use these avoidance strategies for some time [57]. Ironically, it can offer a surface sense of feeling safe although there is invisible physical damage taking place inside the body. This avoidant strategy may also be used by those who acquired HIV through traumatic means, such as sexual assault or an abusive relationship. Reminders of the condition may link directly back to these other traumatic memories that feel unman-ageable. Therefore, distress is managed by avoiding all HIV-related triggers [28].

12.5.4   Disengagement from Care

People who have experienced trauma in early care relationships may also avoid con-tact with health professionals [55]. Abuse and neglect can lead to the development of a belief that "people who care for me hurt me" which impacts on how they approach relationships. This understanding of interpersonal interactions is generalised to all people. Compassion from others can be experienced as both uncomfortable and unfamiliar. It can even feel very aversive. This means that the person always antici-pates getting let down, rejected by or treated unfairly by those providing care or sup-port. Therefore, such potentially "damaging" relationships are avoided. Unfortunately, some rigid healthcare systems can feel impersonal and uncaring. Such experiences can sometimes inadvertently reinforce these expectations. Stigma experienced within the healthcare system itself can also create fears that all healthcare professionals will behave in this manner. This can have a negative impact on engagement with all health systems. As engagement in healthcare relationships is central to HIV healthcare delivery, poor health outcomes are a likely outcome [56].

Drawing on information above, we understand that there are a range of other possible reasons for persons to disengage from care and treatment. For instance, some people may fear others finding out about their diagnosis, and do not want to be seen at a clinic or do not feel able to keep medication in their home. There are heightened levels of inter-partner violence within the HIV population [58]. In these cases, options around taking ART may be decided by the abusive and controlling partner. Some may try to keep safe by concealing their diagnosis from their controlling abusive partner but in doing so they may avoid taking their medications. For those with traumatic histories, there may be strong feelings of shame and worthlessness. Not taking ART may be a form of self-harm or self-punishment, due to thoughts that they are a "bad person" and "do not deserve care". Being self-compassionate may be difficult or even impossible as care and compassion have not been experienced and modelled. Also, if a person is struggling to find a way to live in the world with a diagnosis of HIV, they may not see a future worth living and not be motivated to take their medications. All of these avoidance strategies are common to complex trauma [28]. Whatever the psychological and social foundations, prolonged non-adherence of ART can lead to serious morbidity and even mortality. Of course, there are also risks of onward transmission when the viral load is high [55]. The Three Systems Model can be used to understand the impact of psychological process on health outcomes.

Case Example: Thomas
Thomas just received his HIV diagnosis. This was an unforeseen and stressful event. As a result, he is driven to avoid the high levels of distress associated with the stigma of his diagnosis. Taking ART and visiting clinics become direct links to his memories and emotions related to his traumatic diagnosis. This places Thomas into a state of constant threat. Therefore, in order to try to self-soothe and reduce distress, Thomas avoids all reminders of the unwanted reality of his health situation. Avoiding engagement with care and treatment keeps Thomas feeling safe psychologically. However, the potential damage to his body is inevitable in the long term should his engagement with care not change. A lack of HIV-related symptoms can also reinforce his belief that treatment is not required. It might support his denial for his struggles in adjusting to his diagnosis. Even when ill health occurs, it may be easier for Thomas to cope with the impact of his current ill health, but not the trauma associated with his original diagnosis. In extreme cases, the drive to avoid strong feelings of shame may mean that death offers an escape from a situation that feels completely overwhelming and unmanageable.

The traumatising impact of stigma can mean that HIV treatment activates the *THREAT* system. Since Thomas does not feel safe in sharing his diagnosis with others and does not access support from healthcare professionals, his *SOOTHING* system is not sufficiently activated. This means self-care remains unlikely. Over time, as his body deteriorates, the *DRIVE* system will be inadvertently depleted as there will be minimal energy to pursue activity (see Fig. 12.7).

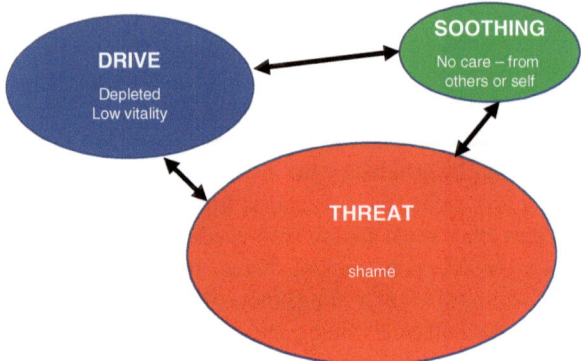

Fig. 12.7 Three systems model example of the influence of trauma on healthcare engagement and health outcomes

12.6 Compassion: How Can it Help in HIV Care?

As we have learned so far, when people are living with high levels of distress, their threat system is frequently in action and becomes highly sensitised. If the threat system is dominating emotional responses, this will limit their ability to pursue goals and activities of importance. Sometimes people go from drive to threat repeatedly with the belief that achievement alone can counteract distress. But in such circumstances, self-criticism begins to prevail as no amount of success with highly activated drive systems will sufficiently reduce threat [2]. This strategy is likely to lead to burn out over time, as it is important to give ourselves time to rest and recuperate [59]. This is where the soothing system comes into play. For people who did not receive adequate care in early life (e.g., neglected, dismissed, criticised), the soothing system may not develop adequately. Compassionate approaches to care can help people to develop ways of accessing their soothing system. People can only care for themselves if they know what "good enough" care looks like.

Self-care is vital when managing long-term health conditions such as HIV [56, 60]. Experiencing and accepting the flow of compassion from others is a starting point for building competencies of self-compassion. Given that HIV is associated with high levels of shame due to societal stigma, the need for compassion is perhaps crucial [61]. Experiencing compassion from others can help people living with HIV to develop self-compassion, which may reduce tendencies to self-attack and reduce shame [56, 60]. When we consider this in the context of the fourth 90 (HIV quality of life), people living with HIV can find ways to develop their compassionate response and access the soothing systems when needed. If possible, this could have positive impacts on emotional states, engagement with healthcare, pursuing valued activities and general wellbeing [33, 62].

12.6.1   Compassionate Communication

How health professionals communicate with people living with HIV is very important when there is a history of trauma. Trauma can lay foundations for vulnerabilities, which are often deeply rooted in shame [63]. The best of intentions can be easily overshadowed by miscommunications that trigger strong emotional responses. Responses that are often tied to previous difficult experiences connected to the threat system [64].

Perhaps the simplest and most effective strategy for health professionals is to give space for someone to talk. Active listening, demonstrated by empathic facial expressions and gestures, words of understanding and use of reflecting back what you are hearing are extremely important to demonstrate to patients. Unfortunately, for some people who have lived through trauma, their stories have been dismissed by others, which can add to distress and shame [43]. Acknowledging any trauma that is shared, followed by normalising and validating any distress associated with it are very powerful compassionate communication strategies. Implicit messages lie within our actions. For example, taking time to listen to a story (*you are worth listening to*), reflecting back what you learn (*I hear you*) and noticing difficult emotions (*you are seen and I will care for you*).

A non-judgemental stance is also essential for compassionate communication [5]. This involves being aware of our responses. For example, being careful not to appear shocked, distressed, or closing down conversations if the details of a patient's conversation become difficult. As well, responses can sometimes leave patients feeling judged or criticised, even with no intention from the health professional. For example, it may be a kind action to tell patients that they should not feel ashamed. However, if they do feel a lot of shame, then they may blame or criticise themselves for failing to free themselves from shame. In essence, they feel more shame for feeling shame [60]. It can also be very helpful to be open, clear, and transparent in talking about HIV treatment recommendations. For instance, in difficult conversations around medication adherence, people living with HIV who have problems in taking their ART can easily feel pressured to comply with the medication adherence advice. Here, it can be useful to make statements such as "I hope you don't feel backed into a corner" and "I am explaining the options so that you can make an informed choice about your care" [56]). "Visible communication" is important, particularly for people living with HIV who have histories of trauma and abuse because they are likely to have been subjected to the hidden agendas of others. Therefore, they may apply this expectation of duplicity or ulterior motives to all relationships. By being visible about intentions, this can remove the need for people living with HIV to "second guess" agendas. It can help them to feel safe and able build trust in relationships with health professionals over time [43].

12.6.2   Building Compassion in HIV

Building compassionate responses to the difficulties of life can be helped by a course of psychological therapy. However, there are other ways for HIV health professionals to help with this process. It is important to give space and time in clinical consultations to the difficult issues of our patients. However, it is equally important for health professionals to bring focus to the strengths, capabilities, and other protective factors of their patients [65]. For example, acknowledging how someone has survived previous trauma or how they are doing their best to cope with an HIV diagnosis can help draw attention to their positive actions [66]. Through this discussion, it might be possible to reduce any tendencies towards shame-related self-blame and self-criticism. It can help patients to develop more self-compassionate language and more helpful and balanced understandings of themselves. It can also help patients to discover aspects of themselves that they can value and appreciate. It is also important to identify activities of interest that can reduce feelings of distress, such as creative hobbies, yoga, and mindful activities. Increasing such positive and affirming activities can help patients to free themselves from their heightened threat system [67].

Again, how a healthcare team delivers support can be integral in strengthening a compassionate response, including the cultivating of the soothing system, when needed. The experience of compassion from others is likely to increase a sense of connectedness and safety, which may have been lacking for people with complex care histories. The delivery of structured, pro-active, and consistent care, where multidisciplinary team members work together from a patient-centred care plan can be effective in creating a secure sense of being cared for. Patients may then begin to build a new framework for relationships. The hope is that by experiencing what it is like to feel cared for, patients may eventually learn how to care compassionately for themselves [56].

For those who want to explore more detailed ways to foster compassionate responses, psychological therapy may be one option. However, there are range of detailed self-help books and courses that can help to start the process of "compassionate mind training" [8, 26, 68].

12.6.3   Connecting with Others

Some people living with HIV can feel isolated, particularly if their very real worries around stigma mean that they choose not to share their HIV diagnosis. Concerns relating to stigma can be an obstacle to building new relationships and can also impact existing ones, if fears around diagnosis discovery result in the avoidance of being around other people. In such cases, relationships may be associated with the threat system [25]. By supporting isolated people living with HIV to begin socially reconnecting in safe contexts, new narratives will gently start to develop.

Relationships can be associated with the soothing system, through a sense of mutual value and support [61].

The HIV community has historically provided an ideal opportunity for developing social connections, as the power of connecting with those with a shared experience in a non-judgemental space cannot be under-estimated. HIV community support services often play a central role in the wellbeing of those living with HIV, and can also provide opportunities for empowerment, which can reduce the impact of stigma and shame [33, 69]. However, some people living with HIV do not feel able, or do not wish to access these services, which reflects the power of anticipated and internalised stigma. When this is the case, it can be important to support people living with HIV to find alternative routes to social re-engagement, based on compassion, acceptance, and with a focus on value-based interests and goals. This can help redevelop aspects of identity outside of an HIV diagnosis [15, 70]. The ultimate aim is to help people living with HIV access their soothing systems by finding ways to feel secure in the company of others (through shared experience and positive feedback) and relate to valued parts of themselves. Reconnecting is healing for trauma. It can reduce the fear of what the world might hold and begin to replace it with experiences of mutual care, respect, and validation. This can help people living with HIV to start feeling safe [71].

12.7   Compassion Fatigue: The Impact of Caring for Traumatised People and Populations

It is well known that there is a high prevalence of trauma in the HIV population [28]. As explored above, people living with HIV will employ a range of coping strategies to try to manage the overwhelming distress when trauma histories are involved. As discussed, these can include avoidance of clinics/treatment, or conversely high contact with clinics, use of alcohol and substances and engagement in sexual risk taking. Such coping behaviours can make care delivery more challenging, and this can have an impact on the relationships between people living with HIV and health professionals. This can be further complicated if the person who is receiving care has already experienced early, unresolved trauma. They might bring expectations of being let down, dismissed, or even hurt by health professionals. The feelings and emotions stemming from unresolved trauma can take many forms; tearfulness, anger, helplessness, and hopelessness, to name a few. If persistent, or overwhelming, these expressions of emotion can feel difficult for health professionals to manage, particularly if their own threat systems are being triggered. For example, staff members who have high standards and expectations of themselves, might struggle if a patient expresses anger about their care not being good enough. The health professionals may become very self-critical (further triggering their own threat systems) and this might send them into over-drive. There are endless examples of how difficult dynamics might occur and play out (see [56]). Without support to make sense of these experiences (e.g., supervision, reflective practice), health professionals might experience compassion fatigue and burnout [72]. Therefore, as well as delivering compassionate care to others within HIV services, it is also of upmost importance for staff to find ways of being compassionate and caring towards themselves.

In the previous section, we discussed how compassion focused approaches can help us understand and respond to those who are struggling and suffering with their HIV diagnosis. We described the importance of maintaining a compassionate stance in our roles as health professionals, and how this is invaluable for the people with whom we work. However, maintaining this stance and an outward flow of compassion is by no means easy. We introduced the Three Systems Model and the various patterns we might see in people we meet in clinic. However, we can also look at how these emotional systems might apply to our own lives as health professionals. How often do we experience drive, soothing, and threat at work? Do one or two system dominate? The next section looks at what can happen when the flows of compassion become unbalanced, when we have to care for others constantly but receive less care from others or ourselves. We then look at some ways of balancing our own emotional systems and strengthening our flows of compassion.

12.7.1   The Potential Cost of Caring

Compassion fatigue (CF) is a relatively easy concept to recognise and appreciate for many of us who work as health professionals. CF has been described as the "cost of caring" [73], when health professionals lose their ability to nurture and empathise. Nursing is a busy and rewarding profession, but it also involves witnessing trauma, working with painful impairment and facing death. According to Dewar et al. [74], the emotional investment of such challenging work can deplete the ability of health professionals to manage the demands of being compassionate, which in turn can have a negative impact on their own health and wellbeing.

Helping others is a primary motivator for most health professionals. However, they can become victims of the continuing and unrelenting stress and hardship of responding to the complicated and complex needs of their patients. CF not only impacts on psychological and physical health, as it can also impact on job satisfaction and work retention [75]. It can also have a negative impact on patient safety and satisfaction [76, 77]. The ongoing experience of threat emotions at work (fear, anxiety, anger) can lead to this system dominating; the drive emotions (enthusiasm and energy) and soothing system (connection and calm) can gradually become very rare in a working day.

Numerous authors have identified and discussed a variety of signs and symptoms of CF. They typically range from work-related problems to both physical and psychological/emotional symptoms. Table 12.1 summarises a number of signs or symptoms of CF.

Table 12.1 Signs and symptoms of compassion fatigue (adapted from [75])

Psychological problems	Physical problems	Occupational problems
• Mood swings • Lack of joy in life • Anxiety • Low mood, depression • Irritability, anger, resentment or cynicism • Poor concentration, reduced focus, memory problems • Problematic use of alcohol, nicotine, or illicit drugs	• Headaches and muscle tension • Digestive problems: diarrhoea, constipation • Sleep disturbance: insomnia, hypersomnia • Fatigue, listlessness • Cardiac symptoms: chest pain, palpitations	• Avoidance or dread of working with certain patient presentations • Reduced ability to feel empathy and sympathy to patients and/or families • Frequent use of sick days • Tension and conflict with co-workers

In helping others, health professionals open their hearts and minds to their patients. Practising compassionate care is rewarding, important, and essential. However, the act of being compassionate is what makes health professionals open to being profoundly affected and even possibly damaged by their work [78]. By nature, humans are hard wired for empathy and concern for others. As discussed in the first part of this chapter, caring (whether for infants or for those in our social groups) has helped us survive. We can be strongly motivated to care for others and can feel a sense of purpose, connection, and satisfaction when we are compassionate to others. However, caregiving can take a toll both emotionally and physically [79]. The stress resulting from helping traumatised or suffering people may result in CF, which some believe develops as a self-protection measure [73].

12.7.2 Is it Another Term for Burnout?

CF is relatively similar to burnout. In fact, they are often confused for each other. However, these two occupational risks are different in some fundamental ways. Burnout is often referred to as a condition that develops when the perceived demands from work outweigh the perceived resources available in the work environment [80]. It is also associated with high patient acuity, overcrowding, and problems with hospital management [79]. Overall, burnout is a condition associated with a variety of negative feelings, such as hopelessness and despair, in addition to work performance problems [81]. These signs of burnout differ from CF, which refers to the profound emotional and physical erosion that takes place when nurses are not able to refuel and regenerate while being surrounded by painfully difficult loss. In fact, CF can develop relatively quickly in reaction to intense and repeated exposure to traumatic situations.

CF refers specifically to when health professionals lose their ability to nurture after being exposed to frequent and intense heartache [82]. Pearlman and Saakvitne [83] have equated CF with *vicarious* or *secondary traumatisation*. They described

CF as a profound shift in world view that occurs when working with patients who have experienced trauma. When this happens, their fundamental beliefs about the world are altered and possibly damaged by being repeatedly exposed to trauma. According to Perregrini [84], CF is sometimes confused with *moral distress*, which occurs when health professionals know the right course of action but are obstructed from acting on it because of institutional or managerial constraints or obstructions.

12.7.3 What Factors Contribute to it?

Saakvitne and Pearlman's book, *Transforming Pain* [83] discusses a number of factors contributing to CF as being a function of the individual and/or the situation. One's personal history, current life circumstances and coping style can all impact on how someone reacts to challenging and demanding work situations. As we discussed earlier, if our own threat and/or drive systems are dominating and our ability to access soothing feelings is depleted, the stress and difficulty encountered at work may well lead to psychological suffering. Many health professionals will have their own personal challenges in their home life and/or difficult previous experiences involving neglect and/or abuse. Some health professionals develop problem-focused coping styles to stress, whereas others may develop more emotion-focused ones, involving denial and/or avoidance. Whatever the case may be, health professionals bring their own personal background and personality to their work—factors which may bode well for being caring and compassionate at work. However, a history of negative experiences and/or problematic personal qualities can also place health professionals at occupational risk for CF.

However, CF is not only a reflection of individual vulnerabilities, as the challenging, complex, and demanding work situation also plays a significant role in how it develops in the workplace [78]. The working environment can be stressful and defined by unhappiness, irritability, pessimism, and cynicism. These negative feelings can develop when dealing with patients who are in crises, living in pain, and facing death. Such negative stressful environments can also develop when working with patients who have their own problems in responding to their own difficult negative feelings, with acting out and angry outbursts. Providing compassionate healthcare in such challenging and sometimes unrewarding circumstances can become difficult to muster and sustain over time, especially when not recognised and addressed by line managers and hospital administrators [85]. Compassion flowing outwards to patients, but not being perceived as flowing inward from managers and organisations can feel like an unbalanced and unstable system.

A recently published study identified a number of individual and institutional factors associated CF [86]. By using the Professional Quality of Life (fifth version) Inventory [81], researchers were able to measure compassion fatigue, compassion satisfaction, and burnout among nearly 300 nurses working in Emergency Departments (ED) across the United States. A clear and significant finding was that lower levels of CF was associated with increasing age and accumulated work experience. Older nurses with more work experience reported relatively lower CF levels compared to younger and/or less work experienced nurses working in ED settings. Higher levels of compassion satisfaction and lower burnout levels were related to increased years in the profession, more years working in ED settings, higher educational qualifications, shorter shift lengths, and adequate reported levels of line manager support. Overall, the researchers discussed how recently qualified and/or younger nurses may be most likely to develop CF in ED settings, especially when line managers are unaware and/or unable to identify and respond to signs of CF and burnout [86].

12.7.4   Is it Blocked Compassion?

From the perspective of CFT, CF is probably associated with competencies of compassion that are underdeveloped and/or when the flows of compassion become blocked (see Fig. 12.3). For example, when health professionals listen to multiple distressing stories from their patients, their *sensitivity to distress* may diminish as a way of coping. They may start to feel unable to tolerate hearing any more pain and distress, with a need to turn away. Remaining *non-judgemental* with a *settled mind* can also take considerable cognitive effort at times. When clinics become rushed and stressful, it can become difficult to remain *concerned for the wellbeing of others* as we become critical and judgemental. It can also become difficult to turn off our critical judgement that we direct towards ourselves should we notice problems in showing compassion to others.

There are numerous ways in which compassion can become blocked for health professionals. However, there can also be fears of what might happen if compassion is *allowed*. As an example, we can become fearful of our capacity to "soldier on" should we let our guard down by becoming "soft" in caring for ourselves. However, being in touch with our own humanity and paying attention to our own emotional needs are extremely important if we want to survive and thrive while working in the challenging field of HIV.

12.7.5   Critique and Conceptual Concerns

There is no doubt that working in healthcare is challenging, especially when working with trauma and/or emotionally provocative situations. Moreover, there is considerable empirical evidence for the role of various work-related and personal factors in the development of occupational risks, such as burnout, stress, and job dissatisfaction and its impact on quality patient care [87, 88]. However, a recently published Canadian meta-narrative review of 90 published studies of CF in healthcare settings recommends that this concept should be examined and redefined because it does not address the significant work-related issues and burnout reported by nurses and other health professionals [89]. The authors note how the original conceptualisation of CF was developed in crisis counselling [73]. However, it has been adapted and applied to other healthcare settings with little empirical scrutiny or theoretical consideration. Most of the research has also used the *Professional Quality of Life Scale* [81], which has appropriate psychometric properties yet it does not differentiate nor measure any of the theoretical aspects of compassion which are supported today [5, 90]. One of the original theoretical propositions of CF in crisis counselling was that it was most likely to occur in practitioners who are highly compassionate and empathetic [73]. However, this has never been tested, nor supported in nursing research [89]. Lastly, none of the studies in this review included the perspectives and reports of patients themselves in receiving compassionate care. In summary, the precise nature of CF in healthcare settings and how it originates out of providing compassionate care appears to have some significant limitations.

The concept of CF has also been challenged as being insufficient or inaccurate in understanding what happens to health professionals after witnessing and working in traumatic and highly distressing conditions. Klimecki and Singer [91] have proposed that CF should be replaced by the term *empathic distress fatigue* to describe and understand the symptoms of withdrawal and burnout in health professionals. According to these researchers, CF is a form of pathological altruism, when health professionals burnout from caring too much for the welfare and wellbeing of their patients. However, it is empathic distress fatigue that underlies the negative consequences of being repeatedly exposed to the suffering of others for health professionals.

According to Klimeck and Singer [91], health professionals strive to relieve the suffering of others because they are motivated by empathic concern. This is a prosocial motivation. However, it can become overwhelming for health professionals should their efforts not succeed. When this happens repeatedly in a relatively short period of time, empathy distress fatigue can develop. Empathy distress motivates health professionals to reduce their *own* negative feelings when witnessing trauma and suffering. This is a self-serving motivation, which propels one to avoid the distressing situation and/or do something to reduce the suffering of others. However, there are difficult circumstances in healthcare settings when there are no interventions that can relieve suffering or reduce pain. When repeatedly exposed and restricted to such circumstances, empathic distress experienced by health professionals will become overwhelming, exhausting, and fatigued. It is in these circumstances when health professionals might lose their capacity for empathic concern [91].

12.8   Importance of Self-Care: Compassion to Self

Self-care is vital in health professions, as it helps to combat the negative impact of work-related stress. It is important for health professionals who spend many hours in caring for patients who may be suffering in pain, struggling with impairment and facing death. Self-care reduces stress, replenishes our capacity to be compassionate, and improves quality of patient care. Simply speaking, if we do not care for ourselves, then we cannot care for others [92]. As noted earlier in this chapter, we might explore which flows of compassion are blocked for our patients. However, we also need to question which flows may be blocked for us in our work and/or home lives. Engaging in compassionate mind training (CMT) can be a way to start noticing and acknowledging these difficulties we face at work (and at home). It can help to develop a better understanding of when more compassionate and self-caring strategies are needed [93].

There are a variety of interventions, strategies, and activities that can promote self-care. A first step may be to note which of your three systems are over or under active and consider which may need to be given more priority. If threat and drive are dominating emotional states at work, then try to think of what activities might foster soothing (e.g., connection and rest). If your drive state is depleted, which activities might generate more feelings of enthusiasm and excitement? Table 12.2 below gives some examples and ideas of interventions at different levels.

In addition to a variety of nourishing and de-stressing self-care activities, Perregrini [84] discussed a variety of other strategies to prevent CF. These ranged from reflective activities such as journaling on the events of the day, noting frustrations, acknowledging barriers, and concluding with an example of something that went well. Coming together as a unit to reflect upon a stressful event, such as an unexpected death could be very helpful as it can help staff members to express themselves and to listen to others. It is one way of utilising the connection we have with our colleagues to manage the difficult emotions that arise in these situations. Setting intentions for the day is another method to prevent CF. Examples include, reminding yourself to get off the unit for lunch, identifying a co-worker to approach when feeling overwhelmed and implementing nourishing rituals to soothe anxieties and recharge batteries.

Table 12.2 Examples of self-care (adapted from Performance Health [94])

Intervention level	Example of self-care
Physical	*Take a walk outside on your lunch break; start cycling on your days off.*
Mental	*Attend workshops on managing stress; listen to podcasts on topics that interest you.*
Emotional	*Write a thank you note to an old mentor; make a playlist of music that brings you joy.*
Spiritual	*Practice mindful activities like meditation; volunteer for a cause that matters to you.*
Social/ Relational	*Eat lunch with your co-workers; spend some time with old friends.*
Personal	*Enjoy a calming bubble bath; take up a new hobby such as pottery.*
Professional	*Stay hydrated with a new colourful water bottle; discuss career goals with a mentor.*

We have suggested a range of strategies that can be helpful in promoting self-care. You may already be doing some of these as part of your weekly routine. However, when things start to get very busy and stressful at work with a risk of CF and burnout, it might become necessary to look more carefully at your situation and focus on your own experience. Understanding which of your three emotional systems may be over or under-regulated and identifying any possible blocks to compassion may be a helpful first step in reducing stress and promoting wellbeing. Compassion-focused therapies, such as CMT may be a helpful intervention for health professionals in developing more genuine and effective self-compassionate responses for themselves [8, 24, 93].

12.8.1 The Workplace and Compassion

The workplace also has a responsibility to promote self-care among its employees, and this is especially the case for healthcare settings where we face a multitude of stressors, challenges, losses, and trauma. Relaxation centres and wellbeing hubs where health professionals can relax, get respite and recharge are becoming a priority for hospitals [95]. Using these resources can stimulate our soothing system in the face of numerous threat triggers at work. Line managers can also play a significant role in reducing the risk of CF by creating an open environment where health professionals can approach each other for support. They can also support training that educates health professionals about CF, burnout, and moral distress. In creating such as environment, line managers should meet regularly with staff members to ensure they can have opportunities to review and discuss

how work is affecting them. Stress management skills-building courses and opportunities to promote resilience should also be encouraged and supported by hospital administrators [96].

12.8.2 Promoting Self-Compassion: Its Vital Role for Health Professionals

The importance of looking after oneself while working as a health professional has been supported and promoted by educators and researchers alike for many years. Self-compassion as a facilitator of psychological wellbeing and resilience in health professions such as nursing is now promoted by many professional bodies, training programmes, and healthcare settings [97]. However, research investigating the role of self-compassion and its impact on occupational risks such as work-related stress, burnout, and CF is still in its infancy. Based on a meta-narrative review of 26 published studies, self-compassion does appear to moderate the impact of these occupational risks in a variety of healthcare providers, such as nurses, medical trainees, and psychologists. Some research also suggests that relatively high levels of self-compassion is associated with positive workplace relationships and higher levels of self-confidence in providing compassionate care [97].

As for interventions to promote self-compassion in health professions, mindfulness training, and mindfulness-based cognitive therapy appear to have a positive impact on stress management and general wellbeing in nurses and other health professionals [98, 99]. However, the impact of such interventions to promote self-compassion have yet to be established as having a measurable impact on the practice of compassionate care, as reported by patients themselves [97].

12.8.3 Promoting Self-Compassion in HIV Health Settings

There is no doubt that working in HIV can be a rewarding, satisfying, and meaningful specialty for health professionals. This is documented by the *Health Care Workers in HIV: An oral history in the UK Aids era,* a project that captures the lived experience of nurses, psychotherapists, medical doctors, and charity sector workers in providing HIV care and support over the years [100]. While working in HIV is rewarding, the role of looking after oneself while working in this challenging field has also been promoted by educators and supported by researchers since the beginning of the epidemic [101].

As discussed in the introduction section of this chapter, Paul Gilbert's theory of compassion with its application in psychological therapy to improve low mood and reduce ruminative anxiety, self-criticism, and shame has been gathering considerable empirical support and public attention in recent years [3]. Gilbert's attributes of compassion (e.g., distress tolerance, empathy, concern for wellbeing) and how they can be directed inward, towards oneself to promote mental health and general wellbeing have also become the cornerstone of a growing number of self-help workshops and books [8, 26, 68].

The application of these theoretical principles to promote self-compassion in health settings can be illustrated in the following case example of Elise who works as a nurse in an HIV outpatient clinic:

> *Elise has been working in an HIV outpatient clinic for more than 30 years. She has witnessed the transformation of HIV care from the early 1990s when the health of HIV-positive patients declined rapidly with multiple deaths to today's potential for a long healthy life with ART. Elise believes her resilience for working in such a challenging specialty was initially developed during these adverse, challenging and traumatic times in the early 1990s.*
>
> *However, Elise has started to struggle at work. The recent lockdown with Covid-19 with a 4-week redeployment to a step-down ward for patients transferred from intensive care was hard. Even though she was proud of herself for facing these challenges and contributing to the "greater good", she has started to dread coming into work, feels tired all day long and has lost her ability to care very much about her patients and colleagues back in the HIV clinic.*
>
> *In fact, her line manager recently commented on how she has noticed that Elise is not spending very much time with her patients during consultations and has been abrupt with some patients over the telephone. Even though it was difficult for Elise to receive such feedback from her manager, she readily admitted that she just doesn't feel much enthusiasm*

for her job at the moment, nor does she feel much sympathy or empathy for many of her patients. In fact, she admitted to transferring some relatively challenging and difficult patients to her colleague's waiting stacks, as a way to avoid them.

After discussing her situation with her manager, Elise agreed to look for some skills-building workshops or short courses that she could take to assist her. She discovered that the Employee Wellbeing Service at her hospital offered a 6-week Promoting Self-Compassion workshop during the lunch hour. Elise was initially sceptical of this idea of "looking after oneself" by focussing on self-compassion. She thought this concept of "self-compassion" as being a bit self-indulgent and a bit too "touchy, feely". But as the weeks went by, Elise started to realise the benefits of paying attention to her difficult emotions and started to find ways to soothe and reassure herself when feeling stressed and upset. Elise also really appreciated the positive feedback from her colleagues after she took the lead in implementing some self-care activities and rituals in the unit. With support from her line manager, Elise was able to convert a disused consultation room to a "wellbeing hub" with comfortable furniture, soft lighting, and aromatherapy. They also began to start their MDT meetings with a 3-minute mindful breathing exercise, which even the medical doctors started to attend!

12.9 Conclusion

This chapter introduced CFT with the goal of improving our understanding and compassion for the psychological difficulties that humans can face. Since this approach aims to normalise and de-shame psychological suffering, CFT appears useful for people living with HIV where stigma and discrimination leading to psychological distress and shame prevail. On understanding the role of individual histories, it is clear that difficult early lives characterised by a lack of love and support can place people at higher risk of falling into detrimental patterns of coping. As negative views of the self can be central to these patterns, we considered how compassionate approaches to supporting people living with HIV might begin to increase self-worth, relieve distress, and improve coping. We looked at different "flows of compassion": providing compassion to others, receiving it from others, and directing compassion towards oneself (self-compassion). Additionally, we discussed the role of compassion for health professionals, as working in the complex area of HIV can be as challenging as it is rewarding. We discussed the concept of compassion fatigue with its negative impact on health professionals and highlighted the importance of self-care.

By building compassion in its many forms, we propose that people living with HIV will feel more cared for, experience less distress, care for themselves better, and improve their health outcomes. If this can happen, then working in HIV will become a more satisfying experience for health professionals who work in this field. It can help to reduce compassion fatigue and enable the ongoing delivery of compassionate care. There is increasing interest in building compassion in HIV services with a hope that it will improve the quality of life and wellbeing for both people living with HIV and health professionals. However, research in this area is just beginning. Further work is now needed to investigate interventions at different levels to build compassion and to translate the theory into helpful future practice.

References

1. England, N. H. S. Compassion in practice strategy and the 6Cs values. 2012.
2. Gilbert P. Introducing compassion-focused therapy. Adv Psychiatr Treat. 2009;15(3):199–208.
3. Gilbert P. The origins and nature of compassion focused therapy. Br J Clin Psychol. 2014;53(1):6–41.
4. Gilbert P. The compassionate mind. Hachette, UK; 2009: 333.
5. Gilbert P. Compassion: conceptualisations, research and use in psychotherapy. London, Routledge; 2005. 417 p.
6. Ayano G, Duko B, Bedaso A. The prevalence of post-traumatic stress disorder among people living with HIV/AIDS: a systematic review and meta-analysis. Psychiatr Q. 2020;91(4):1317–32.
7. Brief DJ, Bollinger AR, Vielhauer MJ, Berger-Greenstein JA, Morgan EE, Brady SM, et al. Understanding the interface of HIV, trauma, post-traumatic stress disorder, and substance use and its implications for health outcomes. AIDS Care. 2004;16(sup 1):97–120.
8. Irons C, Beaumont E. The Compassionate Mind Workbook: a step-by-step guide to developing your compassionate self. Hachette UK; 2017. 419 p.
9. Gilbert P, Irons C. A pilot exploration of the use of compassionate images in a group of self-critical people. Memory. 2004;12(4):507–16.
10. Goss K, Allan S. Compassion focused therapy for eating disorders. Int J Cogn Ther. 2010;3(2):141–58.
11. Heriot-Maitland C, Vidal JB, Ball S, Irons C. A compassionate-focused therapy group approach for acute inpatients: feasibility, initial pilot outcome data, and recommendations. Br J Clin Psychol. 2014;53(1):78–94.
12. Penlington C. Exploring a compassion-focused intervention for persistent pain in a group setting. Br J Pain. 2018;2018:2049463718772148.
13. Leaviss J, Uttley L. Psychotherapeutic benefits of compassion-focused therapy: an early systematic review. Psychol Med. 2015;45(5):927–45.
14. Haj Sadeghi Z, Yazdi-Ravandi S, Pirnia B. Compassion-focused therapy on levels of anxiety and depression among women with breast cancer: a randomized pilot trial. Int J Cancer Manag. 2018; [cited 2020 Dec 8]. https://sites.kowsarpub.com/ijcm/articles/67019.html#abstract.
15. Skinta MD, Lezama M, Wells G, Dilley JW. Acceptance and compassion-based group therapy to reduce HIV stigma. Cogn Behav Pract. 2015;22(4):481–90.
16. Ogueji AI, Okoloba MM. Compassion-focused therapy (CFT) as an intervention against suicidal ideation in newly diagnosed people living with HIV/AIDS (PLWHA) attending a Nigerian maternity teaching hospital. Glob Psychiatry. 2020;3(1):104–12.
17. Bridgham JT, Ortlund EA, Thornton JW. An epistatic ratchet constrains the direction of glucocorticoid receptor evolution. Nature. 2009;461(7263):515.
18. Panksepp J. Affective neuroscience: the foundations of human and animal emotions. London: Oxford University Press; 2004. 481 p.
19. Gilbert P. Explorations into the nature and function of compassion. Curr Opin Psychol. 2019;28:108–14.
20. Porges S. The polyvagal theory: new insights into adaptive reactions of the autonomic nervous system. Cleve Clin J Med. 2009;76(Suppl 2):S86–90.
21. Depue RA, Morrone-Strupinsky JV. A neurobehavioral model of affiliative bonding: implications for conceptualizing a human trait of affiliation. Behav Brain Sci. 2005;28(3):313–50; discussion 350–395.
22. Gilbert P, Catarino F, Duarte C, Matos M, Kolts R, Stubbs J, et al. The development of compassionate engagement and action scales for self and others. J Compassionate Health Care. 2017;4(1):4.
23. Gilbert P. Compassion: concepts, research and applications. Oxon: Routledge; 2017. 498 p.

24. Kolts R, Bell T, Bennett-Levy J, Irons C. Experiencing compassion focused therapy from the inside out: a self-practice/self-reflection workbook for therapists. 2018.

25. Lee D, James S. The compassionate mind approach to recovering from trauma: using compassion focused therapy. Hachette UK; 2012. 199 p.

26. Welford M. The compassionate mind approach to building self-confidence: Series editor, Paul Gilbert. Hachette UK; 2012. 214 p.

27. Chaponda M, Aldhouse N, Kroes M, Wild L, Robinson C, Smith A. Systematic review of the prevalence of psychiatric illness and sleep disturbance as co-morbidities of HIV infection in the UK. Int J STD AIDS. 2018;29(7):704–13.

28. LeGrand S, Reif S, Sullivan K, Murray K, Barlow ML, Whetten K. A review of recent literature on trauma among individuals living with HIV. Curr HIV/AIDS Rep. 2015;12(4):397–405.

29. Nightingale VR, Sher TG, Mattson M, Thilges S, Hansen NB. The effects of traumatic stressors and HIV-related trauma symptoms on health and health related quality of life. AIDS Behav. 2011;15(8):1870–8.

30. Watkins-Hayes C. Intersectionality and the sociology of HIV/AIDS: past, present, and future research directions. Annu Rev Sociol. 2014;40(1):431–57.

31. Campbell T. The seemingly intractable problem of HIV-related stigma: developing a framework to guide stigma interventions with young people living with HIV. In: Croston M, Rutter S, editors. Psychological perspectives in HIV care: an inter-professional approach. London: Routledge; 2020.

32. Eller LS, Rivero-Mendez M, Voss J, Chen W-T, Chaiphibalsarisdi P, Iipinge S, et al. Depressive symptoms, self-esteem, HIV symptom management self-efficacy and self-compassion in people living with HIV. AIDS Care. 2014;26(7):795–803.

33. Williams SL, Fekete EM, Skinta MD. Self-compassion in PLWH: less internalized shame and negative psychosocial outcomes. Behav Med. 2019;0(0):1–9.

34. Lupton D. Risk. London: Routledge; 1999.

35. Ainsworth MS, Bowlby J. An ethological approach to personality development. Am Psychol. 1991;46(4):333–41.

36. Bowlby J. Attachment and loss: Volume II: separation, anxiety and anger. Int Psycho-Anal Libr. 1973 [cited 2021 Jan 14]; https://www.pep-web.org/document.php?id=IPL.095.0001A.

37. Richards MPM. Attachment and loss. Vol. 3. Loss, Sadness and Depression. By John Bowlby. (Hogarth Press and Institute of Psychoanalysis, 1980.). J Biosoc Sci. 1981;13(3):369–73.

38. Ross ND, Kaminski PL, Herrington R. From childhood emotional maltreatment to depressive symptoms in adulthood: the roles of self-compassion and shame. Child Abuse Negl. 2019;92:32–42.

39. MacGinley. A scoping review of adult survivors' experiences of shame following sexual abuse in childhood—Health & Social Care in the Community—Wiley Online Library. 2019. [cited 2021 Jan 14]. https://onlinelibrary.wiley.com/doi/full/10.1111/hsc.12771.

40. Thibodeau M-E, Lavoie F, Hébert M, Blais M. Pathways linking childhood maltreatment and adolescent sexual risk behaviors: the role of attachment security. J Sex Res. 2017;54(8):994–1005.

41. Senn TE, Braksmajer A, Hutchins H, Carey MP. Development and refinement of a targeted sexual risk reduction intervention for women with a history of childhood sexual abuse. Cogn Behav Pract. 2017;24(4):496–507.

42. Weiss NH, Peasant C, Sullivan TP. Avoidant coping as a moderator of the association between childhood abuse types and HIV/sexual risk behaviors. Child Maltreat. 2019;24(1):26–35.

43. Warner S. Understanding the effects of child sexual abuse: feminist revolutions in theory, research and practice. London: Routledge; 2009. 300 p.

44. Collins RL, Ellickson PL, Orlando M, Klein DJ. Isolating the nexus of substance use, violence and sexual risk for HIV infection among young adults in the United States. AIDS Behav. 2005;9(1):73.

45. Berg RC, Amundsen E, Haugstvedt Å. Links between chemsex and reduced mental health among Norwegian MSM and other men: results from a cross-sectional clinic survey. BMC Public Health. 2020;20(1):1785.

46. Halkitis PN, Singer SN. Chemsex and mental health as part of syndemic in gay and bisexual men. Int J Drug Policy. 2018;55:180–2.
47. Theuninck AC, Lake N, Gibson S. HIV-related posttraumatic stress disorder: investigating the traumatic events. AIDS Patient Care STDs. 2010;24(8):485–91.
48. Association AP. Diagnostic and statistical manual of mental disorders (DSM-5®). American Psychiatric Pub; 2013. 1520 p.
49. Hutchinson P, Dhairyawan R. Shame, stigma, HIV: philosophical reflections. Med Humanit. 2017;43(4):225–30.
50. Skinta MD, Brandrett BD, Schenk WC, Wells G, Dilley JW. Shame, self-acceptance and disclosure in the lives of gay men living with HIV: an interpretative phenomenological analysis approach. Psychol Health. 2014;29(5):583–97.
51. Dale S, Pierre-Louis C, Bogart L, O'Cleirigh C, Safren S, Still I. Rise: the need for self-validation and self-care in the midst of adversities faced by black women with HIV. Cult Divers Ethn Minor Psychol. 2018;24(1):15–25.
52. Vitale A, Ryde J. Exploring risk factors affecting the mental health of refugee women living with HIV. Int J Environ Res Public Health. 2018;15(10):2326.
53. 'We are Not Fresh': HIV-Positive Women Talk of Their Experience of Living with Their 'Spoiled Identity'—Poul Rohleder, Kerry Gibson, 2006. [cited 2021 Jan 14]. https://journals.sagepub.com/doi/abs/10.1177/0081246306036001003.
54. 90-90-90: treatment for all I UNAIDS. [cited 2021 Jan 15]. https://www.unaids.org/en/resources/909090.
55. British Psychological Society. BPS response—APPG inquiry into HIV and mental health. https://www.bps.org.uk/news-and-policy/bps-response-appg-inquiry-hiv-and-mental-health. 2019.
56. Warner SRS. Traumatic beginnings, complicated lives: attachment styles, relationships and HIV care. In: Croston M, Rutter S, editors. Psychological perspectives in HIV care: an interprofessional approach. London: Routledge; 2020.
57. Langford SE, Ananworanich J, Cooper DA. Predictors of disease progression in HIV infection: a review. AIDS Res Ther. 2007;4(1):11.
58. Siemieniuk RAC, Krentz HB, Gill MJ. Intimate partner violence and HIV: a review. Curr HIV/AIDS Rep. 2013;10(4):380–9.
59. Salmond E, Salmond S, Ames M, Kamienski M, Holly C. Experiences of compassion fatigue in direct care nurses: a qualitative systematic review. JBI Database System Rev Implement Rep. 2019;17(5):682–753.
60. Gilbert P, Procter S. Compassionate mind training for people with high shame and self-criticism: overview and pilot study of a group therapy approach. Clin Psychol Psychother. 2006;13(6):353–79.
61. Skinta MD, Fekete EM, Williams SL. HIV-stigma, self-compassion, and psychological well-being among gay men living with HIV. Stigma Health. 2019;4(2):179–87.
62. Lazarus JV, Safreed-Harmon K, Barton SE, Costagliola D, Dedes N, del Amo Valero J, et al. Beyond viral suppression of HIV—the new quality of life frontier. BMC Med. 2016;14(1):94.
63. Wagner AC, Bartsch AA, Manganaro M, Monson CM, Baker CN, Brown SM. Trauma-informed care training with HIV and related community service workers: short and long term effects on attitudes. Psychol Serv. 2020;No Pagination Specified-No Pagination Specified.
64. Sweeney A, Clement S, Filson B, Kennedy A. Trauma-informed mental healthcare in the UK: what is it and how can we further its development? Ment Health Rev J. 2016;21(3):174–92.
65. Narrative reconstruction and post-traumatic growth among trauma survivors: the importance of narrative in social work research and practice—Sarah L Jirek, 2017. [cited 2021 Jan 14]. https://journals.sagepub.com/doi/full/10.1177/1473325016656046.
66. Yuen A. Less pain, more gain: exploration of responses versus effects when working with the consequences of trauma. Explorations: E-J Narrat Pract. 2009;1:1–16.
67. Wong CCY, Yeung NCY. Self-compassion and posttraumatic growth: cognitive processes as mediators. Mindfulness. 2017;8(4):1078–87.

68. Welford M. Compassion focused therapy for dummies. New York: John Wiley & Sons; 2016. 336 p.
69. National AIDS Trust. Why we need HIV support services. https://www.nat.org.uk/sites/default/files/publications/NAT_WHY%20WE%20NEED%20HIV%20SUPPORT%20SERVICES_2017_56%20pages_FINAL%20WEB_SINGLE%20PAGE. 2017.
70. Luoma JB, Platt MG. Shame, self-criticism, self-stigma, and compassion in acceptance and commitment therapy. Curr Opin Psychol. 2015;2:97–101.
71. Schultz K, Cattaneo LB, Sabina C, Brunner L, Jackson S, Serrata JV. Key roles of community connectedness in healing from trauma. Psychol Violence. 2016;6(1):42–8.
72. Baverstock AC, Finlay FO. Maintaining compassion and preventing compassion fatigue: a practical guide. Arch Dis Child Educ Pract Ed. 2016;101(4):170–4.
73. Figley CR. Compassion fatigue: coping with secondary traumatic stress disorder in those who treat the traumatized. London: Routledge; 2013. 291 p.
74. Clarifying misconceptions about compassionate care—Dewar—2014—Journal of Advanced Nursing—Wiley Online Library. [cited 2021 Jan 14]. https://onlinelibrary.wiley.com/doi/full/10.1111/jan.12322.
75. Lombardo B, Eyre C. Compassion fatigue: a nurse's primer. Online J Issues Nurs. 2011;16(1):3.
76. Hooper C, Craig J, Janvrin DR, Wetsel MA, Reimels E. Compassion satisfaction, burnout, and compassion fatigue among emergency nurses compared with nurses in other selected inpatient specialties. J Emerg Nurs. 2010;36(5):420–7.
77. Burtson PL, Stichler JF. Nursing work environment and nurse caring: relationship among motivational factors. J Adv Nurs. 2010;66(8):1819–31.
78. Tend Academy. What is compassion fatigue? 2018. https://www.tendacademy.ca/wp-content/uploads/2018/05/what-is-compassion-fatigue-2018-05-20.pdf.
79. Flarity K, Gentry JE, Mesnikoff N. The effectiveness of an educational program on preventing and treating compassion fatigue in emergency nurses. Adv Emerg Nurs J. 2013;35(3):247–58.
80. Potter P, Deshields T, Divanbeigi J, Berger J, Cipriano D, Norris L, et al. Compassion fatigue and burnout. Clin J Oncol Nurs. 2010;14(5):E56–62.
81. Stamm BH. The concise ProQOL manual (2nd Edition). Pocatello, ID: ProQOL.org; 2010.
82. Joinson C. Coping with compassion fatigue. Nursing (Lond). 1992;22(4):118–20.
83. Saakvitne KW, Pearlman LA, Traumatic Stress Institute. A Norton professional book. Transforming the pain: a workbook on vicarious traumatization. New York: W. W. Norton & Co.; 1996.
84. Perregrini M. Combating compassion fatigue. Nursing. 2019;49(2):50–4.
85. Henshall LE, Alexander T, Molyneux P, Gardiner E, McLellan A. The relationship between perceived organisational threat and compassion for others: implications for the NHS. Clin Psychol Psychother. 2018;25(2):231–49.
86. Factors that influence the development of compassion fatigue, burnout, and compassion satisfaction in Emergency Department Nurses—Hunsaker—2015—Journal of Nursing Scholarship—Wiley Online Library. [cited 2021 Jan 14]. https://sigmapubs.onlinelibrary.wiley.com/doi/full/10.1111/jnu.12122.
87. Compassion fatigue in nurses: a metasynthesis—Nolte—2017—Journal of Clinical Nursing—Wiley Online Library. [cited 2021 Jan 14]. https://onlinelibrary.wiley.com/doi/full/10.1111/jocn.13766.
88. Zhang Y-Y, Han W-L, Qin W, Yin H-X, Zhang C-F, Kong C, et al. Extent of compassion satisfaction, compassion fatigue and burnout in nursing: a meta-analysis. J Nurs Manag. 2018;26(7):810–9.
89. Sinclair S, Raffin-Bouchal S, Venturato L, Mijovic-Kondejewski J, Smith-MacDonald L. Compassion fatigue: a meta-narrative review of the healthcare literature. Int J Nurs Stud. 2017;69:9–24.
90. Neff K. Self-compassion: an alternative conceptualization of a healthy attitude toward oneself. Self Identity. 2003;2(2):85–101.

91. Klimecki O, Singer T. Empathic distress fatigue rather than compassion fatigue? Integrating findings from empathy research in psychology and social neuroscience. 10.1093/acprof: oso/9780199738571.003.0253

92. Importance of Self-Care for Nurses and How to Put a Plan in Place. Purdue Global. [cited 2021 Jan 15]. https://www.purdueglobal.edu/blog/nursing/self-care-for-nurses/.

93. McVicar A, Pettit A, Knight-Davidson P, Shaw-Flach A. Promotion of professional quality of life through reducing fears of compassion and compassion fatigue: application of the compassionate mind model to specialist community public health nurses (Health Visiting) training. J Clin Nurs. [cited 2021 Jan 13];n/a(n/a). https://onlinelibrary.wiley.com/doi/abs/10.1111/jocn.15517.

94. Self-Care for Nurses: At Work and At Home | Performance Health. [cited 2021 Jan 15]. https://www.performancehealth.com/articles/self-care-for-nurses-at-work-and-at-home/.

95. Blum CA. Practicing self-care for nurses: a nursing program initiative. Online J Issues Nurs. 2014;19(3):3.

96. Portnoy D. Burnout and compassion fatigue: watch for the signs. Health Prog St Louis Mo. 2011;92(4):46–50.

97. Sinclair S, Kondejewski J, Raffin-Bouchal S, King-Shier KM, Singh P. Can self-compassion promote healthcare provider well-being and compassionate care to others? Results of a systematic review. Appl Psychol Health Well-Being. 2017;9(2):168–206.

98. Boellinghaus I, Jones FW, Hutton J. The role of mindfulness and loving-kindness meditation in cultivating self-compassion and other-focused concern in health care professionals. Mindfulness. 2014;5(2):129–38.

99. Raab K, Sogge K, Parker N, Flament MF. Mindfulness-based stress reduction and self-compassion among mental healthcare professionals: a pilot study. Ment Health Relig Cult. 2015;18(6):503–12.

100. Health Care Workers in HIV Project. Health Care Workers in HIV: an oral history in the UK Aids era. 2014. Health Care Workers in HIV Project. https://www.healthcareworkersinhiv.org.uk. 2014.

101. Gibson S, Plotnick A. Grief at work: helping organizations cope with AIDS-related loss. Oral Abstract. 12th World AIDS Conference, Geneva, Switzerland. 1998

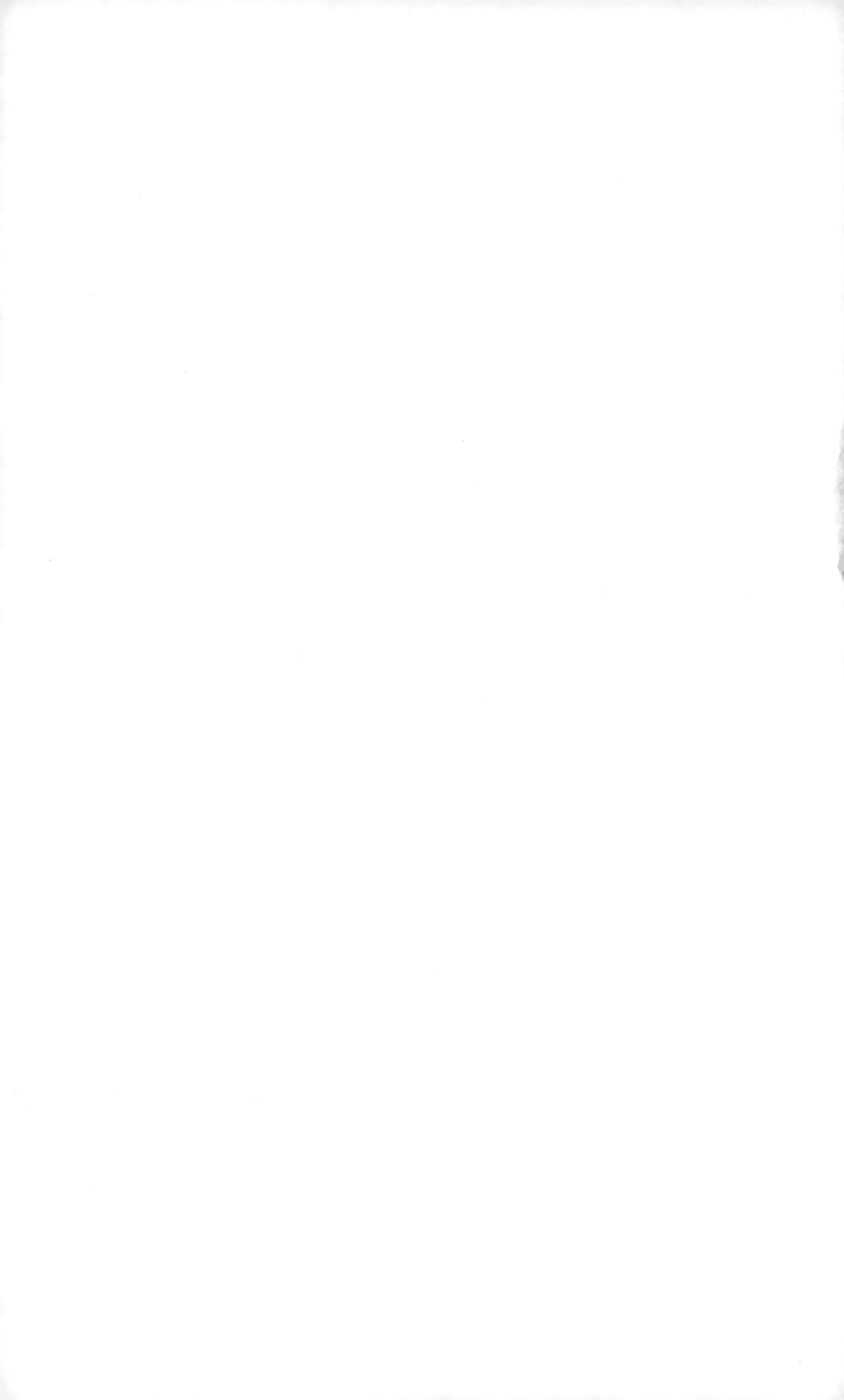

Chapter 13
Wounded Healers in a Shared Traumatic Reality: Why and How We Should Engage in Stepped-Care, Self-Care for Ourselves

Alexander Margetts and Michelle Croston

13.1 Introduction

13.1.1 The Importance of Staff Wellbeing

This could be the most important chapter you've ever read, for you, your colleagues, and your patients. A bold statement to start with, but why might this be?

In order to help others, we must be well ourselves, and there is a clear relationship between improved staff experiences (e.g., staff engagement, motivation, satisfaction, morale, work pressure, stress, and intention to leave) and improved patient care and safety [1]. Whilst it would be hoped that it is enough to frame staff health and wellbeing in its own right, should further argument be needed beyond this and patient care performance, from a commissioning and organisational performance perspective, recruitment, retention, sickness absence, and agency spend costs can all be improved by healthy working environments [2]. Thus, there is individual, patient, and organisational benefit from maintaining our wellbeing.

A. Margetts
Chelsea and Westminster Hospital, London, UK

M. Croston (✉)
Manchester Metropolitan University, Manchester, UK
e-mail: m.croston@mmu.ac.uk

© The Author(s), under exclusive license to Springer Nature Switzerland AG 2021
M. Croston, I. Hodgson (eds.), *Providing HIV Care: Lessons from the Field for Nurses and Healthcare Practitioners*,
https://doi.org/10.1007/978-3-030-71295-2_13

13.1.2 Work Satisfaction and Attendance

From the most recently published data available from the UK 2019 National Health Service (NHS) staff survey, 40.3% reported feeling unwell as a result of work-related stress in the last 12 months. What is more this figure has been steadily increasing since 2016 (when it was at 36.8%). This has led over half (56.6%) of NHS workers to report going to work in the last 3 months despite not feeling well enough to perform their duties. In total, nearly one-fifth (19.6%) of people are thinking of leaving the NHS (be it retiring or taking a career break or moving to a job outside healthcare, or in healthcare but outside the NHS) [3].

13.2 Nursing Practice and Role of Nurses

Specific to UK nursing is the Royal College's employment survey [4]. This found 3/5 nurses (61%) saying they were "too busy to provide the level of care to patients that they would like", only half (51%) were happy with their working hours, 29% had suffered physical abuse from patients or relatives in the past year, and 65% had experienced verbal abuse. Approximately 10% of nurses are seriously thinking of leaving, with job satisfaction, stress, and burnout having significant correlation with this [5].

So, what impact does this have? NHS nurses have a slightly above average sickness absence rate (4.5%) compared to all NHS staff (4.2%), and higher than across the wider public sector (2.9%) and private sector (1.7%) [6]. Furthermore, 7.3% of NHS staff reported stress or depression as their reason for sickness absence. However, just as concerning, many more nurses are working when unwell (known as "presenteeism"), with 84% surveyed reporting going to work at least once in the past year despite feeling too ill to do so [4].

> **Reflection Point**
> In the past 12 months, had you gone into work feeling unwell? What was your thought process that encouraged you to go into work? What might you consider doing differently if the situation should arise again?

13.2.1 Occupational Health

A quantitative survey of Canadian nurses found that 86% (277/323) responding met criteria for "burnout syndrome", described as emotional exhaustion, depersonalisation, and lack of personal accomplishment in response to interpersonal and emotional stressors experienced in the workplace [7]. Furthermore, 18% (61/322) met criteria for Post-Traumatic Stress Disorder (PTSD).

The UK has one of the highest rates of nurses reporting burnout across Europe, 42% compared to a European average of 28% [5]. At the other end of the scale regarding stress is the concept of "rust out" in nursing, in which we find ourselves bored and demotivated due to a lack of challenge or utilisation of our skillset within our role or position [8]. These can be conceptualised on a work pressure continuum, as explored by the Royal College of Nursing [9]. Here, the relationship between performance and pressure can be seen as a bell-shaped curve, starting with "rust out" and progressing through six stages: sleepy, tired, relaxed, energised (where performance is maximised) and then struggling, shattered, and, finally, burnout, where performance is seriously impeded.

Compassion fatigue is another term used in nursing occupational health, sometimes used synonymously with burnout, and often characterised as a loss of emotional connectedness with patients. However, there are subtle differences [10, 11]. Valent [12] argues that burnout is concerned following difficulties with "assertiveness–goal achievement" and a failure to achieve desired results, whilst compassion fatigue relates to guilt and distress when a "rescue–caretaking" mode cannot be enacted, and we are unable to save or rescue individuals from harm. Burnout is also viewed as occurring and declining more slowly than compassion fatigue, which can be faster to originate or subside. More recent research has also drawn on the concept of "moral injury" from military literature, in which difficult decisions that might go against our values cause distress (e.g., who to allocate limited life-supporting resources to during covid-19 [13]). There are also movements to recognise the positive impact of such work also, with "compassion satisfaction" being the pleasure, satisfaction, and achievement derived through working in the helping profession [14].

13.2.2   Nurses' Mental Health

Work-related stress can lead to more general mental health difficulties. For example, in a study of American hospital-employed nurses, depression rates were found to be twice that of the general population (18% to 9.4% [15]). This added to the global literature indicating healthcare professionals (and in some cases specifically nurses) had difficulties with depression, including Finland, France, Sweden, and Taiwan [16–19]. The relationship with work can be bi-directional, with strong evidence for associations between common mental disorders and general errors, medication errors, near misses, patient safety, and patient satisfaction [20].

Whilst the majority of literature has focused on burnout and depression, anxiety when studied, has been found to be even more prevalent. For example, in a study of Chinese nurses, 43.4% reported anxiety symptoms against a general population baseline of 5.6% [21]. Whilst this could vary culturally and by specific nursing group, it was consistent with findings of anxiety usually being higher within nurses than the local general population (e.g., Iran = 43.2%; Japan = 7%; Singapore = 21%; the USA = 20%) [22–25].

In extreme cases, this leads to mental health deterioration, and even suicide. Between 2011 and 2017, at least 305 NHS nurses took their own lives, with a suicide rate estimated as 23% above the national average for female nurses [26, 27]. This equates on average to a nurse dying by suicide every 1–2 weeks. These upsetting statistics are not a UK exclusive phenomena, with higher suicide rates relative to either general population or occupation-matched controls also reported in America, Australia, Canada, Denmark, Iceland, and Norway [28–33].

It is important that the debate and finesse around precise language, nomenclature, and diagnosis does not distract or prevent us from action. Clearly, there is an urgent need to both understand and intervene with regard to nursing wellbeing and mental health.

Reflection Point
You are invited to think about a time in your career when you may have experienced a range of emotions from rust out to burnout. Take some time to consider your experience and how it made you feel, what impact did it have on you and how did it make you feel? How might you recognise these experiences in others?

13.2.3   Non-work Stress and Wellbeing

Firstly, it is important to acknowledge that nurses are human beings! This relates to their likelihood of experiencing mental health difficulties for *non*-work-related reasons. For example, the UK "Time to Change" campaign has been effective in helping reduce stigma regarding mental illness [34], which notes that one-fourth of us will experience mental health difficulties in any given year. When examined in more detail, in the past week, 1 in 6 adults reported concerns or symptoms, the most prevalent being mixed anxiety and depression (8.8%), then generalised anxiety disorder (4.4%), with other issues such as depressive episodes, phobias, obsessive compulsive disorder, and panic ranging from 2.6% to 0.7% [35].

We should therefore not always scapegoat the nursing role as being complicit in this; indeed, many nurses report good job satisfaction, giving a positive sense of achievement, pride, and identity [4]. Thus, for some it will be a source of coping, and it is therefore important to consider how this can be maintained. However, for others it may also or instead be a source of stress, and so this must also be considered in tandem.

Table 13.1 Factors influencing nursing stress (adapted from [4])

Factor	Aspects	Issues
Working patterns and workloads	Workload, work-life balance, presenteeism	Feeling overworked and overloaded; intense pressure from increased demand and staffing shortages; pervasive blame culture; lack of working hours flexibility. Moral distress when struggle to provide quality of care wishing to deliver
Pay, earnings, and additional work	Satisfaction with pay, pensions, additional working	Wages not increased in line with workload and work intensity. Additional levels of responsibility, skill, and years of experience seen as poorly rewarded
Nature of work and views re: nursing	Intention to leave, job satisfaction, emotional demands, voice, and value	Satisfaction strongly related to job design, task allocation, autonomy level/control, development opportunities, resources and support from colleagues/ managers, feeling valued, work being meaningful. Many derive satisfaction from nursing career however becoming less likely would recommend it to others
Physical and verbal abuse and bullying	Experiences of physical/verbal abuse, bullying; reporting	Workplace conflict common, many subject to physical/ verbal abuse by patients/relatives or bullying from a colleague; if issues likely to be seeking new job
Education and training	Mandatory training and appraisals	Training and personal development central to advancement of individuals; staffing shortages, reduced funding, opportunities and time; threatens patient safety, organisational productivity and effectiveness, risks motivation, and likelihood of nursing staff leaving

13.2.4 Nursing-Related Stress

Nursing generally is recognised as having various possible stress factors within the role. The UK Royal College of Nursing noted all levels of nursing staff reported being overworked and lacking resources to perform the job to the level they wished [4]. They reported being dedicated to protecting patients, but often at a personal cost, with various factors and aspects highlighted (Table 13.1).

There are also interesting ideas about the "type" of person who chooses nursing as a career. For most motivation appears to be from an altruistic perspective; however, personal and self-development have been found to be equally as important as the desire to care, including self-esteem and social status [36]. Whilst the idea of "wounded healer" has been applied to nursing in terms of the impact of the job [37], it may be that some people who are attracted to the role of nurse hope it may help them better navigate pre-existing difficulties.

13.2.5 HIV Nursing-Specific Challenges

Nurses will choose different clinical areas and career paths based upon a variety of factors. This chapter is written in the context of HIV nursing, and so this domain will be briefly considered now. This is not to try and argue that HIV nursing is "more" stressful than other types (which would be a most unenviable competition), more that each field of nursing has its own unique facets and challenges (and of course accompanying rewards and growth).

Being HIV+ continues to carry a great stigma worldwide [38]. For some, this stigma is also applied to working in the field. Within the UK and other Western settings, this was especially apparent in the earlier days of the epidemic, with healthcare staff often hiding their vocation from friends and family [39]. Whilst public perceptions may be (slowly) changing, this continues to be found globally also, especially in low-resource settings, such as China and various African countries [40, 41]. Various other studies have also found issues with wellbeing, job satisfaction, burnout, and retention amongst HIV nurses around the world, such as Brazil, Canada, Italy, Russia, and South Africa [42–46].

Within this there is the concept of vicarious/secondary traumatisation and "survivor's guilt" for those working with people who are HIV+, the witnessing of trauma to and of others having a cumulative and negative impact on oneself [47]. This arises as some patients have found (or continue to find) becoming and/or being HIV+ a traumatic experience [48]. Lastly, some nurses are HIV+ themselves ("the other side of the pill bottle" [49], and/or will have close friends and family who are HIV+, and will need to consider their boundaries and beliefs regarding what it means to be HIV+ and how these might be shaped by the interplay of their personal vs. professional experiences. This leads to the concept of "shared traumatic reality", whereby staff are exposed to a traumatic event both by their patient's experiences and their own direct exposure [50]. Whilst usually applied to experiences of war, violence, and natural disasters, it is also being applied to health settings including pandemics [51].

13.2.6 Impact of Covid-19

Finally, it is important to acknowledge the impact that covid-19 has had, to both the general mental health and wellbeing of the population, and to nursing roles. This will continue to evolve, however at the time of writing it is estimated that at least 500,000 more people in the UK may experience mental ill health as a result of covid-19 [52]. However, above and beyond that is the extra stress endured by the healthcare system and its workers [53], with nursing stressors of:

- Working in an (even further) depleted workforce (e.g., due to infection, self-isolation, and/or family caring responsibilities),
- Increases in intensity and volume of work alongside new protocols and restrictive practice (e.g., services rapidly transforming from face-to-face to virtual/remote; end-of-life care more frequent with rapid deterioration and isolation rules prohibiting bedside presence of family),

- Reorganisation of established nurse–patient ratios (e.g., ITU one-to-one chang-ing to one ITU nurse to six or more patients),
- Staff recruitment changes: fast-tracking of final-year nursing students; retired or part-time colleagues encouraged to return,
- Redeployment to work in new specialities or higher acuity areas, with new teams,
- Concern for personal and/or family health from own potential contact with covid-19 vs. ethical/professional obligations of continuing care provision,
- Lack of staff-testing, shortages and variability of access to personal protective equipment (PPE), fatigue, discomfort, injury, and communication barriers, when it is available,
- Moral distress from treatment decisions based on finite resources (e.g., whom to allocate ventilator access to),
- A lack of organisational support (be this actual or perceived),
- Guilt and/or shaming of those unable to contribute to direct patient care (e.g., due to own vulnerability/risk re: covid-19).

Another important factor to note is the disproportionate impact of covid-19 on B.A.M.E. (Black and Minority Ethnic) healthcare workers in the UK, with two-third of those that died being from B.A.M.E. background, rising to 71% of the 35 nurses and midwives who had died at the time of the report [54–56]. Given that approximately 20% of nurses, midwives, and health-visitors in the NHS identifies as being from a B.A.M.E. background, it is important that this, alongside other racial inequalities within nursing such as regarding pay-banding and career progres-sion, are addressed [57].

13.2.7 Individual and Organisational Accountability

Clearly then, now more than ever, there is an imperative for us to think about our own wellbeing. It is important not to place blame or onus within individuals if sys-temic factors such as workload, pay conditions, or a global pandemic are the main (or sole) contributor. In addition to any individual "resilience" building work, pres-sure from organisational policy and practices (e.g., unhealthy work environments, poor communication, stigma) will require system-level solutions to address root causes. Otherwise, we risk pathologising individual nurses and healthcare profes-sionals and their understandable and rational responses to issues such as intense emotional work and understaffing [58, 59]. Whilst the focus of this chapter is what individual action one can take to safeguard wellbeing, this should not be read as implying it is therefore always or solely the responsibility of the affected individual to instigate change. Neither should it be read that self-care means doing things alone, indeed the majority of self-care is likely to be most beneficial when engaged with others, be they peers or professionals depending on the level of help needed.

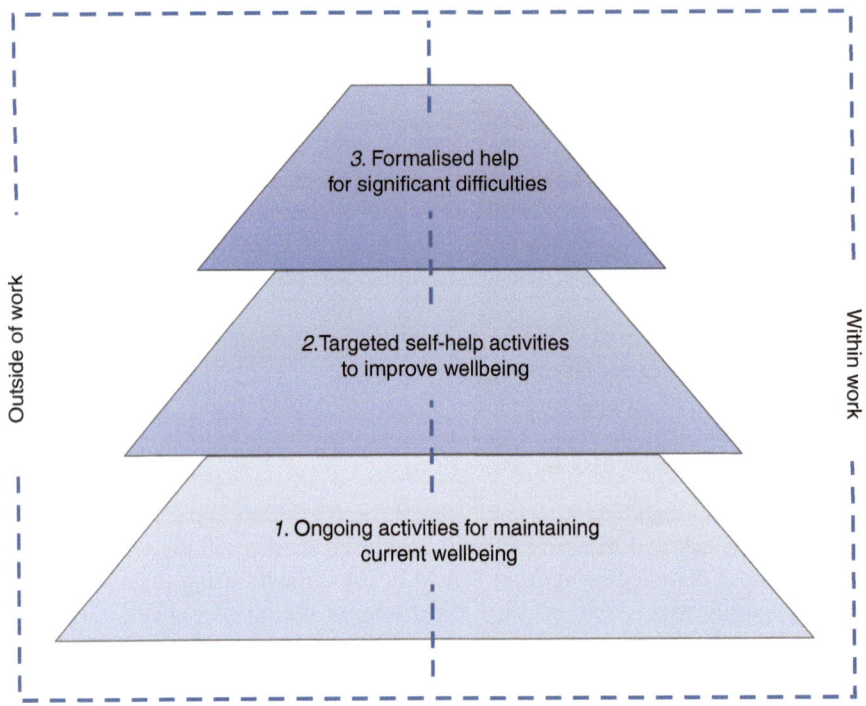

Fig. 13.1 A self-care, stepped-care model

13.2.8 Stepped-Care Model of Self-Care

Most of us are aware of stepped-care models within healthcare, and this chapter proposes one specifically for healthcare workers *themselves* and their own wellbeing, with actions to be taken both outside and within work (Fig. 13.1).

13.2.9 Terminology

Various different terms have been used to describe occupational wellbeing and self-care, such as "Mental Health First Aid", "Psychological PPE", "Self-Practice Self-Reflection", "Stress Management and Resilience Training", and "Wellness Recovery Action Plan" [60–65]. Rather than align itself to a particular training programme, this chapter focuses more on the *process* of self-care than the content and methodology of the different packages. Instead, what is more important is how we define and assess wellbeing within ourselves.

13.3   Recommendations for Nursing Practice

13.3.1   Assessment of Wellbeing

In order to decide where on the stepped-care model we are best placed (with greater severity of difficulties/need moving us up the steps), we must be able to self-assess where we are currently. A "good" and "bad" day will look different to everybody depending on their personal definitions and values [66] and the spiritual, religious, and cultural context which they are within (Task 1). For example, important values to me include being a good uncle to my nephew and nieces, mentor to my students, and partner to my husband. However, values can also exist outside of relationships, for example for myself I enjoy exercise, the arts, intellectual stimulation, and creativity (tennis, theatre, boardgames, and building Lego dinosaurs being specific enjoyable hobbies that help me achieve these in goal-orientated format).

Task 1
What does wellness mean and look like for you? What are your values? How does your culture and any spirituality or faith interplay with this? What specific hobbies and goals do you enjoy?

Informal self-assessment would include noting both our current state and what our "early warning" signs are that our wellness or mood is being negatively affected. Again, these will be individual to each of us and could be emotional, cognitive, physiological, or behavioural (Task 2). For example, for myself if I notice that I've become overly emotional in response to banal adverts, irritable with my other half at life-long habits of his that I should have adjusted to and accepted by now, extra forgetful at work, or dehydrated, these are signs that I'm starting to feel drained! Another form of informal self-assessment would be idiosyncratic scales of daily general mood, for example, on a 0–10 scale, with pictures, symbols, or colours.

Task 2
What are your "early warning signs" that things are not going well for you? What do you start to do (or stop doing)? What emotions "leak" out? Physically how do you feel? What thoughts do you have?

Formal assessment would involve the use of questionnaires to assess mood and wellbeing. These could be self-administered, or by professionals, depending on the issue, public access, and step required. For example, the PHQ-9 and GAD-7 are widely used in the UK healthcare system as indicators of low mood and anxiety, respectively, and are freely available for people to self-administer and score [67, 68]. There are also occupational stress-specific measures, such as Maslach Burnout Inventory, Compassion Fatigue Self Test, and Copenhagen Burnout Inventory [69–71].

Furthermore, some scales have been developed specifically to the nursing context, such as the Nursing Stress Scale, Expanded Nursing Stress Scale, Nurse Stress Index, Nursing Burnout Scale, and Nursing Job Stressor Scale [72–76]. In keeping with the reminder that one should not solely think about individuals, the nursing context itself can also be measured, for example, by the Revised Nursing Work Index [77].

Whilst many of these rely upon self-observation and introspection, feedback from others (colleagues and managers at work, and friends and family from home) is equally as valuable, as we are not always able to spot signs and symptoms ourselves, or have a higher tolerance of what we think of as "acceptable" stress. In order to make this most effective, it is important to give people permission in advance (Task 3). This might be at regular appraisals (in work), or on a reactive basis. For example, for myself following a significant bereavement I wished to continue to work as a coping strategy, but I asked my manager (whom I had a very positive relationship with) to let me know if she felt I was "not coping", as I was aware my insight was limited, and we reviewed my caseload more regularly during this period. At the other end of the scale, my other half on an ongoing basis is used to gently pointing out that I said I'd "only be 30 min" about 2 h ago when writing from home, and that I really need to stop!

Task 3
Who in your work and home life could you ask to provide feedback on your wellbeing for you?

The last consideration for assessment is when to do this. This will depend slightly on the level at which assessment is occurring, with more informal ongoing self-assessment at Step 1, and less frequent and more formalised assessment by others at Step 3. Specific stressors or trigger points will vary for individuals, but challenging patient situations (e.g., unexpected patient death, formal complaints), unusual work stress (e.g., work inspection, crisis planning), and times of major life events and transitions (e.g., job promotion, moving house, wedding, illness, bereavement) would be especially important times to monitor.

13.3.2 Disclosure of Difficulties

Should wellbeing issues be detected and self-identified with, we then need to decide to whom, if anyone, we share this with (both personally and professionally: Task 4). Interestingly, we might assume that given as healthcare professionals we are more adept to working with mental health issues, we might hold less stigma about these. However, this is not always the case. In Canada, for example, a "web of silence" from stigmatisation regarding mental health and wellbeing amongst healthcare professionals has been found [78]. Within the NHS, interviews of 24 NHS healthcare professionals (13 from within mental health, 11 from other health fields) found those outside of mental health noted that mental health at best was not discussed, or worse seen as not a "proper" illness [79]. Most reported concern of negative views from colleagues, despite having positive views themselves, often borne from personal as well as professional experiences. The role of manager was seen as crucial for examples of good practice; for those of us in managerial roles therefore we must reflect on our views, as well as consider if and how we might approach our own managers should we have such difficulties. As when we are able to disclose (rather than assume everyone "is in the same boat"), advantages reported included understanding from colleagues and support.

Task 4
Who in your work and home life would you feel able to talk to about wellbeing issues and why? Who wouldn't you want to, and why not?

13.3.3   Wellbeing Interventions

The type of intervention(s) required will depend on the person, their difficulties, available resources, and which Step they are at Table 13.2; Task 5. Step 1 is concerned with ongoing general wellbeing and applies to us all. Even if we identify as "not having any problems", it is important to ensure this is actively maintained, rather than taken for granted. Step 2 is enacted when we note specific but relatively minor difficulties, or upcoming potential triggers that may threaten these, and involves actions that help us gain low-level support. Should this not be sufficient, or

Table 13.2 Examples of different interventions for wellbeing

Step		Within work	Outside of work
1	Ongoing activities for maintaining current wellbeing	Reflective practice (diaries, groups); supervision; appraisals and job plans; team support; taking annual leave; delegating, saying "no"; work gardens	Sleep; diet; socialising; exercise; mindfulness; flow activities; hobbies; spirituality/faith
2	Targeted self-help activities to improve wellbeing	Speak to supervisor and/or line manager; "emergency work toolkit"; targeted role plays/simulations; specific training; professional guidelines; Schwartz rounds; "wobble" rooms	Planning specific events; talking to family/friends about work and mood issues
3	Formalised help for significant difficulties	Occupational health; union support; professional body support; whistle blowing	General practitioner; own therapy; legal advice

Table 13.3 An example of a self-care plan

Daily self-care needs	
Consider your physical, emotional, spiritual, and professional needs	
Area of self-care	What do I need to do?
Emergency self-care needs	
Consider, relaxation, how do you stay calm, what helps your mood, how will you manage your self-talk, support needed	
When I am/need/feel/have ……….	What would be helpful
Insert name **Top Coping skills**	
1.	
2.	
3.	
Support Networks	
Contact numbers, email addresses, websites I might need	
Something else	

we be in crisis, then Step 3 is warranted. This involves invoking professional input and support. Importantly at each Step, there are likely to be activities and relationships that are helpful both in a work context, and outside of this. Some aspects of the Steps will require more support from others (especially the higher ones), and so self-care in this context is about identifying the difficulties and allowing oneself to seek and utilise such support. This is in keeping with the philosophy discussed earlier that the onus must not always be on us as individuals to "fix" or "solve" everything with regard to our own wellbeing, especially when organisational or systemic factors are involved (Table 13.3).

> **Task 5**
> What would your personalised stepped-care plan look like? What can you access within work at the different stages, and how could you get help outside of work?

13.4 Conclusion

HIV nursing and healthcare, like all nursing and healthcare roles, can be stressful. For most this is usually outweighed by the benefits and satisfaction of the role, and it is enough to engage in normal work and home activities to maintain a sense of wellbeing. At times for all of us, however, this will be compromised, either by work or life events. It is essential that we (and others) can help highlight when this occurs, and think about what available support options are most helpful, both within and outside of work. Actions and solutions can be found at individual and organisational levels, no matter the cause or severity of distress, which can lead not only to recovery but growth and development beyond this too.

Please note this chapter has been adapted from an article written by the lead author as a continuing professional development paper on self-care for HIV nurses (**Margetts A. Self-care for HIV Nursing Staff. HIV Nursing. 2020. 20. 4**).

References

1. Dawson J. Staff experience and patient outcomes: what do we know? A report commissioned by NHS Employers on behalf of NHS England. 2014.
2. RCN. Healthy Workplace, Healthy You. R Coll Nurs. 2017. http://www2.rcn.org.uk/newsevents/campaigns/healthy-workplace?_ga=1.47296295.1083312183.1489072682.
3. NHS England. NHS Staff Survey 2019 National results briefing. 2019;(February):1–42. http://www.nhsstaffsurveyresults.com/wp-content/uploads/2020/01/P3255_ST19_National-briefing_FINAL_V2.pdf.
4. RCN. RCN Employment Survey 2019. RCN Prof Dev. 2019;1–91. https://www.rcn.org.uk/professional-development/publications/pub-007927.
5. Health Education England. Growing Nursing Numbers: literature review on nurses leaving the NHS. 2014;1–28.
6. Moberly T. Sickness absence rates across the NHS. BMJ. 2018;2018:361.
7. Mealer M, Burnham EL, Goode CJ, Rothbaum B, Moss M. The prevalence and impact of post traumatic stress disorder and burnout syndrome in nurses. Depress Anxiety. 2009;26(12):1118–26.
8. Moustaka E, Constantinidis TC. Sources and effects of work-related stress in nursing. Health Sci J. 2010;4(4):210.
9. RCN. Stress and you: a guide for nursing staff. R Coll Nurs. 2015.
10. Peters E. Compassion fatigue in nursing: a concept analysis. Nurs Forum. 2018;53(4):466–80.
11. Yoder EA. Compassion fatigue in nurses. Appl Nurs Res [Internet]. 2010;23(4):191–7. https://doi.org/10.1016/j.apnr.2008.09.003.
12. Valent P. Diagnosis and treatment of helper stresses, traumas, and illnesses. Treat Comp Fatig. 2002;1:17–38.
13. Borges LM, Barnes SM, Farnsworth JK, Bahraini NH, Brenner LAA. Commentary on moral injury among health care providers during the COVID-19 pandemic. Psychol Trauma Theory Res Pract Policy. 2020;12:138–40.
14. Stamm BH. Measuring compassion satisfaction as well as fatigue: developmental history of the compassion satisfaction and fatigue test. In: Figley CR, editor. Psychosocial stress series, no 24 Treating compassion fatigue. London: Brunner-Routledge; 2002. p. 107–19.
15. Letvak BS, Ruhm CJ, Mccoy T. Depression in hospital-employed nurses. Clin Nurse Spec. 2012;26(3):177–82.
16. Virtanen M, Pentti J, Vahtera J, Ferrie JE, Stansfeld SA, Helenius H, et al. Overcrowding in hospital wards as a predictor of antidepressant treatment among hospital staff. Am J Psychiatry. 2008;165(11):1482–6.
17. Jolivet A, Caroly S, Ehlinger V, Kelly-Irving M, Delpierre C, Balducci F, et al. Linking hospital workers' organisational work environment to depressive symptoms: a mediating effect of effort–reward imbalance? The ORSOSA study. Soc Sci Med. 2010;71(3):534–40.
18. Peterson U, Demerouti E, Bergström G, Samuelsson M, Åsberg M, Nygren Å. Burnout and physical and mental health among Swedish healthcare workers. J Adv Nurs. 2008;62(1):84–95.
19. Lin H, Probst JC, Hsu Y. Depression among female psychiatric nurses in southern Taiwan: main and moderating effects of job stress, coping behaviour and social support. J Clin Nurs. 2010;19(15-16):2342–54.

20. Gärtner FR, Nieuwenhuijsen K, Van Dijk FJH, Sluiter JK. The impact of common mental dis-orders on the work functioning of nurses and allied health professionals: a systematic review. Int J Nurs Stud. 2010;47(8):1047–61. https://doi.org/10.1016/j.ijnurstu.2010.03.013.
21. Gao YQ, Pan BC, Sun W, Wu H, Wang JN, Wang L. Anxiety symptoms among Chinese nurses and the associated factors: a cross sectional study. BMC Psychiatry. 2012;12(1):141.
22. Ardekani ZZ, Kakooei H, Ayattollahi SM, Choobineh A, Seraji GN. Prevalence of mental disorders among shift work hospital nurses in Shiraz, Iran. Pak J Biol Sci. 2008;11(12):1605.
23. Kawano Y, Association of job-related stress factors with psychological and somatic symptoms among Japanese hospital nurses. Effect of departmental environment in acute care hospitals. J Occup Health. 2008;50(1):79–85.
24. Chan AOM, Chan YH. Influence of work environment on emotional health in a health care setting. Occup Med (Chic Ill). 2004;54(3):207–12.
25. Mealer ML, Shelton A, Berg B, Rothbaum B, Moss M. Increased prevalence of post-traumatic stress disorder symptoms in critical care nurses. Am J Respir Crit Care Med. 2007;175(7):693–7.
26. ONS. Suicide deaths among nurses aged 20 to 64 years, deaths registered in England and Wales between 2011 and 2017. 2018. https://www.ons.gov.uk/peoplepopulationandcommu-nity/birthsdeathsandmarriages/deaths/adhocs/009209suicidedeathsamongnursesaged20to64y earsdeathsregisteredinenglandandwalesbetween2011and2017.
27. ONS. Suicide by occupation, England: 2011 to 2015. Health Stat Q. 2017;1–16. https://www.ons.gov.uk/peoplepopulationandcommunity/birthsdeathsandmarriages/deaths/articles/suicidebyoccupation/england2011to2015.
28. Davidson JE, Proudfoot J, Lee K, Terterian G, Zisook S. A longitudinal analysis of nurse suicide in the United States (2005–2016) with recommendations for action. Worldviews Evid-Based Nurs. 2020;17(1):6–15.
29. Kõlves K, De Leo D. Suicide in medical doctors and nurses: an analysis of the Queensland Suicide Register. J Nerv Ment Dis. 2013;201(11):987–90.
30. King AS, Threlfall WJ, Band PR, Gallagher RP. Mortality among female registered nurses and school teachers in British Columbia. Am J Ind Med. 1994;26(1):125–32.
31. Hawton K, Agerbo E, Simkin S, Platt B, Mellanby RJ. Risk of suicide in medical and related occupational groups: a national study based on Danish case population-based registers. J Affect Disord. 2011;134(1–3):320–6.
32. Gunnarsdóttir H, Rafnsson V. Mortality among Icelandic nurses. Scand J Work Environ Health. 1995:24–9.
33. Hem E, Haldorsen T, Aasland OG, Tyssen R, Vaglum P, Ekeberg Ø. Suicide rates accord-ing to education with a particular focus on physicians in Norway 1960–2000. Psychol Med. 2005;35(6):873.
34. Evans-Lacko S, Corker E, Williams P, Henderson C, Thornicroft G. Effect of the time to change anti-stigma campaign on trends in mental-illness-related public stigma among the English population in 2003–2013: an analysis of survey data. Lancet Psychiat. 2014;1(2):121–8. https://doi.org/10.1016/S2215-0366(14)70243-3.
35. Singleton N, Bumpstead R, OBrien M, Lee A, Meltzer H. Psychiatric morbidity among adults living in private households , 2000 London : the stationery office. Int Rev Psychiatry. 2000;15(1–2):65–73.
36. McLaughlin K, Moutray M, Moore C. Career motivation in nursing students and the perceived influence of significant others. J Adv Nurs. 2010;66(2):404–12.
37. Conti-O'Hare M. The nurse as wounded healer: from trauma to transcendence. Burlington: Jones & Bartlett Learning; 2002.
38. Friedland BA, Gottert A, Hows J, Baral SD, Sprague L, Nyblade L, et al. The people living with HIV stigma index 2.0: generating critical evidence for change worldwide. Philadelphia: LWW; 2020.
39. Bennett L. The experience of nurses working with hospitalized AIDS patients. Aust J Soc Issues. 1992;27(2):125–43.

40. Li L, Lin C, Wu Z, Wu S, Rotheram-Borus MJ, Detels R, et al. Stigmatization and shame: consequences of caring for HIV/AIDS patients in China. AIDS Care. 2007;19(2):258–63.
41. Chirwa ML, Greeff M, Kohi TW, Naidoo JR, Makoae LN, Dlamini PS, et al. HIV stigma and nurse job satisfaction in five African countries. J Assoc Nurses AIDS Care. 2009;20(1):14–21.
42. Benevides-Pereira AMT, Alves RDN. A study on burnout syndrome in healthcare providers to people living with HIV. AIDS Care—Psychol Socio-Medical Asp AIDS/HIV. 2007;19(4):565–71.
43. Murphy GT, Stewart M, Ritchie J, Viscount PW, Johnson A. Telephone support for Canadian nurses in HIV/AIDS care. J Assoc Nurses AIDS Care. 2000;11(4):73–88.
44. Bellani ML, Furlani F, Gnecchi M, Pezzotta P, Trotti EM, Bellotti GG. Burnout and related factors among HIV/AIDS health care workers. AIDS Care. 1996;8(2):207–22.
45. Hamama L, Tartakovsky E, Eroshina K, Patrakov E, Golubkova A, Bogushevich J, et al. Nurses' job satisfaction and attitudes towards people living with HIV/AIDS in Russia. Int Nurs Rev. 2014;61(1):131–9.
46. Makhado L, Davhana-Maselesele M. Knowledge and psychosocial wellbeing of nurses caring for people living with HIV/AIDS (PLWH). Heal SA Gesondheid. 2016;21:1–10. https://doi.org/10.1016/j.hsag.2015.10.003.
47. Jonsson G, Davies N, Freeman C, Joska J, Pahad S, Thom R, et al. Guideline: management of mental health disorders in HIV-positive patients. South Afr J HIV Med. 2013;14(4):155–65.
48. Theuninck AC, Lake N, Gibson S. HIV-related posttraumatic stress disorder: investigating the traumatic events. AIDS Patient Care STDs. 2010;24(8):485–91.
49. Jones SH, Akers N, Eaton J, Tyler E, Gatherer A, Brabban A, et al. Improving access to psychological therapies (IAPT) for people with bipolar disorder: summary of outcomes from the IAPT demonstration site. Behav Res Ther. 2018;111:27–35. https://doi.org/10.1016/j.brat.2018.09.006.
50. Freedman SA, Mashiach RT. Shared trauma reality in war: mental health therapists' experience. PLoS One. 2018;13(2):1–13.
51. Durcan G, Shea NO, Allwood L. Covid-19 and the nation's mental health: forecasting needs and risks in the UK: May 2020. 2020.
52. Sinclair C, Durcan G, O'Shea N. Covid-19 and the nation's mental health Forecasting needs and risks in the UK: July 2020. 2020.
53. Maben J, Bridges J. Covid-19: supporting nurses' psychological and mental health. J Clin Nurs. 2020;29(15–16):2742–50.
54. Rimmer A. Covid-19: two thirds of healthcare workers who have died were from ethnic minorities. London: British Medical Journal Publishing Group; 2020.
55. Rimmer A. Covid-19: disproportionate impact on ethnic minority healthcare workers will be explored by government. London: British Medical Journal Publishing Group; 2020.
56. Cook T, Kursumovic E, Lennane S. Exclusive: deaths of NHS staff from covid-19 analysed. Health Serv J. 2020;2020:22.
57. NHS England. Workforce race equality standard: an overview of workforce data for nurses, midwives and health visitors in the NHS. 2019.
58. Kelly L. Burnout, compassion fatigue, and secondary trauma in nurses: recognizing the occupational phenomenon and personal consequences of caregiving. Crit Care Nurs Q. 2020;43(1):73–80.
59. Traynor M. What's wrong with resilience? J Res Nurs. 2008;23(1):5–8.
60. Kitchener BA, Jorm AF. Mental health first aid manual. Canberra: Centre for Mental Health Research; 2002.
61. Hardacre J, Margetts A. Psychological PPE: survival kit for creating a safer culture in the Covid-19 context by Dr Jeanne Hardacre & Dr Alexander Margetts—The official blog of BMJ Leader. BMJ Lead. 2020. https://blogs.bmj.com/bmjleader/2020/04/15/psychological-ppe-survival-kit-for-creating-a-safer-culture-in-the-covid-19-context/.

62. Kitto C, Bakhai K. Psychological PPE—the space between signposting and action. BMJ Opin. 2020; https://blogs.bmj.com/bmj/2020/08/14/psychological-ppe-the-space-between-signposting-and-action/.
63. Bennett-Levy J, Thwaites R, Haarhoff B, Perry H. Experiencing CBT from the inside out: a self-practice/self-reflection workbook for therapists. New York: Guilford Publications; 2014.
64. Magtibay DL, Chesak SS, Coughlin K, Sood A. Decreasing stress and burnout in nurses: efficacy of blended learning with stress management and resilience training program. JONA J Nurs Adm. 2017;47(7/8):391–5.
65. Copeland ME. Wellness recovery action plan. Occup Ther Ment Heal. 2002;17(3–4):127–50.
66. Hayes SC, Strosahl KD, Wilson KG. Acceptance and commitment therapy: the process and practice of mindful change. 2nd ed. New York: Guildford Press.
67. Kroenke K, Spitzer RL, Williams JBW. The PHQ-9: validity of a brief depression severity measure. J Gen Intern Med. 2001;16(9):606–13.
68. Spitzer RL, Kroenke K, Williams JBW, Löwe BA. brief measure for assessing generalized anxiety disorder: the GAD-7. Arch Intern Med. 2006;166(10):1092–7.
69. Maslach C, Jackson SE, Leiter MP. MBI: Maslach burnout inventory. Incorporated Sunnyvale, CA: CPP; 1996.
70. Figley CR. Compassion fatigue: coping with secondary traumatic stress in those who treat the traumatized. London: Brunner/Mazel, Publishers; 1995.
71. Kristensen TS, Borritz M, Villadsen E, Christensen KB. The Copenhagen burnout inventory: a new tool for the assessment of burnout. Work Stress. 2005;19(3):192–207.
72. Gray-Toft P, Anderson JG. The nursing stress scale: development of an instrument. J Behav Assess. 1981;3(1):11–23.
73. French SE, Lenton R, Walters V, Eyles J. An empirical evaluation of an expanded nursing stress scale. J Nurs Meas. 2000;8(2):161–78.
74. Harris PE. The nurse stress index. Work Stress. 1989;3(4):335–46.
75. Moreno B, Garrosa E, González-Gutiérrez JL. El desgaste profesional de enfermería. Desarrollo y validación factorial del CDPE. Arch Prev Riesgos Labor. 2000;3(1):18–28.
76. Higashiguchi K. The job stressor experienced by hospital nurses; Development of the nursing job stressor scale and examination of psychometric properties. Jap J Heal Psychol. 1998;11:64–72.
77. Aiken LH, Patrician PA. Measuring organizational traits of hospitals: the revised nursing work index. Nurs Res. 2000;49(3):146–53.
78. Moll SE. The web of silence: a qualitative case study of early intervention and support for healthcare workers with mental. London: BMC Public Health; 2014.
79. Waugh W, Lethem C, Sherring S, Henderson C. Exploring experiences of and attitudes towards mental illness and disclosure amongst health care professionals: a qualitative study. J Ment Health. 2017;26(5):457–63.